Clinics in Developmental Medicine No. 138
BEHAVIOURAL PHENOTYPES

© 1995 Mac Keith Press
526/529 High Holborn House, 52–54 High Holborn, London WC1V 6RL

Senior Editor: Martin C.O. Bax
Editor: Pamela A. Davies
Managing Editor: Michael Pountney
Sub Editor: Pat Chappelle

Set in Times and Avant Garde on QuarkXPress

First published in this edition 1995

British Library Cataloguing-in-Publication data:
A catalogue record for this book is available from the British Library

ISSN: 0069 4835
ISBN: 0 898683 06 9

Printed by The Lavenham Press Ltd, Water Street, Lavenham, Suffolk
Mac Keith Press is supported by **Scope** (formerly The Spastics Society)

Clinics in Developmental Medicine No. 138

Behavioural
Phenotypes

Edited by

GREGORY O'BRIEN
Northgate Hospital
Morpeth, Northumberland

WILLIAM YULE
Institute of Psychiatry
London

with a Foreword by
WILLIAM L. NYHAN
University of California, San Diego
San Diego

1995
Mac Keith Press

Distributed by ▓ **CAMBRIDGE**
UNIVERSITY PRESS

CONTENTS

AUTHORS' APPOINTMENTS

Jennifer Dennis, DM, MSc, DCH

Associate Specialist (Childhood Mental Handicap), Park Hospital for Children, Oxford, England.

Jonathon Flint, BM, BCh, MRCPsych

Senior Registrar in Psychiatry, Institute of Molecular Medicine, John Radcliffe Hospital, Oxford, England.

Randi Hagerman, MD

Professor of Child Health, Child Development Unit, The Children's Hospital, Denver, CO, USA.

Gregory O'Brien, MB, ChB, MRCPsych, MA

Consultant Psychiatrist, Northgate Hospital, Morpeth, Northumberland, England.

Sarah-Jane Richards, PhD

MRC Senior Research Fellow in Molecular Biology, Department of Medicine, Addenbrooke's Hospital, Cambridge, England.

Orlee Udwin, MPhil, PhD, CPsychol, AFBPsS

Consultant Clinical Psychologist in Child Health, West Lambeth Community Care (NHS) Trust; *and* Honorary Senior Lecturer in Child Psychology, Institute of Psychiatry, London, England.

William Yule, MA, Dip Psychol, PhD, FBPsS, CPsychol

Professor of Applied Child Psychology, Institute of Psychiatry, London, England.

FOREWORD

Behavioral phenotypes are recognizable patterns of behavior—syndromes, if you will, of behavior. The genetic determinants of behavior have continued to intrigue me since my initial observations on two boys with the Lesch–Nyhan syndrome reported in 1964. On the other hand, when I coined the term 'behavioral phenotypes' in the course of my presidential address to the Society for Pediatric Research in 1971 I had in mind the fact that recognizable patterns of human morphogenesis, the syndromes that launched the discipline of dysmorphology, are valuable to clinicians in coming to diagnoses, to investigators, leading to elucidation of etiology, and to parents, particularly in the area of prognosis. Conceptually, just as dysmorphic syndromes may result from environmental causes such as rubella as well as from genetic determinants, it seemed reasonable that a behavioral phenotype could be acquired as well as genetic. Isolation-reared monkeys seemed to me to be relevant examples in 1971.

Biologists formerly tended to think of phenotype in terms of its visible characteristics, whereas today we would also refer to a level of enzyme activity or a pattern of organic acids in the urine as phenotypic characteristics—in fact, any characteristics besides the genotype. The word 'phenotype' comes from the Greek *phainein*, to show, and the *Oxford English Dictionary* defines phenotype as 'an organism distinguishable from others by observable features' but goes on to generalize it as 'the sum of the attributes of an individual' and acknowledges environmental as well as genetic etiologies. These issues are considered in detail in the present text. The working definition, set out on page 2, is of a characteristic pattern consistently associated with a biologic disorder.

The importance of the recognition that a stereotyped or reproducible pattern of behavior accompanies a disease deserves emphasis. Recognition of the pattern of the behavior may permit the clinician to make the diagnosis. More than 30 years ago, when the disease was little known I made a diagnosis of the Tourette syndrome, as a visiting professor on rounds prior to seeing the patient, from the nature of the utterances heard. We have more recently confirmed the diagnosis of Angelman syndrome made initially by parents who recognized the behavioral phenotype from the description of one of our patients in a newspaper. Often of more importance to families is prognosis. In the practice of clinical medicine we are constantly reminded that what parents want most is to know what their child will be like as the years go on. Of course, the health and illness aspects with which clinicians are familiar are important, but more important are the behaviors that must be lived with day-to-day. It is behavior that can destroy a family or lead to admission to institution, not IQ or cytogenetic or enzymatic status. Appropriate counseling as to what to expect, and introduction to parent support groups and to others with children with the same phenotype lead to the development of realistic ways of coping with an unusual child.

Advances in genetics and molecular biology have clarified many of the genetic underpinnings of some behavioral phenotypes. Appropriately, in Chapter 2 the nature of this new genetics is reviewed, providing the background for an understanding of what is for most of the phenotypes the result of research to come. The usefulness of the transgenic mouse or other animal for the study of the *in vivo* function of a single modified gene is discussed. Mouse models of the Lesch–Nyhan syndrome have been engineered by the creation of mutations in the hypoxanthine guanine phosphoribosyl transferase (HPRT) gene in mouse stem cells, but it is now possible to make transgenic animals in which a single copy of a defective gene is inserted into the embryo and carried in every cell of the adult. Quite recently, Chen and colleagues at the Massachusetts Institute of Technology have created a behavioral phenotype by creating an autosomal dominant mutation in the gene for α-calcium calmodulin kinase II. The α-CaMKII knockout mouse has a lack of fear and remarkable defensive aggression.

The pathway from genotype to behavioral phenotype is seldom clear, as is reviewed in Chapter 6, but the power of the search for abnormal behavior in populations of individuals of known genetic abnormality is very great. If a reproducible pattern of unusual behavior is established in patients with a defect in a single gene, then one knows that that gene in some way controls the behavior. This is in contrast to the kind of linkage analysis that has been undertaken to localize genes determining common psychiatric disorders. It may not be surprising that few needles have been found in such haystacks. An interesting example of the pathway from the gene is the behavioral phenotype that results from a deficiency in the gene for monoamine oxidase A (*MAOA*). An X-linked pattern of violent behavior, such as rape, arson and attempted murder, was linked to a region of the short arm of the X chromosome (Xp11.4–11.3). A mutation in the *MAOA* gene at this locus led to a stop codon and a truncated nonfunctional enzyme. Insight into the biological basis of violent aggression is exciting.

Chapter 7 is a compendium of the individual disorders in which behavioral phenotypes have been described—each disease section providing alternative names, history, incidence, genetics, physical phenotype and behavioral or psychological phenotype— and a separate chapter (5) is devoted to lessons learned from the fragile X syndrome. The behavior of the fragile X syndrome is increasingly well characterized. The striking gaze-avoidance behavior alone permits a clinical diagnosis. The molecular biology is complex, and in each suspected patient the size of the trinucleotide repeat should be determined. The knowledge of what goes on in the DNA is so intricate, it carries with it the expectation that one day the details of the link with behavior will be clear.

This volume represents a coming of age for the field of behavioral phenotypes. It should stimulate us as clinicians to seek out and observe with precision the behavioral features of our patients. The tools of molecular biology permit us increasingly to decide exactly what genotype underlies the phenotype. The future should bring elucidation of the mechanisms by which the genotype is etiologic and more effective methods of treatment.

WILLIAM L. NYHAN, MD, PhD
Professor of Pediatrics
University of California, San Diego

1
WHY BEHAVIOURAL PHENOTYPES?

Gregory O'Brien and William Yule

The aim of this chapter is to provide a general introduction to behavioural phenotypes. The chapter opens with an account of the concept of the behavioural phenotype and its history and place in behavioural genetics and developmental medicine. A definition is proposed, and its implications are outlined. In discussion of the historical background we examine how a wide variety of schools of thought have contributed to the concept as it is now understood. These contributions come not only from the genetics of behaviour, learning and psychopathology, but also from certain principles enshrined in psychological thinking, and from other such diverse sources as sociology, philosophy, mythology and modern history. The two principle lines of enquiry in behavioural phenotypes research, the genomic and the phenomic, are described, and various aspects of phenomic research are discussed in greater detail. (Chapter 7 of the present text concentrates mostly on genomic research.) Throughout, the intention is to promote clarity of thought and rigorous enquiry in the developing field of behavioural phenotypes.

The behavioural phenotype: one concept or many?

The behavioural phenotype concept was introduced to contemporary thinking by Nyhan (1972) in his presidential address to the Society for Pediatric Research. This paper focused on a vivid description of the aggressive self-mutilation that characterizes the condition to which his name is attached—the Lesch–Nyhan syndrome. The title of the lecture in which he made this pivotal contribution indicates Nyhan's view of the nature of the behavioural phenotype—'Behavioral phenotypes in organic genetic disease.' Clearly, he used the term 'behavioural phenotype' to refer to the behaviours which are an integral part of certain genetic disorders, and emphasized the role of organic factors in the development of such behaviours. In Nyhan's view, therefore, the genetic disorder gives rise to a set of behaviours, whether by biochemical, neurophysiological or other means. In concentrating his thinking on 'organic genetic disease' in this way, Nyhan was taking what we now refer to as a genomic viewpoint (see below).

Other writers have suggested different models of what a behavioural phenotype might comprise. One view which has attracted some considerable interest is that of Harris (1987), who proposed that behavioural phenotypes are the 'unlearned behaviour disorders'. In Harris' approach, the Lesch–Nyhan syndrome and Prader–Willi syndrome —two major genetic disorders which clearly have substantial behavioural consequences —are discussed alongside a rather different kind of contender for 'behavioural phenotype' status, that of infantile autism. In the cases of Lesch–Nyhan and Prader–Willi syndromes we have identifiable biological disorders which *include* behavioural features,

1

while in infantile autism we have a disorder which is largely *defined* on basis of behaviour. As will be seen when we come to discuss the phenomic approach to behavioural phenotypes, there is some support for this suggestion.

An even wider view has been taken by Plomin (1990, 1991) in stating that 'behaviour is a phenotype'. In this context, 'behaviour' includes observations of mental illness, learning skills and even intelligence, in addition to manifest behaviour problems— essentially, any observable event or interaction in which an organism participates. While this is of course applicable to some behavioural studies, it is a more all-encompassing interpretation of behaviour than most workers in the behavioural phenotypes field would make. At its inaugural meeting in 1990 the Society for the Study of Behavioural Phenotypes adopted the statement that 'some of the behaviours exhibited by children with biologically based mentally handicapping disorders are organically determined' (SSBP 1990). This proposal emphasizes that, although organic factors are clearly implicated in behavioural phenotypes, only 'some' are. In other words, it is implied that a host of other influences—including both developmental and environmental considerations—also operate. A complex interaction between those behaviours which are a result of 'biologically based mentally handicapping disorders' and such other influences constantly operates, forming and shaping observable behaviour.

Behavioural phenotype: definition
These strands of thought have come together in the definition of behavioural phenotype to be adopted in this text, which is in line with that proposed by Flint and Yule (1994), as follows:

The behavioural phenotype is a characteristic pattern of motor, cognitive, linguistic and social abnormalities which is consistently associated with a biological disorder. In some cases, the behavioural phenotype may constitute a psychiatric disorder; in others, behaviours which are not usually regarded as symptoms of psychiatric disorders may occur.

The inter-relationship of these elements is illustrated schematically in Figure 1.1.

It is useful to consider this definition carefully, and to explore what is being proposed. First, it is suggested that there is such an entity as a 'behavioural phenotype'. The next phrase, 'a characteristic pattern' refers to the observation that there are certain behaviours which commonly co-occur, and comprise the behavioural phenotype. This pattern is 'characteristic' in that a frequent and significant association is apparent between, on the one hand, the set of behaviours, and, on the other, the 'biological disorder' in question. We then read on to see that there are a variety of different types of behaviour which feature in the behavioural phenotype: 'motor, cognitive, linguistic and social abnormalities'. In this definition, therefore, the behavioural phenotype is an umbrella term for a host of developmental and psychological observations. These extend from problem behaviour 'disorders' through to specific patterns of language functioning. Indeed, as we shall see in consideration of certain biological disorders (*e.g.* fragile X syndrome), the 'characteristic pattern' commonly includes both such behavioural features.

2

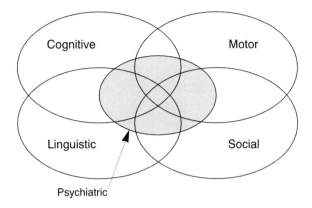

Fig. 1.1. Inter-relationship of the four cardinal elements of the behavioural phenotype as defined in text: cognitive, linguistic, social and motor. It is apparent that in any one behavioural phenotype any one or a selection of these four elements may figure more highly. Some behavioural phenotypes are largely accountable by cognitive and linguistic factors, while others feature prominent motor anomalies and/or characteristics of social dysfunction. In a minority of behavioural phenotypes, diagnosable psychiatric disorders occur.

The definition next says that these characteristics of behaviour and functioning are 'consistently associated with a biological disorder'. This is crucially important, for in stating that these findings are 'consistently associated' it is asserted that the behavioural phenotype should only be assumed to be present in a biological disorder where there is clear 'consistent' evidence, in the form of clinical and scientific observation. To be 'consistent' is to be so common as to comprise the rule. However, as in other medical disorders where certain findings are 'consistently' made, this is not to say that the behaviours in question occur in all cases, or with the same degree of severity in different cases. The issue of the association with a 'biological disorder' indicates that there is assumed to be a causal link between the behavioural characteristics observed and some biological disorder. In some such disorders, there is now substantial insight into the mechanisms by which these associations operate (*e.g.* see sections on Williams syndrome, tuberous sclerosis and Down syndrome). In general, however, we are at an early stage in our understanding of the apparently complex mechanisms by which behavioural phenotypes arise in different biological disorders.

The definition ends with reference to two findings. First, that the behavioural phenotype might be so well-elaborated and clear-cut as to amount to a recognizable and diagnosable psychiatric disorder. This seems to be true for only a minority of behavioural phenotypes. It is the second possibility—that 'behaviours not usually regarded as symptoms of psychiatric disorders may occur'—which seems to be the more common situation. There are further ramifications of this important characteristic of behavioural phenotypes, since, from the point of view of detection and measurement, it means that conventional psychiatric diagnostic schedules may be of little applicability. (If a behavioural phenotype does not constitute a diagnosable psychiatric disorder, then schedules designed for the detection and measurement of such disorders are unlikely to be useful. This issue and its implications are elaborated extensively in the chapter on behavioural measurement.) It also begs the question of whether there may be present in these biological disorders hitherto unrecognized psychiatric disorders, which might in turn shed other insights into other behaviours or behaviour disorders which are 'not usually regarded as symptoms of psychiatric disorders'.

Finally, in this definition it is not proposed that there is a simple, one-to-one or universal relationship between the behavioural phenotype and the associated biological disorder. On the contrary, it is anticipated by the present authors that the relationships here are likely to be complex and varied.

Phenotype and behavioural phenotype

A class of medical students was recently asked to describe their understanding of the term 'phenotype'. The responses from the group were very much in keeping with such definitions as 'an observable characteristic we can measure' (Plomin 1991), 'the physical expression of genes throughout the lifecycle of the individual' (Tsuang 1993) and 'the sum-total of the observable or detectable characteristics of an individual or group, as determined by its genotype and by genetic or environmental factors' (*Oxford English Dictionary*), albeit phrased in a more roundabout manner. Interestingly, the students discussed the term 'phenotype' in relation to their knowledge and understanding of certain genetic conditions. When they were pressed further to give examples of just which 'individual characteristics' comprise the phenotype of a given condition, three distinctive themes emerged. First of all, dysmorphology. It was clearly understood by the group that certain characteristics—such as the typical facies of Down syndrome— are good examples of features of the phenotype of a condition. Next, descriptions of specific medical problems and physically disabling conditions were mentioned—again, students were quick to recount some of the congenital cardiac anomalies found in Down syndrome and so on. Finally, the fact that the group had chosen to illustrate its understanding of 'phenotype' by referring to conditions which cause some degree of mental retardation showed that they knew that specific or generalized cognitive impairments comprised the third member of the classic triad of the medical phenotype (Flint and Yule 1994). In summary, the student group was describing the long accepted three cardinal features of the clinical phenotype by which congenital conditions have traditionally been described—dysmorphology, medical conditions, and cognition—as illustrated in Figure 1.2.

Any group of medical students who had been attached to J. Langdon Down in the 1860s would have described things rather differently. His detailed clinical observations of the children who were affected by the syndrome which was later named after him were rich with accounts of their social behaviour and personality attributes. In his writings he stated, 'They are humorous and a lively sense of the ridiculous often colours their mimicry . . . another feature is their great obstinacy—they can only be guided by consummate tact' (Down 1866).

4

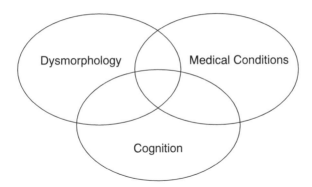

Fig. 1.2. Inter-relationship of the three traditionally recognized elements of the clinical phenotype. In some respects these associations consist of causal links. For example, dysmorphology—abnormal facies—may be due to a particular medical condition, such as in cleft lesions. In other cases the reasons for the co-existence of features of the phenotype in characteristic groupings—such as a given facies with a certain cognitive profile—are as yet unclear. The areas of overlap are not intended to represent the extent of co-associations or causal interactions, merely to illustrate that these factors do exert some influence upon each other.

Not that Down's observations were lost—far from it. His behavioural descriptions found their way into medical textbooks with widespread acceptance, and the picture of sociability and musicality of the Down syndrome child has been persistently quoted for as long as the condition has been recognized as a discrete entity.

The rather more interesting issue is the question: why has behavioural description not been a constant feature of other disabling syndromes? In other words, although this chapter is entitled 'Why Behavioural Phenotypes?', the discussion is equally concerned with the complementary question, 'Why not?' This somewhat flippant-sounding comment conceals over 2000 years of argument and controversy. The proposition that certain individuals are born genetically predisposed to certain characteristic patterns of behaviour and temperament has a history as long as the written word, as can be seen in Plato's *Republic*. Here, according to the 'Myth of Metals', some individuals (the Philosopher Kings) were born 'Gold'. Status, success and wisdom were their birthright. That there could be such very substantial consequences of genetic endowment for the lifestyle of the Philosopher Kings seems to have been due in part to the expectations held of them by others. This in turn naturally had a major impact on their subsequent development and behaviour. Viewed in this way, Plato's Myth of Metals was an early attempt to bring together genetic and environmental factors in an interactive model which gives an account of the development of certain exceptional individuals. In fact, it was more of an apologia for the status quo, in which the Philosopher Kings retained their privileged position in society. Ever since then, different reviewers and commentators on the genetic contribution to human behaviour have adopted even more extreme stands.

Most approaches to human development and behaviour have concentrated solely on either 'nature' or 'nurture' effects in attempting to explain group similarities and individual differences. Indeed, some have focused exclusively on one view or the other. Even today, certain writers seem to find difficulty appreciating that genetic factors are important contributors to behaviour, preferring instead to emphasize the role of other influences and to dismiss the role played by genetics. This polarized thinking has a history. It is informative therefore to carry out a brief review of the background and development of the behavioural phenotype idea, and to examine how different schools of thought have not so much contributed to the emergence of the concept but rather have impeded it.

On one side of this divide, certain schools of thought at times overplay the 'nature' hand. Claims have been made of links between genetic endowment and behaviour and/or development which have been overstatements or even wildly speculative theories which have been subsequently seen to be quite incorrect. This in turn has had a stifling effect on further advancement in the field, or in some cases has resulted in a backlash of (quite justifiable) objection against the principles being proposed.

On the other hand, approaches which concentrate on the influence of 'nurture' have also played a part. Whether in the broadest consideration of the impact of environment on development, or in the detailed study of the effects of specific therapeutic influences on particular behaviours, it has become commonplace to give little or no attention to genetic influences. At first sight this may seem as ludicrous as those schools of thought which have over-emphasized genetic or somatic influences on behaviour and development. In fact, clinical and educational programmes which are based entirely on 'nurture' principles have been enormously successful—so much so that their proponents quite rightly question the importance of the behavioural phenotype concept, and indeed see it as potentially harmful, for reasons we shall shortly explore.

Overplaying the 'nature' hand
Somatotypes
The notion of somatotypes was widely held, and can still be found in some spheres of psychiatric thinking. This school, which was pioneered by Kretschmer (1936) and further elaborated by Sheldon and Stephens (1942), held that genetic endowment affected the development of personality according to the relative distribution in the body of the three primitive embryonic cell layers, the endoderm, the mesoderm and the ectoderm. Sheldon's types were therefore the endomorph, the mesomorph and the ectomorph. The endomorphic body shape was rounded, contained massive and highly developed viscera, and had a high content of endodermal tissue. This build—which Kretschmer referred to as pyknic—was said to be associated with a 'viscerotonic' temperament, in which love of comfort, affection and sociability figured highly (Sheldon and Stephens 1942). The mesomorph, in whom mesoderm was particularly prominent, was characterized by muscle and bone, with broad shoulders, a slim waist and well developed musculature. Kretschmer referred to this constitution as 'the athletic type'; Sheldon and Stephens held that it was associated with 'somatotonic' temperament, in which energy, assertiveness and concentration on action for 'here and now' issues featured highly. The ectomorphic build was linear and fragile, and corresponded to Kretschmer's asthenic or leptosomatic

types. It was said to be associated with a 'cerebrotonic' temperament, characteristically restrained, inhibited and socially withdrawn.

If there is any truth in these archetypes, it is probably not that body shapes as such represent any biological predisposition to some kind of temperamental or personality phenotype, or proneness to psychiatric disorder. For example, the widely held belief that fat people are happy, jovial and exuberant is still endemic today, and there are obvious reasons for this. Here we are probably seeing reactions to circumstances and environmental outcomes to predispositions, rather than any result of body shape (Freeman 1983). An outward-going, exuberant person may well lead a self-indulgent and expansive lifestyle, with natural consequences on body shape. Also, it has long been held that an individual who for other reasons is obese may well attempt to compensate for this attribute by developing a sociable and extrovert attitude.

This is all very well, but does such a discussion have any bearing on our thoughts concerning the expression of behavioural phenotypes? The answer is very definitely yes. For, as will be discussed in detail throughout this chapter and elsewhere in this text, the behavioural phenotypes we observe are the result of myriad complex interactions of genetic endowment and environmental factors, where a host of variables exert influences upon the manifest behaviours (Harris 1987).

The main lesson to be learnt from the somatotype school of thought is that the simplistic direct relationships between embryonic tissue and personality which were suggested are a far cry from our concept of the behavioural phenotype. It was entirely appropriate that the approach was heavily criticized (Humphreys 1957) and that non-genetic influences on the development of personality were given far more prominent consideration in the two to three decades which immediately followed Sheldon and Stephen's work.

'Clinical personalities'
Another factor which prevented behavioural phenotypes from attaining earlier the prominence in developmental and clinical thinking that they now enjoy was the reaction engendered by the concept of 'clinical personalities' or 'clinical stereotypes'. According to this idea, specific personality types do occur in identifiable medical disorders. There are numerous examples. Many were widely believed, in some cases until very recently. Indeed, there is something of a resumption of interest in some of these stereotypes in certain quarters, although they are generally regarded as over-simplistic, unhelpful and probably misleading.

One of the most-cited 'clinical personalities' is the epileptic personality. This stereotype was often described as truculent, evasive, 'sticky', 'touchy', 'circumstantial' and generally irritable in nature (Fenwick 1987). This notion has now been largely rejected. For example, in an extensive survey by Pond and Bidwell (1960), only 4 per cent of epileptic patients displayed these characteristics. It is now accepted that other factors are implicated in the genesis of such attributes (Tizard 1962). A similar example is the case of the XYY personality. An aggressive, anti-social psychopathy was proposed to occur in individuals affected by the XYY anomaly (double Y chromosome male), as described by Jacobs *et al.* (1965). However, those studies were carried out in a high security hospital setting and have subsequently been strongly refuted on grounds of sample bias (*e.g.* Borgaonkar and Shah 1974). It is now accepted that the original observations were the result of a combination of factors. First, there is indeed the nature of the population investigated (Billings *et al.* 1992). Second, the tendency for XYY men to be of lower intelligence is thought to contribute to their criminality (Witkin *et al.* 1976). Third, other effects of the extra Y chromosome, particularly large stature, may well for social reasons exert an interactional effect on their development (Borgaonkar and Shah 1974). On this basis there is no clear evidence for a simple predisposition to a specific personality type among XYY males. Apparently, though, through intervening biological and social mechanisms such individuals may be prone to develop certain attributes of personality and to exhibit certain behaviours. So, the notion of a simple relationship between double Y chromosome status and aggressive criminality is clearly erroneous; however, would it be stretching the remit of our concept to regard the preceding discussion as evidence for a behavioural phenotype in the XYY anomaly?

The eugenics movement

In the second and third decades of the 20th century, there was an increasing interest in the genetic basis of a host of human attributes and in the possibility that natural experiments in breeding might result in advantage for populations. This was in some respects a logical extension of the thinking of early 20th century physicians and thinkers such as the great British psychiatrist Henry Maudsley (1905) (see Turner 1988). The eugenics movement held great hopes for the benefits to mankind offered by the possibility of steadily increasing intelligence, height, physical fitness and mental well-being through genetic manipulation. The movement's enthusiasm extended to experiments in selective breeding and other forms of population control (Tsuang 1993). However attractive these theories may have been and however tenaciously they were believed, intrinsic problems of the philosophy became apparent through the eventual implementation of genocide which occurred in Western Central Europe in the late 1930s and early 1940s.

The abhorrent manner in which these principles have been exercised is anathema to all members of civilized society. What has been less clear until fairly recently has been that in rejecting these repellant ideologies, the medical and scientific community has failed to pursue an important line of enquiry. For there has been a reluctance to probe further into the extent to which genetic susceptibility is important in the development of personality, the functioning of intelligence and the aetiology of psychiatric disorders (Tsuang 1993). In effect, the reaction against the eugenics movement has contributed to the failure to advance further enquiry into behavioural genetics. Moreover, this reluctance is most apparent with respect to the proposition that people with certain genetically determined disabilities might also have even more socially undesirable natural characteristics. That is, in such people there may occur behavioural problems which have some basis in their genetic condition (O'Brien 1992). Moreover, clinical science and practice which have been informed by learning theory and behavioural ecology have further strengthened this situation.

By various means, overplaying the nature hand has resulted in a strong reaction of rejection. Consequently, until very recently there has been little consideration given to the possibility of genetic influences on behaviour in people affected by disabling congenital conditions.

Overemphasizing the influence of nurture
Behavioural ecology
Contemporary thinking in behavioural ecology makes consideration of the interaction of the genotype with the *environmentype*, which is a shorthand term for the product of the various factors in the individual's environment which affect behaviour and development (Bronfenbrenner 1977). However, it is true to say that most clinicians in learning disability (mental retardation) practice who would describe themselves broadly as behaviourists pay rather more attention to environmental determinants of behaviour than to the genetic propensities which are clearly regarded as being important by theorists in this school of thought. Indeed, the first lesson most such clinicians learn as an introduction to behavioural theory is to construct an 'a–b–c' analysis. By this simple approach, a problem behaviour is considered in close detail with respect to : (i) *a*ntecedents, or putative environmental precipitants; (ii) the form or type of *b*ehaviour itself; and (iii) the *c*onsequences of the behaviour, for the individual and others, which may in some way promote or shape the behaviour. It is therefore common practice for the antecedents and the consequences of the behaviour—the factors in the environment which are important in maintaining that behaviour—to be given more attention than the form of behaviour itself. This approach to clinical practice has clearly had immense benefits for many individuals, and in no field is this more apparent than in investigation and management of the myriad behavioural problems of people with severe learning disabilities. Clearly, many of the behaviours seen in this patient group are environmentally determined, and are consequently substantially ameliorated by this kind of approach.

There are two potential major drawbacks of a–b–c behavioural analysis applied in this way. The first is that it concentrates too much on the here and now. As outlined above, in planning behavioural interventions it is crucial to take account of genetic and constitutional factors such as temperament and personality (Yule 1987). Experience and common sense tell us that when this is not done, unrealistic goals may be set. The other problem with this approach is at first sight less obvious. Certainly, through the application of interventions and different management strategies indicated by a–b–c analysis, many parents learn to enable their children to behave more appropriately and to acquire new skills. However, this suggests a disquieting corollary. Some parents come to believe that because they have been able to modify their child's behaviour and improve her/his functioning, it follows that their previous handling of the child was the cause of the problem. In fact, many parents have been told this by professionals and clinicians with whom they have come in contact. The behavioural phenotype concept is something of a challenge to this kind of approach. In clarifying that some of these behaviours are to some extent genetically determined, we also hope to alleviate the guilt which so many parents in this situation have experienced.

9

Similarly, those 'behaviourists' who are themselves involved in work on behavioural phenotypes caution of the great danger of over-emphasizing the importance of genetic factors in the development and maintenance of behavioural problems in such individuals. The dangers in question are particularly important, and are therefore elaborated at greater length later in this chapter. In brief, the themes of the perceived dangers in behavioural phenotypes include: (i) accepting the behaviour as inevitable and therefore doing nothing about it; (ii) anticipating the occurrence of the behaviour, and in this way potentially contributing to its occurrence and maintenance; and (iii) the possibility of additional stigmatization of people with learning disabilities because of the expectation of such behavioural problems.

Learning theory
The past four or five decades have seen enormous strides in our understanding of the capacity of people with learning disabilities to learn and develop in ways which previously were not envisaged. Indeed, there has been continuous debate over the appropriateness of such labels as 'mental retardation' and 'learning disability' because of the self-fulfilling prophecy by which such individuals may not acquire learning because it is not expected of them. One of the most extreme examples of the power of terminology in this connection was the use of the technical term 'ineducable' with respect to people with very severe learning disabilities. The result of this policy was that such severely learning-disabled individuals did not receive any real education, with consequent adverse impact on their development (Nelkin and Tancredi 1991).

This situation has shaped attitudes to behavioural phenotypes. It seems to work in the following way. It is known and widely recognized that a programme constructed for an individual which focuses on learning a task will often result in a reduction of a behavioural problem (*e.g.* Gow *et al.* 1990). Also, there is good evidence that the limits of such work have not yet been reached. Approaches which concentrate on learning theory therefore question the value of the exploration of behavioural phenotypes. Some would argue that because we have not yet reached the limits of the possible impact of learning approaches in the management of learning disabled individuals, it follows that we should not be creating for ourselves limitations based on our supposed knowledge of their genetic endowments in the realm of behaviour problems. However, it is now appropriate to redress this position and to accept that, just as there are plateaux of ability which are unlikely to be exceeded in some individuals (Hodapp *et al.* 1990), so are there some individuals whose behavioural problems are best understood by other means than by insights from learning theory.

Diagnostic inertia
If inertia is defined as 'the property by which matter continues in its existing state of rest or uniform motion' (*Oxford English Dictionary*), then a 'diagnostic inertia' can be identified in the reluctance of clinicians in some quarters to include consideration of behavioural phenotypes in their diagnostic formulations. For in seeking to understand the behavioural problems which so often present in people with congenital developmen-

tal disabilities, many clinicians focus their attention only on life events, current stressors in the environment and the various means by which environmental experiences and developmental capacities shape behaviour. True, most authorities recognize that there are a few genetic disorders—notably Prader–Willi syndrome (Clarke *et al.* 1989) and Lesch–Nyhan syndrome (Nyhan 1972)—which have obvious and major behavioural features in their phenotype, but there is a widespread assumption that these are exceptions and that most genetically determined biological disorders do not have behavioural concomitants. It is often generally assumed that any behaviours which do appear in a given condition relate more to the severity and/or type of the learning disability present in affected probands. However, as the detailed descriptions of the behavioural phenotypes in Chapter 7 show, there is a rapidly accumulating body of evidence which suggests that, far from being exceptions, it may be that these disorders represent the norm in this sense. In other words, for any given cause of learning disability or developmental disability it may be that certain behavioural features are more likely to occur. It is our experience that this suggestion is commonly met with scepticism, and sometimes with emphatic denial, but is rarely accepted for what it is: an hypothesis which is as yet untested in many disorders, but for which there is some support.

An example of diagnostic inertia is seen in the fragile X story, as detailed by Randi Hagerman in Chapter 5. Here it is striking to see how much questioning and discussion there has been over the possibility that the fragile X syndrome might have a behavioural phenotype. However, as many others have commented, many of the early claims made in respect of the behavioural phenotype of fragile X have subsequently been shown to be erroneous (Einfeld and Hall 1994). While we naturally concur with other authorities who stress that discrete genetic disorders which demonstrate high penetrance in respect of their behavioural manifestations are particularly rare (Plomin 1991, Billings *et al.* 1992), we would assert that it is important in the present state of our knowledge to be open to the possibility of the description and elaboration of many further behavioural phenotypes.

These different factors, as outlined above, all seem to play a part in the reluctance which is still found in some quarters to accept the behavioural phenotype concept. Although we may take issue with the emphases, interpretations or conclusions drawn, in all of these matters there is some element of truth. From the experience of others and from the reactions which their schools of thought have engendered, we must learn to proceed with caution in a spirit of rigorous scientific enquiry.

Having reviewed the roots of the reservations which have been expressed concerning the nature and scope of behavioural phenotypes, we will now look at the routes which have led to the concept.

Behavioural phenotypes—toward a coherent concept
Myths and folklore: cheeky imps and charming cherubs
Certain aspects of folklore, with origins lost in historical time, probably represent the earliest exposition of the behavioural phenotype concept. These were more recently revisited in J.R.R. Tolkien's Middle Earth sagas (*The Hobbit* and *Lord of the Rings*)

where a particularly strong association was seen between the abilities and temperaments of the different races. Hobbits were short and fat, with a fondness for fine ale, good food and song, set against a background of a rather reclusive, isolated lifestyle. Elves were tall, fair, articulate and active sportsmen, with particular skills in the area of woodmanship and archery. However, within these different races the impact of natural selection and the interaction of gene and environment are apparent when one remembers that hobbits lived in holes in the ground, and elven folk lived in woodland. A closer look at our own folklore reveals that there may be some basis to some of these notions. For example, the skull shape, stature and prominent eyebrows of the imp character in popular folklore, coupled with its mischievousness, might well be based on observations of certain forms of dwarfism, notably de Lange syndrome or achondroplasia. However, the intervening variables between cause of dwarfism and manifest behaviour in these two conditions are very different, as are the associated levels of intellect. The comical behaviour which is so often ascribed to people affected by achondroplasia is clearly a piece of playacting on their part when carried out professionally in a circus setting. This seems to be based on the premise that their very body shape is held by some to be an amusing parody of more conventional human shape. However, the rather more aggressive and self-injurious behaviours which commonly occur in de Lange syndrome appear to be more directly related to the impairment underlying the syndrome, although the intervening variables are as yet not fully understood (Johnson *et al.* 1976).

A rather different approach to the notion that there are specific character types to be observed in people affected by different syndromes is seen in certain Renaissance paintings. For example, Mantegna's *Madonna and Child* at Mantua in Italy features a Christ Child who appears to be affected by Down syndrome. This attempt to portray the condition in such a positive light is particularly dramatic.

There are many other examples in mythology of the supposed personality or temperament of races, or of breeds of different sorts of human beings, and in all of these there is probably some foundation in observation, compounded by fanciful thinking. Whether we are considering giants, cyclops, people with appendages to their skulls, or even a different characteristic that has been ascribed to the major races of human beings which are currently manifest on the planet, the circumstances in which these people live clearly play a massive part in the selective breeding of advantageous genes.

The genomic approach

The genomic approach to behavioural phenotypes is one which studies genetically identifiable conditions and seeks to identify to what extent they have behavioural characteristics. It was work of this type which first led Nyhan to ascribe a severely mutilating and refractory form of self-injurious behaviour directly to the cause of the other disabilities inherent in the Lesch–Nyhan syndrome (Nyhan 1972). An account of the current knowledge of the condition is given in Chapter 7. This approach has many attractions, in that discrete, identifiable groups are the starting point, usually defined by genetic investigations. This in turn is currently driving a major area of enquiry into the role of various biological mechanisms in the genesis of the manifest behaviours (*e.g.* see

Harris 1987, Pfadt 1990, Turk 1992). Indeed, there have now been several extensive studies of some quite rare conditions. Some of the most important findings are given in Chapter 7; other examples include such diverse studies as the work on Aarskog syndrome (Fryns 1992); sex aneuploidies such as 48,XXYY syndrome (Borghraef *et al.* 1991) and 49,XXXXY syndrome (Lomelino and Reiss 1991, Jancar 1992); inborn metabolic errors such as argininosuccinic aciduria (Lågas and Ruokonen 1991); and Sturge–Weber syndrome (Lee 1990). The fruits of this approach are seen in the syndromic descriptions which comprise Chapter 7, and by the references to the behavioural phenotypes of the many conditions which are cited throughout this book. One of the most important features of this approach is its capacity to indicate the likely strength of environmental contributions to behaviours identified (Rutter *et al.* 1990a,b, Billings *et al.* 1992). Whenever a behaviour is identified as being present in a proportion of people but not universally among those who are affected with a given condition, then there is the need to consider other aetiologies of behaviour. A good example is the peculiar skin-picking of Prader–Willi syndrome. This behaviour is common in Prader–Willi subjects but not ubiquitous (Clarke *et al.* 1989). Most important in all these situations is the need to consider some environmental contribution (Plomin 1991). One attraction of the genomic approach therefore is its capacity to identify the strength of genetic influence on behaviour, and so in turn to indicate how much of the variance might be due to environmental factors.

The phenomic approach
The phenomic approach to the study of behavioural phenotypes, while being complementary to the genomic one, takes a somewhat different starting point. Whereas the reference point in the genomic approach is a discrete and genetically identifiable condition, *e.g.* Down syndrome, the line of enquiry taken by the phenomic approach begins with observations of the behavioural phenotype itself. The process works in the following way. A group of individuals is observed to have certain behavioural characteristics in common. This behavioural profile may be unusual, but is not as yet known to be due to any identifiable biological condition. However, there are good reasons to group these subjects together, such as only one sex being affected, or the recognition of a common predictable natural history. A good example of a disorder which has been identified by the phenomic approach is Rett syndrome. This condition presents only in girls, and includes a pathognomonic combination of symptoms including a movement disorder, an idiosyncratic social regression and longitudinal changes over time in motor, cognitive and social functioning (see Chapter 7).

Several areas of inquiry have employed this approach, with varying degrees of success. From these studies, a great deal has been learned about research into the behavioural phenotypes field. Also, through consideration of these studies, the behavioural phenotype concept has been elaborated and clarified.

Phenomic research—findings in general psychiatry
Genetic studies in adult and general psychiatry have a long history and, indeed, there is scarcely a psychiatric disorder which has not been the subject of rigorous genetic

enquiry. Most notably, the major psychoses have been found to have, at the very least, substantial genetic predisposition (McGuffin and Thapar 1992, Tsuang 1993). These studies are of crucial importance to the present area of enquiry for a variety of reasons. First of all, many of the principles of behavioural genetics as they apply to the developmental disabilities have been elaborated through this field of research (Plomin 1990). Consideration of these studies in many cases therefore suggests models for inquiry in behavioural phenotypes research. Equally, many studies serve as cautions and pitfalls for the unwary. Also, because psychiatric disorder is now known to be more common in people with mental retardation (*e.g.* Bouras and Drummond 1992), the findings in these studies must be borne in mind when proposing the possibility of any link between a major mental illness and a particular condition, as has been proposed for both Down syndrome (Myers and Pueschel 1991, Cooper and Collacott 1993) and fragile X syndrome (Reiss *et al.* 1989). The explanations for any such putative associations need to include consideration of the genetics of a specific psychiatric disorder, *e.g.* schizophrenia, as a phenotype *per se*, in order to clarify the basis of any co-association of that disorder with another cause of disability (such as fragile X or Down syndrome). Finally, in consideration of the definition and nature of the behavioural phenotype (see above) it was anticipated that in only a minority of cases would a behavioural phenotype include or indeed comprise symptoms of a diagnosable psychiatric disorder. However, the fact that psychiatric disorder is more common among people with mental retardation seems to pose yet another important question. To what extent might this excess of mental illness be linked to the discrete causes of mental retardation?

Schizophrenia
Genetic studies in schizophrenia have revealed a genetic contribution, but have also emphasized the importance of environmental influences. The risk of developing schizophrenia among first degree relatives of affected probands is currently estimated at 8 per cent (Gottesman and Shields 1982). The risk for identical twins, including those adopted away, is estimated at 30 per cent (Kendler and Robinette 1983). This is far below the 100 per cent rate which would occur if the condition were entirely genetic (Plomin 1990). Moreover, even the superficially convincing evidence of the findings among separately adopted identical twins has been questioned in some quarters (Hrubec and Robinette 1984, Billings *et al.* 1992). One important issue here is the well-documented policy of adoption agencies to place siblings within settings which are socioeconomically and environmentally similar to their natural families, thus questioning the assumption that any similarities which develop in the behaviour of such individuals are likely to be of genetic rather than environmental origin. However, most authors do accept that there is a genetic component to schizophrenia (for a review, see Plomin 1986).

The major initiative of the World Health Organization in schizophrenia has been pivotal in clarifying the important contribution made by genetic susceptibility, this being constant across virtually all cultures and environments (WHO 1973). The same WHO study demonstrated that, although the genetic susceptibility as revealed in the incidence of new cases was similar in the different countries and cultures studied, the outcome was substantially better in certain developing countries, emphasizing again the complex manner in which environmental and genetic influences interact to produce the phenotype. In addition, a few regions of the world, including Croatia and western Ireland, have been found to have higher incidence rates of schizophrenia, and these studies have indicated the importance of environmental stressors such as migration in the aetiology of the disease.

With the advent of molecular biology, linkage studies employing RFLP (restriction fragment length polymorphisms—see Chapter 2) have sought to identify single gene(s) responsible for schizophrenia (Sherrington *et al.* 1988), but with equivocal results to date (Kennedy *et al.* 1988, St Clair *et al.* 1989). However, one proposition is of particular interest to the present area of inquiry. This is the possibility that certain extended families may have 'their own unique major gene responsible for a disorder' (Plomin 1990). A recent suggestion from Boerwinkle *et al.* (1986) is also pertinent. These authors maintain that a useful starting point in the study of behavioural genetics is the group of single genes implicated in neurological or centrally debilitating disorders. It follows that studies of the occurrence of major disorders such as schizophrenia in individuals with mental retardation syndromes of single-gene origin is most timely (Reid 1994).

Major affective disorder
Studies on the genetics of major affective disorder have been at least as revealing as those in schizophrenia. Most writers agree that there are certain subtypes of affective disorder which show particularly high rates of genetic susceptibility (McGuffin and Katz 1989). In general, it appears that affective or depressive disorders of minor severity are more environmentally determined, while more severe variants display greater genetic causality. This is most pronounced in the more severe condition of manic–depressive psychosis. However, studies of a recently described subtype of manic–depressive psychosis, rapid cycling manic–depressive disorder, have found that this illness is no more likely to show genetic loading than other forms of manic–depressive disorder (Cole *et al.* 1993). Studies employing brain scanning techniques have reported that this condition often occurs in the presence of some identifiable brain lesion (Berney and Jones 1988).

These studies have major implications for the application of the phenomic approach to behavioural phenotype studies. Populations of patients with major psychiatric disorders have been identified, often with many similarities to other conditions, yet differing only in certain respects (severity of mood change but not frequency of any such changes, as in the case of rapid cycling disorder). Even on the basis of comparatively minor differences, therefore, some disorders are found to have discrete genetic bases, while other more substantial variations in behavioural phenotype may share a common genotype. The message conveyed by this work is clear. Meticulous behavioural observation and description of clinical state may be instrumental in detecting the presence of different genetic disorders.

Other psychiatric disorders
Studies have suggested that there is some genetic basis to disorders across the whole

spectrum of psychopathology, from alcoholism and anorexia nervosa to personality disorders and phobias (Bohman 1978, Carey and Gottesman 1981, McGuffin and Thapar 1992). In many of these disorders, the evidence is far from convincing. Indeed, critics of genetic approaches to human behaviour have identified methodological flaws which lay behind many of the over-enthusiastic claims made by some early genetic psychiatric studies (Billings *et al.* 1992). Several of these issues remain contentious. Many writers have claimed that genetic studies all too often pay insufficient attention to environmental influences (*e.g.* Waller and Muthén 1992; see the above section on schizophrenia for an account of one potential problem in the very widely quoted twin studies of genetic predisposition to major mental illness.) Still other criticisms have centred on genetic research which has employed heterogenous samples rather than tightly defined diagnostic groups.

The principal lesson to be learned from these studies seems to be one of avoiding over-inclusion in diagnostic groupings of behavioural phenotypes. Just as research on the genetic basis of different aspects of personality functioning can only proceed on the foundation of a valid and coherent model of personality and its disorders (McGuffin and Thapar 1992), so is it crucial to focus on reliable and clearly defined behaviours when it comes to consideration of behavioural phenotypes.

Phenomic research—findings in mental retardation syndromes

One of the most striking sets of findings indicating the utility and power of the phenomic approach has been the ability of this approach to highlight conditions which have subsequently been shown to have a discrete biological basis. It has been routine practice for many decades for clinicians to begin with detailed observations of the phenotype, in terms of intellectual disability and dysmorphology. These observations have then been grouped together, the aim being the eventual identification of common aetiologies. In this way, a replication of the obligate region of chromosome 21 was found to be responsible for Down syndrome. However, much more recently, it has been through observations of a common behavioural phenotype that populations have been grouped together. In some cases this has already resulted in the identification of causative genes.

One of the most notable examples of this has been Prader–Willi syndrome. This syndrome has been recognized for many years as a separate condition, equally common in males and females. It is characterized by a particular pattern of insatiable carbohydrate over-eating, and includes hypogonadism and tissue laxity. More recent reports have also identified mood disorders and anxiety regulation problems (Whitman and Accardo 1987, Whitman and Greenswag 1991). Within the past few years a gene has been identified on chromosome 15: a deletion at the 15q site (Butler *et al.* 1986). Among individuals who on clinical phenomic diagnosis have Prader–Willi syndrome, the proportion found to have this gene is currently rising. Chapter 7 gives a more detailed account of the clinical features of this condition. It is as yet unknown whether the different affective features of the disorder are linked to different genetic lesions. Conversely, it is as yet unclear whether more rigid phenomic definition including other behavioural characteristics such as these mood anomalies will result in even closer correspondence between clinical and genetic diagnosis of the condition. Ongoing animal studies which suggest that genetic factors play some part in choice of food in omnivorous species (Runyan and Koschorreck 1990) may well indicate the direction to be taken by future research. In any case, the need for detailed structured behavioural studies of the condition remains as urgent as does further elucidation of the mechanisms which cause and bring about the expression of the deletion.

Another disorder which has been the subject of extensive inquiry but which as yet has not been found to have a discrete biological cause is Rett syndrome (Hagberg 1985, 1993). This condition is characterized by midline repetitive hand movements, with onset early in life. There is an idiosyncratic pattern of an evolution of changing symptoms over time, with a period of autistic-type regression in early childhood, followed by the re-emergence of the capacity for social learning later. Throughout childhood into adult life, there is increasing muscle tone, resulting in an eventual picture of a flexed posture with generalized spastic paresis and mental retardation. It is most striking that only females have as yet been described with this condition. This strongly suggests that the disorder has a genetic basis. (For a full description of current findings, see Chapter 7).

In different ways, the study of these two disorders illustrates the strength of the phenomic approach. In the case of Prader–Willi syndrome, the gene has now been identified. In the case of Rett syndrome, the identification of a biological cause is still awaited but is made possible because of the available descriptions of the behavioural phenotype. In both cases, meticulous behavioural observation has been crucial in the initial delineation of the syndrome. This has in turn paved the way for investigation of aetiology and pathogenesis.

Phenomic research—intelligence and learning

Genetics of intelligence

There is an immense amount of literature on the genetics of intelligence, yet still the subject remains highly controversial. Most recent reviewers have concluded that there is a powerful genetic contribution to intelligence (Plomin 1990). The heritability of intelligence is now estimated at around 50 per cent, and a polygenic model is most widely accepted (Thapar *et al.* 1994). However, environmental factors obviously play a major part in development and shaping of intelligence, through nutrition, education, social experience, parental factors and a host of other influences (Tizard 1975, Schiff and Lewontin 1986). All authorities therefore agree that intelligence has multiple aetiologies: multiple both in terms of the genes and environmental influences operating, and in the manner of their mutual interactions. Interestingly, it is now understood that parental and family environmental factors operate most powerfully in this connection early in life. Also, it appears that genetic predisposition is less important in the determination of intelligence in early childhood, but becomes more important as the child grows older (Plomin and Rende 1991). Insights from animal experiments on temporal–genetic analysis, which have shown that when behaviours do vary across time the temporal profile of some behaviours may be genotype dependent, lend some support to this view (Vadasz *et al.* 1992). This suggestion, however, has enormous implications.

One proposal which flows from these insights into the genetic and environmental origins of intelligence is that education systems and structures should take account of genetic endowment. Putting it simply, some might claim that the educational opportunities given to an individual should depend on genetic endowment. Others fear such a scenario, let alone propose that such policies should be pursued. Their fear is that the insights derived from this work might be over-enthusiastically applied. It is conceivable that this might even extend to setting the agenda for education, with possibly even different levels of expectation according to genetic endowment (Nelkin and Tancredi 1991). It is hardly surprising to note that the current international initiative which comprises the human genome project has raised alarm in certain quarters (Waller 1991).

Consideration of the genetics of intelligence as applied to people with mental retardation can both inform and be informed by these debates. First of all, there is the issue of the heritability of mental retardation. In the case of single gene disorders this is—at first sight—a comparatively straightforward matter. However, in many cases, notably of milder forms of mental retardation, the cause is as yet unknown. Most authorities agree that many such cases will, in time, prove to be due to single genes (McKusick and Amberger 1993). However, if it is accepted that many multiple interacting genes will eventually be identified as responsible for a substantial proportion of the population with mental retardation (Bregman and Hodapp 1991, McGuffin et al. 1994) and that these genes interact in some fashion with environmental influences, then it seems likely that people with mental retardation whose intelligence is determined by this model will fall into two groups (Thapar et al. 1994). First, there are those who are essentially at the extreme end of normal variation. As described above, this is the model which prevails in our understanding of the genetics of normal intelligence. In fact, Plomin (1990) has estimated that something of the order of 20 genes will be found to be implicated in this connection. It has long been accepted that a substantial number of individuals with mild mental retardation should be viewed in this way. This genetic model lends strength to this assumption, and supplies a mechanism for its operation. The remainder of cases of mental retardation which might be due to gene combinations remains somewhat conjectural. The possibility is that some types of mental retardation will be found to be due to a small number of deleterious genes, whose impact is mutually dependent through complex mechanisms and 'switches'. It may be that cases determined in this way will be of more severe mental retardation.

Those who are involved in the debate surrounding the possible educational repercussions of genetic investigations of intelligence might do well to consider the experience yielded, and the lessons which have been learned, through the education of individuals with mental retardation. First and foremost, educational classification no longer employs such language as 'ineducable'—a term which was used until quite recently to describe children with severe mental retardation (see 'Learning theory', p. 10). Many such individuals go on acquiring skills, and gaining in academic ability, well into adult life. Despite the real insights yielded by genetic studies of intelligence, and particularly the observation that environmental factors become less important while genetic factors increase in importance with age (Plomin and Rende 1991), it does not necessarily follow that a genetically determined 'ceiling' in terms of intelligence and educational attainment should be anticipated for any one individual. On the contrary, it seems that education planning must look to give all individuals maximal opportunity, rather than anticipate educational failure by some, for to follow the latter course is both to plan for and bring about such failure, with the inevitable adverse developmental consequences. This is in line with long-established mainstream educational thinking (Goacher *et al.* 1988, Haskell and Barrett 1989).

Yet another issue is that of phenotypic heterogeneity of single gene disorders. This is the capacity for one single genetic lesion, such as a deletion or replication, to be variable in its manifest clinical phenotype. This phenomenon is widespread. In addition, where a single gene produces one commonly identifiable phenotype, the severity of mental retardation associated with the condition can be variable. This is apparent even in Down syndrome, where most affected individuals have moderate or severe retardation, but a minority have only mild retardation. Other disorders including de Lange and Prader–Willi syndromes are far more diverse in their associated degrees of intellectual disability. It seems logical that this variability is due not only to gene/environment interactions, but also to the other genes which so powerfully determine intelligence in all humans (Plomin 1990). The implication of this line of thinking for behavioural phenotypes research is that when we perform genetic investigations of family pedigrees we should not only be looking for dilute forms of severe disorders and 'carriers', but also seek to study other 'intelligence genes', since these are likely to exert a powerful influence on the eventual level of intelligence of the affected individual, and in turn upon disability.

Concluding comment

In all considerations and studies of behavioural phenotypes, one powerful factor must be borne in mind. This is the severity of the intellectual or developmental disability present (Siggers 1977). A host of studies of psychiatric disorders in people with mental retardation has demonstrated that the patterns of disorder which occur change with differing degrees of retardation: some psychiatric disorders which are commonly encountered in the general population, *e.g.* depression, take on different forms in people with mental retardation; others, such as anorexia nervosa, rarely occur; and some types of behaviour disorder which are seldom seen in the general population—*e.g.* some of those associated with autism—are quite common in people with severe mental retardation (Corbett 1979, Gillberg *et al.* 1986, O'Brien and Whitehouse 1990, Campbell and Malone 1991). Clearly, the general level of severity of intellectual disability exerts a profound influence on the psychiatric and behaviour disorders which occur. One of the greatest challenges for behavioural phenotypes research therefore lies in clarifying which behaviours are more dependent on degree of intellectual disability rather than reflecting a specific causal gene.

REFERENCES

Berney, T.P., Jones, P.M. (1988) 'Manic depressive disorder in mental handicap.' *Australian and New Zealand Journal of Developmental Disabilities*, **14**, 219–225.

Billings, P.R., Beckwith, J., Alper, J.S. (1992) 'The genetic analysis of human behavior: a new era?' *Social Science and Medicine*, **35**, 227–238.

Boerwinkle, E., Chakraborty, R., Sing, C.F. (1986) 'The use of measured genotype information in the analysis of quantitative phenotypes in man. 1. Models and analytical methods.' *Annals of Human Genetics*, **50**, 181–194.

Bohman, M. (1978) 'Some genetic aspects of alcoholism and criminality. A population of adoptees.' *Archives of General Psychiatry*, **35**, 269–276.

—— Cloninger, R., Sigvardsson, S., von Knorring, A-L. (1982) 'Predisposition to petty criminality in Swedish adoptees. I. Genetic and environmental heterogeneity.' *Archives of General Psychiatry*, **39**, 1233–1241.

Borgaonkar, D.S., Shah, S.A. (1974) 'The XYY chromosome. Male—or syndrome?' *Progress in Medical Genetics*, **10**, 135–222.

Borghgraef, M., Fryns, J-P., Van den Bergh, E. (1991) 'The 48,XXYY syndrome. Follow-up data on clinical characteristics and psychological findings in 4 patients.' *Genetic Counseling*, **2**, 103–108.

Bouras, N., Drummond, C. (1992) 'Behaviour and psychiatric disorders of people with mental handicaps living in the community.' *Journal of Intellectual Disability Research*, **36**, 349–357.

Bregman, J.D., Hodapp, R.M. (1991) 'Current developments in the understanding of mental retardation. Part 1: biological and phenomenological perspectives.' *Journal of the American Academy of Child and Adolescent Psychiatry*, **30**, 707–719.

Bronfenbrenner, U. (1977) 'Toward an experimental ecology of human development.' *American Psychologist*, **32**, 513–531.

Butler, M.G., Meaney, F.J., Palmer, C.G. (1986) 'Clinical and cytogenetic survey of 39 individuals with Prader–Labhart–Willi syndrome.' *American Journal of Medical Genetics*, **23**, 793–809.

Campbell, M., Malone, R.P. (1991) 'Mental retardation and psychiatric disorders.' *Hospital and Community Psychiatry*, **42**, 374–379.

Carey, G., Gottesman, I.I. (1981) 'Twin and family studies of anxiety, phobic and obsessive disorders.' *In:* Klein, D.F., Rabkin, J. (Eds.) *Anxiety: New Research and Changing Concepts.* New York: Raven Press, pp 117–135.

Clarke, D.J., Waters, J., Corbett, J.A. (1989) 'Adults with Prader–Willi syndrome: abnormalities of sleep and behaviour.' *Journal of the Royal Society of Medicine*, **82**, 21–24.

Cole, A.J., Scott, J., Ferrier, I.N., Eccleston, D. (1993) 'Patterns of treatment resistance in bipolar affective disorder.' *Acta Psychiatrica Scandinavica*, **88**, 121–123.

Cooper, S-A., Collacott, R.A. (1993) 'Mania and Down's syndrome.' *British Journal of Psychiatry*, **162**, 739–743.

Corbett, J.A. (1979) 'Psychiatric morbidity and mental retardation.' *In:* James, F.E., Snaith, R.P. (Eds.) *Psychiatric Illness and Mental Handicap.* London: Gaskell Press, pp. 11–25.

Dolan, C.V., Molenaar, P.C., Boomsma, D.I. (1992) 'Decomposition of multivariate phenotypic means in multigroup genetic covariance structure analysis.' *Behavior Genetics*, **22**, 319–335.

Down, J.L. (1866) 'Observations on an ethnic classification of idiots.' *London Hospital Reports*, **3**, 259–262. (Reprinted in Down, J.L. *Mental Affectations of Childhood and Youth*, republished by Mac Keith Press, London, 1990, pp. 127–131.)

Einfeld, S.L., Hall, W. (1994) 'When is a behavioural phenotype not a phenotype?' *Developmental Medicine and Child Neurology*, **36**, 467–470. *(Annotation.)*

Fenwick, P. (1987) 'Epilepsy and psychiatric disorders.' *In:* Hopkins, A. (Ed.) *Epilepsy.* Cambridge: Chapman & Hall, pp. 511–552.

Flint, J., Yule, W. (1994) 'Behavioural phenotypes.' *In:* Rutter, M., Taylor, E., Hersov, L. (Eds.) *Child and Adolescent Psychiatry, 3rd Edn.* Oxford: Blackwell Scientific, pp. 666–687.

Freeman, C. (1983) 'Personality disorders.' *In:* Kendal, R.E., Zuyie, A.K. (Eds.) *Companion to Psychiatric Studies.* Edinburgh: Churchill Livingstone, pp. 355–373.

Fryns, J-P. (1992) 'Aarskog syndrome: the changing phenotype with age.' *American Journal of Medical Genetics*, **43**, 420–427.

Gillberg, C., Persson, E., Grufman, M., Themner, U. (1986) 'Psychiatric disorders in mildly and severely mentally retarded urban children and adolescents: epidemiological aspects.' *British Journal of Psychiatry*, **149**, 68–74.

Goacher, B., Evans, J., Welton, J., Wedell, K. (1988) *Policy and Provision for Special Educational Needs.* London: Cassell.

Gottesman, I.I. Shields, J. (1982) *Schizophrenia: the Epigenetic Puzzle.* Cambridge: Cambridge University Press.

Gow, L.P., Balla, J., Butterfield, E. (1990) 'The relative efficacy of cognitive and behavioural approaches in instruction in promoting adaptive capacity.' *In:* Fraser, W.I. (Ed.) *Key Issues in Mental Retardation Research.* London: Routledge, pp. 366–376.

Hagberg, B. (1985) 'Rett's syndrome: prevalence and impact on progressive severe mental retardation in girls.' *Acta Paediatrica Scandinavica*, **74**, 405–408.

—— (1993) *Rett Syndrome—Clinical and Biological Aspects. Clinics in Developmental Medicine No. 127.* London: Mac Keith Press.

Harris, J.C. (1987) 'Behavioural phenotypes in mental retardation: unlearned behaviours.' *Advances in Developmental Disorders*, **1**, 77–106.

Haskell, S.H., Barrett, E.K. (1989) *The Education of Children with Motor and Neurological Disabilities. 2nd Edn.* London: Chapman & Hall.

Hodapp, R.M., Burack, J.A., Zigler, E. (1990) 'The developmental perspective in the field of mental retardation.' *In:* Hodapp, R.M., Burack, J.A., Zigler, E. (Eds.) *Issues in the Developmental Approach to Mental Retardation.* Cambridge: Cambridge University Press, pp. 3–76.

Hrubec, Z., Robinette, C.D. (1984) 'The study of human twins in medical research.' *New England Journal of Medicine*, **310**, 435–441.

Humphreys, L.G. (1957) 'Characteristics of type concepts with special reference to Sheldon's typology.' *Psychological Bulletin*, **54**, 218–228.

Jacobs, P.A., Brunton, M., Melville, M.M, Brittain, R.P., McClemont, W.F. (1965) 'Aggressive behaviour, mental sub-normality and the XYY male.' *Nature*, **208**, 1351–1352.

Jancar, J. (1992) '49,XXXXY syndrome: behavioural and developmental profiles.' *Journal of Medical Genetics*, **29**, 357. *(Letter.)*

Johnson, H.G., Ekman, P., Friesen, W., Nyhan, W.L., Shear, C. (1976) 'A behavioral phenotype in the de Lange syndrome.' *Pediatric Research*, **10**, 843–850.

Kendler, K.S., Robinette C.D. (1983) 'Schizophrenia in the National Academy of Sciences—National Research Council Twin Registry: a 16-year update.' *American Journal of Psychiatry*, **140**, 1551–1563.

Kennedy, J.L., Giuffra, L.A., Moises, H.W., Cavalli-Sforza, L.L., Pakstis, A.J., Kidd, J.R., Castiglione, C.M., Sjogren, B., Wetterberg, L., Kidd, K.K. (1988) 'Evidence against linkage of schizophrenia to markers on chromosome 5 in a northern Swedish pedigree.' *Nature*, **336**, 167–170.

Kretschmer, E. (1936) *Physique and Character. 2nd Edn.* London: Routledge & Kegan Paul.

Lågas, P.A., Ruokonen, A. (1991) 'Late onset argininosuccinic aciduria in a paranoid retardate.' *Biological Psychiatry*, **30**, 1229–1232.

Lee, S. (1990) 'Psychopathology in Sturge–Weber syndrome.' *Canadian Journal of Psychiatry*, **35**, 674–678.

Lomelino, C.A., Reiss, A.L. (1991) '49,XXXXY syndrome: behavioural and developmental profiles.' *Journal of Medical Genetics*, **28**, 609–612.

Maudsley, H. (1905) 'Medicine, present and prospective.' *British Medical Journal*, **2**, 227–231.

McGuffin, P., Katz, R. (1989) 'The genetics of depression and manic–depressive disorder.' *British Journal of Psychiatry*, **155**, 294–304.

—— Thapar, A. (1992) 'The genetics of personality disorder.' *British Journal of Psychiatry*, **160**, 12–23.

—— Owen, M.J., O'Donovan, M.C., Thapar, A., Gottesman, I.I. (1994) *Seminars in Psychiatric Genetics.* London: Gaskell.

McKusick, V.A., Amberger, J.S. (1993) 'The morbid anatomy of the human genome: chromosomal location of mutations causing disease.' *Journal of Medical Genetics*, **30**, 1–26.

Myers, B.A., Pueschel, S.M. (1991) 'Psychiatric disorders in persons with Down syndrome.' *Journal of Nervous and Mental Disease*, **179**, 609–613.

Nelkin, D., Tancredi, L. (1991) 'Classify and control: genetic information in the schools.' *American Journal of Law and Medicine*, **17**, 51–73.

Nyhan, W.L. (1972) 'Behavioral phenotypes in organic genetic disease. Presidential address to the Society for Pediatric Research, May 1, 1971.' *Pediatric Research*, **6**, 1–9.

O'Brien, G. (1992) 'Behavioural phenotypy in developmental psychiatry. Measuring behavioural phenotypes, a guide to the available schedules.' *European Child and Adolescent Psychiatry*, Suppl. 1, 1–61.

—— Whitehouse, A.M. (1990) 'A psychiatric study of deviant eating behaviour among mentally handicapped adults.' *British Journal of Psychiatry*, **157**, 281–284.

21

Pfadt, A. (1990) 'Diagnosing and treating psychopathology in clients with a dual diagnosis: an integrative model.' *In:* Dosen, A., Van Gennep, A., Zwanikken, G.J. (Eds.) *Treatment of Mental Illness and Behaviour Disorder in the Mentally Retarded. Proceedings of the International Congress, 3 and 4 May, 1990, Amsterdam, the Netherlands.* Leider, the Netherlands: Logon, pp. 217–224.

Plomin, R. (1986) *Development, Genetics and Psychology.* Hillsdale, NJ: Lawrence Erlbaum.

—— (1990) The role of inheritance in behavior.' *Science*, **248**, 183–188.

—— (1991) 'Behavioral genetics.' *In:* McGugh, P.R., McKusick, V.A. (Eds.) *Genes, Brain and Behavior.* New York: Raven Press, pp. 165–180.

—— Rende, R. (1991) 'Human behavioral genetics.' *Annual Review of Psychology*, **42**, 161–190.

Pond, D.A., Bidwell, B.H. (1960) 'A survey of epilepsy in fourteen general practices. II. Social and psychological aspects.' *Epilepsia*, **1**, 285–299.

Reid, A.H. (1994) 'Psychiatry and learning disability.' *British Journal of Psychiatry*, **164**, 613–618.

Reiss, A.L., Freund, L., Vinogradov, S., Hagerman, R., Cronister, A. (1989) 'Parental inheritance and psychological disability in fragile X females.' *American Journal of Human Genetics*, **45**, 697–705.

Runyan, T.J., Koschorreck, R. (1990) 'Evidence for genetic determination of specific food choices of rats.' *Journal of the American College of Nutrition*, **9**, 623–629.

Rutter, M., Bolton, P., Harrington, R., Le Couteur, A., MacDonald, H., Simonoff, E. (1990*a*) 'Genetic factors in child psychiatric disorders—I. A review of research strategies.' *Journal of Child Psychology and Psychiatry*, **31**, 3–37.

—— Macdonald, H., Le Couteur, A., Harrington, R., Bolton, P., Bailey, A. (1990*b*) 'Genetic factors in child psychiatric disorders—II. Empirical findings.' *Journal of Child Psychology and Psychiatry*, **31**, 39–83.

Schiff, M., Lewontin, R. (1986) *Education and Class: the Irrelevance of IQ Genetic Studies.* Oxford: Clarendon Press.

Sheldon, W.H., Stephens, S.S. (1942) *The Varieties of Temperament: a Psychology of Constitutional Difficulties.* New York: Harper.

Sherrington, R., Brynjolfsson, J., Petursson, H., Potter, M., Dudleston, K., Barraclough, B., Wasmuth, J., Dobbs, M., Gurling, H. (1988) 'Localization of a susceptibility locus for schizophrenia on chromosome 5.' *Nature*, **336**, 164–167.

Siggers, D.C. (1977) 'Human Behavioural Genetics.' *Developmental Medicine and Child Neurology*, **19**, 818–820.

SSBP (1990) *Behavioural Phenotypes Study Group Symposium. Abstracts and Syndrome Information.* (Available from Dr Gregory O'Brien, Northgate Hospital, Northumberland.)

St Clair, D., Blackwood, D., Muir, W., Baillie, D., Hubbard, A., Wright, A., Evans, H.J. (1989) 'No linkage of chromosome 5q11–q13 markers to schizophrenia in Scottish families.' *Nature*, **339**, 305–309.

Thapar, A., Gottesman, I.I., Owen, M.J., O'Donovan, M.C., McGuffin, P. (1994) 'The genetics of mental retardation.' *British Journal of Psychiatry*, **164**, 747–758.

Tizard, B. (1962) 'The personality of epileptics: a discussion of the evidence.' *Psychological Bulletin*, **59**, 196–210.

Tizard, J. (1975) 'Race and IQ: the limits of probability.' *New Behaviour*, **1**, 6–9.

Tsuang, M.T. (1993) 'Genotypes, phenotypes, and the brain. A search for connections in schizophrenia.' *British Journal of Psychiatry*, **163**, 299–307.

Turk, J. (1992) 'The fragile-X syndrome. On the way to a behavioural phenotype.' *British Journal of Psychiatry*, **160**, 24–35.

Turner, T. (1988) 'Henry Maudsley—psychiatrist, philosopher and entrepreneur.' *Psychological Medicine*, **18**, 551–574.

Vadasz, C., Kobor, G., Lajtha, A. (1992) 'Motor activity and the mesotelencephalic dopamine function. 1. High-resolution temporal and genetic analysis of open-field behaviour.' *Behavioural Brain Research*, **48**, 29–39.

Waller, M.J.C. (1991) 'Selfish psycho-darwinism.' *Nature*, **351**, 264. *(Letter.)*

Waller, N.G., Muthén, B.O. (1992) 'Genetic Tobit factor analysis: quantitative genetic modeling with censored data.' *Behaviour Genetics*, **22**, 265–292.

Whitman, B.Y., Accardo, P. (1987) 'Emotional symptoms in Prader–Willi syndrome adolescents.' *American Journal of Medical Genetics*, **28**, 897–905.

—— Greenswag, L.R. (1991) 'The use of mood and behavior altering drugs in persons with Prader–Willi syndrome.' *Pediatric Research*, **29**, 126A. *(Abstract.)*

Witkin, H.A., Mednick, S.A., Schulsinger, F., Bakkestrøm, E., Christiansen, K.O., Goodenough, D.R.,, Hirschhorn, K., Lundsteen, C., Owen, D.R., *et al.* (1976) 'Criminality in XYY and XXY men. The elevated crime rate of XYY males is not related to aggression. It may be related to low intelligence.' *Science*, **193**, 547–555.

WHO (1973) *Report of the International Pilot Study of Schizophrenia*. Geneva: World Health Organization.

Yule, W. (1987) 'Identifying problems: functional analysis and observation and recording techniques.' *In:* Yule, W., Carr, J. (Eds.) *Behaviour Modification for People with Mental Handicaps*. London: Croom Helm, pp. 8–27.

2
THE NEW GENETICS

Sarah-Jane Richards

Genetic linkage—an historical perspective

The model for a double helical structure for deoxyribonucleic acid (DNA) proposed by Crick and Watson in 1953 became the accepted basis for the transmission of genetic information and heralded the birth of molecular biology. While Crick and Watson were busy cracking the genetic code, Fred Sanger, also based in Cambridge, was developing a technique for sequencing amino acids, the building blocks for proteins. This study and his later work on the nucleotide sequence of nucleic acids not only gave him the accolade of being awarded two Nobel prizes but also provided the climate in the 1980s for spurring on a plethora of scientific endeavour toward increasing our understanding of genetic information.

Molecular genetics today is distinctly more complex than in the late 1980s when this pioneering research amounted almost exclusively to the search for disease genes through genetic linkage analysis. Single gene disorders such as Huntington's disease (Tagle *et al.* 1993), Duchenne muscular dystrophy (Kunkel 1986) and cystic fibrosis (Rommens *et al.* 1989) were particularly aptly investigated by this technique which represented the real possibility of tracking down disease genes. This novel approach to understanding the causes of single gene disorders led to the formation of large and powerful research groups in which significantly large sums of research monies were invested. Successes, failures and scurrilous practices associated with the race for disease genes were part of the strength and weakness of this newly discovered and exciting molecular technology.

The search for a specific disease gene locus and for the defective gene itself involved the identification of families suffering from these autosomal dominant disorders. Blood samples were obtained from affected and non-affected family members across as many generations as possible and their DNA extracted. Young scientists and clinicians, keen to apply these new techniques, were harnessed to the research bench in the great linkage race. Day and night, DNA would be extracted from blood samples, digested with restriction enzymes and bound to membranes for screening. In this way, Southern blots comprising DNA from entire families would be screened for any unusual arrangements of the DNA markers used (Southern 1975). Such rearrangements in affected family members and absent in the non-affected relatives provided information about how close the markers used were to the disease locus. In an attempt to increase the pedigree membership for whom a DNA profile was available, wax embedded post-mortem histology samples were assessed as a viable source of information about deceased family members. Unfortunately, most laboratories succeeded in isolating only small fragments of mainly degraded DNA.

In other laboratories techniques were developed to collect and analyse discrete populations of chromosomes. Fluorescent Activated Chromosome Sorting (FACS) permitted the pooling of individual chromosomes according to their fluorescent peak which in turn was determined by their size (Young *et al.* 1981). This technique was dependent on the affinity of DNA to bind the fluorescent ethidium bromide. Thus, chromosome 1 being a much larger chromosome than 21 would produce a distinctly higher peak value. By fluorescent labelling of all of the chromosomes within the human genome, individual chromosomes could be collected by high pressure liquid chromatography according to their peak value. Specific chromosomes, especially those associated with a single gene disease locus, would be collected and digested with restriction enzymes into more manageably sized fragments for cloning and subsequent amplification. Exploiting this technology, Davies *et al.* (1981) constructed their X chromosome specific genomic library for isolating flanking polymorphic markers in the race to identify the Duchenne muscular dystrophy gene.

In parallel, cloning vector technology was also rapidly developing. Gene libraries incorporating fragments of either whole chromosomes or human genomic DNA were constructed using suitable vectors for amplification. These became the resources from which new chromosomal markers were generated, and always the aim was to flank the disease gene locus and with new polymorphic markers to move closer to the disease locus.

Chromosomal libraries tended to exploit Yeast Artificial Chromosomes (YACs) as the host vector system, which offered the advantage of accepting large fragments of up to 10,000 kilobases of chromosomal DNA (Burke *et al.* 1987). Chromosomes identified and sorted by FACS were restriction enzyme digested into smaller fragments before being ligated into these YACs. Using known DNA markers already associated with specific regions of the known chromosome, it was possible to align the various YACs so that a complete chromosome was covered by a series of overlapping YACs containing chromosomal DNA.

Genomic libraries were constructed using genes associated with a specific genome, and these were mainly human genomic libraries. The major part of genomic DNA comprises intronal DNA which provides information pertaining to splice sites, regulatory sequences and other elements important to the genes being expressed within specific tissues at a specific time. As in the case of YAC library construction, genomic DNA was restriction enzyme digested into smaller fragments and ligated into a suitable host vector. Cosmids, being able to accept up to ~45 kilobases of foreign DNA, provided an ideal vector system for these genomic libraries (Collins and Hohn 1978).

Over the years a range of libraries has been constructed—both 'in house' and commercially available. These resources have been invaluable in identifying new markers for flanking disease gene loci. Furthermore, by using existing markers it has been possible to identify a single YAC or cosmid containing both flanking markers and, by virtue of this, the disease gene itself. Once a YAC or cosmid was identified as containing the disease gene, the DNA was excised from the vector, digested, and fragments sub-cloned into a vector suitable for sequencing,

Initially, sequencing involved sub-cloning the DNA of interest into M13, a single-stranded vector. In order to be able to sequence both orientations of the cloned DNA, a number of clones had to be screened to ensure both orientations were obtained (Sanger *et al.* 1977). Later, Bluescript, a versatile and stable double-stranded plasmid vector, facilitated sub-cloning double-stranded DNA of up to 4 kilobase pairs. Thus, having successfully sub-cloned the sequence of interest into Bluescript, it could be amplified, labelled and sequenced without further treatment. Furthermore, this vector had the distinct advantage of being ideal for automated sequencing. Sequencing by hand involved the use of radioactive isotopes, a six hour polyacrylamide gel run, overnight film development, and reading the sequence into a computer data base. Each step provided plenty of opportunity for human error, and a good run would generate only a few hundred bases of identifiable sequence. The advent of the automated sequencer dramatically changed this process. Fluorescent tags, an overnight run and the automatic installation of as much as a kilobase of novel sequence directly into the computer data base vastly increased the speed at which data could be analysed.

Molecular biology, even its more elementary form, has led to the discovery of variable length trinucleotide repeats within the intronal region of patients suffering with Huntington's disease, variable deletions in Duchenne muscular dystrophy, and mutations in the calcium channel gene associated with cystic fibrosis. However, the diseases to have benefited from this type of genetic linkage analysis have had a very unambiguous diagnosis. In situations where diagnosis may not be confirmed by hard physiological data, the assumptions in statistical analysis involved in genetic linkage have been demonstrated as being insufficiently stringent (Sherrington *et al.* 1988).

Today, the fervour associated with racing to isolate disease genes prevalent in the late 1980s has been replaced with a more mature approach to human genetics based on the knowledge that isolating a gene is but the first step to understanding the mechanisms underlying a disease process and several steps away from developing an effective treatment or cure for the disease. Molecular genetics has itself diversified to include several new parameters, the most celebrated being that of mapping human and comparative genomes. The emphasis of this work has in part been determined by national and international financial investment.

Recombinant DNA technology evolves

Inevitably, exposure to molecular techniques, which are now employed within many scientific disciplines, and to the language used to explain the technology has largely demystified molecular biology. Techniques once the domain of biochemists and cytogeneticists are now routinely used in anatomy, psychiatry and pathology departments. Although the technology has become more sophisticated, it has also been developed with the non-specialist in mind. Thus we have seen the emergence of many biotechnology companies which are simplifying procedures and developing kits to minimize the skills and training required by their users. Similarly, concerns about user safety and consequences upon the environment of massive increases in the use of radioisotopes has led to the development of fluorescent labelling systems.

From the initial surge of research on single gene diseases and autosomal dominant disorders, we have compiled a composite picture of the mutations which underlie many of these diseases. Such disease genes have now been cloned and identified using restriction fragment length polymorphisms (RFLPs) derived from these genes, anonymous probes and probes associated with highly variable regions (HVRs). While genetic studies of human disease have successfully identified aberrant genes associated with distinct pathological phenotypes such as Huntington's disease, the current challenge for recombinant DNA technology is the application of genetic analysis to common diseases such as cancer and coronary heart disease and disorders such as schizophrenia and manic depression which appear to have both strong multiple genetic and environmental (non-genetic) components to their aetiology. A quantitative trait loci (QTL) polygenic or multiple gene approach seeks the identification of a number of genes, none of which alone is essential or sufficient to produce the trait.

While genetic linkage has commonly been the method of analysis employed for the single gene–single disease approach, it is frequently insufficiently sensitive to detect QTLs. However, allelic association, otherwise known as linkage disequilibrium, is able to identify correlations within the population between the occurrence of a particular allele and a specific phenotype. An example of this has been the identification of the chromosome 19, ApoE4 allele and its association with late onset Alzheimer's disease (AD) (Corder et al. 1993). Information to date on the aetiology of AD implicates several genes: (i) a gene dosage effect of the chromosome 21 amyloid gene as a risk factor for individuals with trisomy 21 (Down syndrome); (ii) various mutations in the chromosome 21 amyloid gene; (iii) various mutations in the S182 gene on chromosome 14 (Sherrington et al. 1995); (iv) allelic association of the ApoEε4; and (v) other unidentified associations. While a genetic linkage approach yielded only a hint of an implication of ApoEε4 to AD (Pericak-Vance et al. 1991), the more sensitive QTL approach has detected a fairly robust correlation.

In order to begin to understand the problems associated with multifactorial inheritance, molecular genetics has to address extremely complex questions. For example, understanding the contribution of specific genes to normal development may involve getting to grips with genomic imprinting, transcription factors, apoptosis and cell differentiation, to name but a few genetically regulated processes, in addition to external influences such as maternal nutrition status during pregnancy. Molecular techniques employed have also moved on from Southern blotting and library construction to the genetic manipulation of whole organisms, gene delivery systems, cell immortalization, karyotyping by chromosomal painting and many others ranging in complexity. The interaction of genes with environmental factors and the implication of such combinations for human disease is becoming increasingly pertinent to the fields of cancer and heart disease research. Yet the unifying aspect of all of these varied branches of molecular genetics is that to some extent they depend on the isolation of genes which influence and regulate specific processes intrinsic to normal development and behaviour.

In the UK, while the Wellcome Trust, the Medical Research Council (MRC) and many smaller charities concerned with specific diseases are sponsoring such research in universities and clinical schools, the major input to understanding human genetics has been through the massive investment made by the MRC into the Human Genome Mapping Project (HGMP) initiated in 1989.

The Human Genome Mapping Project

Through a range of different programmes undertaken within universities, MRC establishments and other institutes, the HGMP has harnessed the activities of many research projects otherwise being conducted in a piecemeal and uncoordinated fashion throughout the scientific community. Thus, the HGMP has invested in and built upon one of the UK's traditional scientific strengths—that of human genetics research.

Today the initiative is overseen by the MRC's HGMP Coordinating Committee, which has the responsibility of ensuring the programme is developed with the support of other UK sponsors and industry. Furthermore, it liaises with other international organizations over the development of ideas and strategies relating to human genome research. The recently agreed strategy for the next five-year programme of the HGMP in the UK mirrors to a major extent commitment in the USA and encompasses the following main research areas: human and comparative genome mapping; communication and interaction; and training. Within these categories the MRC funds short-term grants and contracts, studentships, training fellowships, conferences, workshops and travel to international single chromosome workshops. 'Users meetings' are annual events designed to keep the community informed of changes in policy and strategy as well as to communicate progress on the UK initiative.

Building on the international discoveries from genetic linkage analysis and the subsequent success in the USA and Canada at identifying disease genes through this approach, the Genetic Approach to Human Health Initiative was established in 1992. This initiative seeks to sponsor the identification of disease genes through to the development of diagnostics and therapies which can be influential in determining clinical practice and application.

The UK programme

While the HGMP is an international concern, the strengths of the UK contribution are in the area of genetic and physical mapping and sequencing of human and other animal genomes. It is in the area of comparative genome mapping that the MRC is making a substantial commitment to expanding the programme. There is similar expansion in the field of bioinformatics.

The construction of *library banks* is a key component of the HGMP. Such libraries may: (i) incorporate genes being expressed by a specific tissue at the time it was taken to generate the library (cDNA libraries); (ii) incorporate fragments of whole chromosomes which are cloned into a suitable vector for amplification (chromosome specific libraries); or (iii) comprise genes cloned from single species genomic DNA (*e.g.* nematode genomic libraries). These libraries have become valuable resources in the identification of specific genes and the subsequent mapping of these genes onto human chromosomes. A range of libraries has been constructed and collated by Dr Hans Lehrach at the Imperial

Cancer Research Fund and also in association with the Human Genome Reference Library in Berlin.

Along with the generation of chromosomal, genomic and cDNA libraries, the UK programme has simultaneously developed robotics by which individual clones may be immobilized on filters in series of arrays for easy screening. Such high density gridding of gene libraries created in different research centres throughout the UK has formed the basis of a European-based resource available to any research group.

As previously mentioned, family pedigrees associated with specific diseases have been identified and their DNA collections used in 'linkage' studies to map the disease gene. Success with mapping these gene loci has been associated with the development of the Jeffrey's probes—micro-satellite genetic markers which span most of the human genome.

Sequence homology between families of genes has permitted genes of similar function to be isolated from cDNA libraries. Their conservation throughout evolution provides information about species diversity and gene manipulation. The technology is in place for cloning such genes, sequencing them and mapping them to a chromosome. Fluorescent *in situ* hybridization (FISH) permits cDNAs or fragments of genomic DNA to be localized to specific chromosomes via metaphase spread analysis. Successful application of FISH has mainly been restricted to situations where the amount of DNA available for labelling exceeds 2–3 kilobases.

Mapping and sequencing the genome of comparative systems has seen the investment by the MRC in the nematode (*Caenorhabditis elegans*) genome project located at the Sanger Centre at Hinxton Park, Cambridge. Sequencing the entire nematode genome is yielding valuable information about the conservation of genetic function through evolution and has beneficial implications for the human as well as other comparative genomes. The mouse genome is an area of increasing interest, and markers covering the entire genome are being mapped and entered into the mouse genome database. Distribution of mouse DNA immobilized on filters is undertaken through the HGMP as part of the European Collaborative Interspecific Mouse Backcross Programme—the largest in the world.

The UK contribution to HGMP has not been determined in isolation. The main initiative for mapping the human genome originated in the USA, and links with the UK project have involved establishing an arm of the USA Genome Database at the Sanger Centre. In particular, the *C. elegans* sequencing and mapping programme is part of a collaborative effort with the USA. Information dissemination is a further responsibility of the HGMP and occurs under the auspices of the Human Genome Organization. Single chromosome workshops and full scientific conferences have been organized on an annual basis and with full participation of European and US scientific counterparts.

Funding the HGMP has represented a major investment by the MRC. During 1989–93, the HGMP received £16.7m in ring-fenced funding. In addition to this sum, £1.5m was invested in comparative mapping in 1993 and a further £1.7m in 1994/5. The nematode sequencing programme being undertaken at the Sanger Centre has been sponsored at the level of £2m per annum for a five year period. Furthermore, the

European Bioinformatics Institute, also located at Hinxton Park, Cambridge, is funded at a total cost of £8m. The Genetic Approach to Human Health Initiative (1992–97) is anticipated to cost in the region of £84m.

The investment of such a high proportion of the MRC's research budget into sequencing the human and other genomes is extremely controversial and indicates the importance placed on gene isolation, sequencing and mapping. Ascribing function to these genes will involve more complex analyses and ones involving the use of *in vivo* and *in vitro* models using comparative systems. It is inevitable that as more information is generated through the current investment in the HGMP then concomitant functional analyses of these genes will be undertaken in whole animals. Work on genetically manipulated organisms is already addressing some of these questions. Transgenesis permits manipulated genes of interest to be inserted into a mouse (or other species) genome, at the single cell stage of development. Similarly, the expression of specific genes may be blocked within gene 'knock out' studies. Thus functional and behavioural consequences of over-expressing or suppressing a gene or manipulating the sequence of a gene may be determined in the whole animal.

Transgenesis

Transgenesis has become a powerful method by which the function of a modified gene may be examined *in vivo*. The technology was initially developed in the early 1970s when SV40 DNA was micro-injected into the pre-implanted mouse blastocyst. However, this resulted in the majority of animals being mosaics (Jaenish and Mintz 1974). One of the early transgenic models of Lesch–Nyhan syndrome was developed through the introduction of mutations of the hypoxanthine–guanosine phosphoribosyl transferase (HPRT) gene into mouse stem cells. Two clonal lines giving rise to chimeras permitted the subsequent generation of a transgenic mouse line carrying the same biochemical defect as Lesch–Nyhan patients (Kuehn *et al.* 1987). However, the outcome of transgenesis was greatly improved when viral DNA was micro-injected into the cytoplasm of single cell embryos with the resulting adults carrying a single copy of the inserted DNA in every cell (Harbers *et al.* 1981). Today, cloned plasmid or YAC DNA is micro-injected into the larger, male pronucleus of the recently fertilized egg (Fig. 2.1). The manipulated embryos are cultured until the blastocyst stage of development is achieved, whereupon they are implanted into a pseudo-pregnant host.

Successful integration of foreign DNA into host chromosomes is usually observed in fewer than 50 per cent of progeny, with little control of the copy numbers of foreign sequences incorporated into the host genome or the chromosomal site of integration. Developments in homologous recombination now permit the insertion site to be predetermined with the advantage of conserving upstream regulatory factors. Invariably, transgenesis has been used to investigate human genetic disorders, and cloned human sequences containing single base mutations, deletions, trinucleotide repeat sequences and other recombination events have been used to generate transgenic strains. Although mice have most commonly been used as the host animal, transgenic rats, rabbits and *Drosophila* have also been raised.

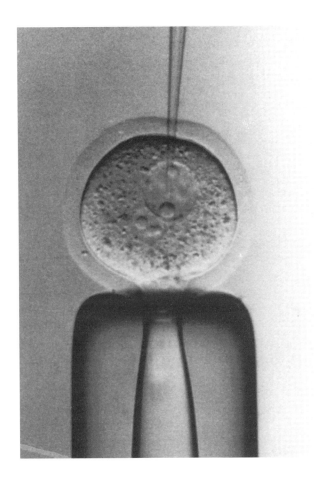

Fig. 2.1. Micro-injection of yeast artificial chromosome (YAC) or plasmid DNA incorporating gene(s) of interest into the male pronucleus of a recently fertilized egg.

Genetic imprinting

One of the key factors to understanding the scientific issues and technologies of a different discipline is mastering the language which can often be confusing. Imprinting, to the majority of psychologists and psychiatrists, is the process by which neonates form an essential parental bond. The process invariably involves a visual image of recognition of a parent by the infant at a critical time after birth. Thus, we have well cited examples of baby ducklings erroneously imprinting on humans or even on footballs. Genetic imprinting to the geneticist has a completely different meaning, and since the mid-1980s it has become a field of expanding research interest. Observations that normal mouse development requires both a maternal and a paternal genome, despite the fact that both genomes contribute similar genes, has raised questions about differences in parental genes. Normal mouse development is dependent on the zygote being euploid, yet in genetically balanced zygotes aberrant development occurs if both copies of certain chromosomal regions are from one parent. This suggests that the expression of at least some alleles is determined by their parental origin.

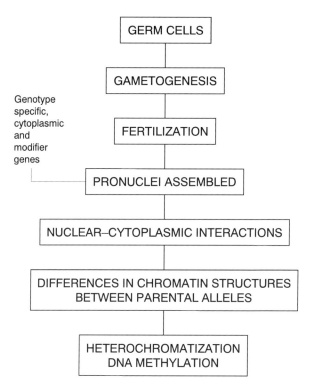

Fig. 2.2. Factors which influence epigenetic modification and imprinting. (Adapted by permission from Surani *et al.* 1990.)

The process of embryonic development begins with the zygote possessing two parental pronuclei and maternally inherited cytoplasmic factors. Imprinting is initiated in the germline and may continue after fertilization with interactions between the oocyte cytoplasmic factors and the parental genomes. Homologous chromosomes or regions of chromosomes may be imprinted with epigenetic information which results in specific functional differences between parental genomes. These chromosomal determinants have been shown to be relatively stable and vital for development (Fig. 2.2).

Studies are currently investigating the forms of genetic modification which render the expression either of most genes independent of their parental origin or of some autosomal genes dependent on whether they are of maternal or paternal origin. Such gene regulation would involve germ line specific modification and the laying down of a memory about the parental origin of imprinted loci. Investigations of the molecular mechanisms of genomic imprinting have gained momentum with the recent identification of some imprinted genes (Surani *et al.* 1990; Surani 1993, 1994). DNA methylation is one of the genetic modification determinants that is both inheritable and reversible. Results from a recent study using the 'restriction landmark' scanning approach combined with the methylation of imprints to detect other imprinted loci, irrespective of where or when they are expressed, identified approximately 100 imprinted loci throughout the genome. Furthermore, 6 per cent of CpG islands (bases frequently associated with methylation) demonstrated parental differences.

Four imprinted genes have recently been identified and reported. Three of the four genes map to the distal region of mouse chromosome 7, which is syntenic to human chromosomes 11 and 15q—areas associated with the human genetic diseases of Beckwith–Wiedemann syndrome, Wilms' tumour, Prader–Willi syndrome and Angelman syndrome. One of the imprinted genes is *Igf2*, which encodes an embryonic growth factor with mitogenic properties and which is involved in the growth and proliferation of many cell types including skeletal muscle during development (De Chiara *et al.* 1991, Ferguson-Smith *et al.* 1991). In Wilms' tumour the paternal chromosome carrying the *Igf2* gene is duplicated (Reeve *et al.* 1985, Scott *et al.* 1985). The maternal allele is repressed when the paternally inherited copy is expressed. However, another imprinted gene in this chromosomal region *H19* demonstrated a reciprocal mode of action to *Igf2* in so far as the maternal gene was active while the paternal gene was repressed. The third imprinted gene identified on mouse chromosome 7, *Snrp*, is believed to be involved with the splicing of mRNA. It is expressed in the brain from birth, reaching peak levels of expression at 4 weeks of life. The gene maps to human chromosome 15q12, and deletion of human, paternal chromosome 15q11–13 or maternal disomy for chromosome 15 results in Prader–Willi syndrome. The fourth imprinted gene maps to the proximal arm of mouse chromosome 17 and is found to have only a maternal effect. The deletion mutation *Tme* is lethal when inherited from the mother but has no detectable effect when inherited from the father.

The contribution of genetic imprinting to human genetic disorders is already attracting greater attention since recent reports indicate that the unstable expansion of the trinucleotide repeats—CAG in Huntington's disease and CGG in the *FMR-1* gene on the X chromosome in fragile X syndrome (Verkerk *et al.* 1991)—demonstrate parent of origin effects.

Future perspectives

Understanding the inheritance of genetic information and determining the expression and interaction of these genes during development through to ageing continues to be a scientific challenge. Yet discovery concerning determinants of human behaviour, performance and abilities does not remain in the scientific domain. Ramifications of understanding gene function on genetic manipulation whether in the context of repairing or replacing disease genes or responding to external influences becomes the concern of each of us. The technology and the pressure for manipulating human genes already exist. Society now has to examine its position and make some very difficult decisions about how it wishes to use the discoveries scientists are daily placing at its door.

REFERENCES

Burke, D.T., Carle, G.F., Olson, M.V. (1987) 'Cloning of large segments of exogeneous DNA into yeast by means of artifical chromosome vectors.' *Science*, **236**, 806–812.

Collins, J., Hohn, B. (1978) 'Cosmids: a type of plasmid gene-cloning vector that is packageable *in vitro* in bacteriophage heads.' *Proceeding of the National Academy of Sciences of the USA*, **75**, 4242–4246.

Corder, E.H., Saunders, A.M., Strittmatter, W.J.,Schmechel, D.E., Gaskell, P.C., Small, G.W., Roses, A.D. Haines, J.L., Pericak-Vance, M.A. (1993) 'Gene dose of apolipoprotein E type 4 allele and the risk of Alzheimer's disease in late onset families.' *Science*, **261**, 921–923.

Davies, K.E., Young, B.D., Elles, R.G., Hill, M.E., Williamson, R. (1981) 'Cloning of a representative genomic library of the human X chromosome after sorting by flow cytometry.' *Nature*, **293**, 374–376.

DeChiara, T.M., Robertson, E.J., Efstratiadis A. (1991) 'Parental imprinting of the mouse insulin-like growth factor II gene.' *Cell*, **64**, 849–859.

Ferguson-Smith, A.C., Cattanach, B.M., Barton, S.C., Beechey, C.V., Surani, M.A, (1991) 'Embryological and molecular investigations of parental imprinting on mouse chromosome 7.' *Nature*, **351**, 667–670.

Harbers, K., Jähner, D., Jacnisch, R. (1981) 'Microinjection of cloned retroviral genomes into mouse zygotes: integration and expression in the animal.' *Nature*, **293**, 540–542.

Jaenisch, R., Mintz, B.(1974) 'Simian virus 40 DNA sequences in DNA of healthy adult mice derived from preimplantation blastocysts injected with viral DNA.' *Proceedings of the National Academy of Sciences of the USA*, **71**, 1250–1254.

Kuehn, M.R., Bradley, A., Robertson, E.J., Evans, M.J. (1987) 'A potential animal model for Lesch–Nyhan syndrome through introduction of HPRT mutations into mice.' *Nature*, **326**, 295–298.

Kunkel, L.M., and co-authors (1986) 'Analysis of deletions in DNA from patients with Becker and Duchenne muscular dystrophy.' *Nature*, **322**, 73–77.

Pericak-Vance, M.A., Bebout, J.L., Gaskell, P.C., Yamaoka, L.H., Hung, W-Y., Alberts, M.J., Walker, A.P., Bartlett, R.J., Haynes C.A., *et al.* (1991) 'Linkage studies in familial Alzheimer disease: evidence for chromosome 19 linkage.' *American Journal of Human Genetics*, **48**, 1034–1050.

Reeve, A.E., Eccles, M.R., Wilkins, R.J., Bell, G.I., Millow, L.J. (1985) 'Expression of insulin-like growth factor-II transcripts in Wilms' tumour.' *Nature*, **317**, 258–260.

Rommens, J.M., Iannuzzu, M.C., Kerem, B-S., Drumm, M.L., Melmer, G., Dean, M., Rozmahel, R., Cole, J.L., Kennedy, D., *et al.* (1989). 'Identification of the cystic fibrosis gene: chromosome walking and jumping.' *Science*, **245**, 1059–1065.

Sanger, F., Nicklen, S., Coulson, A.R. (1977) 'DNA sequencing with chain-terminating inhibitors.' *Proceedings of the National Academy of Sciences of the USA*, **74**, 5463–5467.

Scott, J., Cowell, J., Robertson, M.E., Priestley, L.M., Wadey. R., Hopkins, B., Pritchard, J., Bell, G.I., Rail, L.B., *et al.* (1985) 'Insulin-like growth factor–II gene expression in Wilms' tumour and embryonic tissues.' *Nature*, **317**, 260–262.

Sherrington, R., Brynjolfsson, J., Petursson, H., Potter, M., Dudleston, K., Barraclough, B., Wasmuth, J., Dobbs, M., Gurling, H. (1988) 'Localisation of a susceptibility locus for schizophrenia on chromosome 5.' *Nature*, **336**, 164–167.

—— Rogaev, V.I., Liang, Y., Rogaeva, E.A., Levesque, G., Ikeda, M., Chi, H., Lin, C., Li, G., *et al.* (1995) 'Cloning of a gene bearing missense mutations in early-onset familial Alzheimer's disease.' *Nature*, **375**, 754–760.

Southern, E.M. (1975) 'Detection of specific sequences among DNA fragments separated by gel electrophoresis.' *Journal of Molecular Biology*, **98**, 503–517.

Surani, M.A. (1993) 'Genomic imprinting: silence of the genes.' *Nature*, **366**, 302–303.

—— (1994) 'Genomic imprinting: control of gene expression by epigenetic inheritance.' *Current Opinion in Cell Biology*, **6**, 390–395.

—— Kothary, R., Allen, N.D., Singh, P.B., Fundele, R., Ferguson-Smith, A.C., Barton, S.C. (1990) 'Genome imprinting and development in the mouse.' *Development*, (Suppl.), 89–98.

Tagle, D.A., Blanchard-McQuate, K.L., Valdes, J., Castilla, L., MacDonald, M.E., Guscella, J.F., Collins, F.S. (1993) 'Dinucleotide repeat polymorphism in the Huntington's disease region at the D4S 182 locus.' *Human Molecular Genetics*, **2**, 489.

Young, B.D., Ferguson-Smith, M.A., Sillar, R., Boyd, E. (1981) 'High-resolution analysis of human peripheral lymphocyte chromosomes by flow cytometry.' *Proceedings of the National Academy of Sciences of the USA*, **78**, 7727–7731.

Verkerk, A.J.M.H., Pieretti, M., Sutcliffe, J.S., Fu, Y-H., Kuhl, D.P.A., Pizzuti, A., Reiner, O., Richards, S., Victoria, M.F., *et al.* (1991) 'Identification of a gene (*FMR-1*) containing a CGG repeat coincident with a breakpoint cluster region exhibiting length variation in fragile X syndrome.' *Cell*, **65**, 905–914.

34

3
METHODOLOGICAL ISSUES IN BEHAVIOURAL PHENOTYPES RESEARCH

Gregory O'Brien and William Yule

In this chapter we explore some of the aspects of study design and academic enquiry which are relevant to research in the field of behavioural phenotypes. We describe the experience of working with syndrome based carer support societies at some length, because so many studies in the field are carried out with their help. Two of the topics briefly mentioned, behavioural measurement and choice of genetic model, are covered in greater detail elsewhere in the present text. In making these comments, we wish to acknowledge the contributions made by our many colleagues in the Society for the Study of Behavioural Phenotypes. Their deliberations and discussions (not to mention frustrations) concerning research in our field have been the basis for this review. [For further reading, we recommend the excellent review of research strategies employed in genetic studies of child psychiatric disorders carried out by Rutter *et al.* (1990) and the recent text book on psychiatric genetics by McGuffin *et al.* (1994).]

Starting point
Start with a research question, or at least with a clinical observation which suggests one. This may seem obvious, but we have witnessed many examples of potentially useful studies in behavioural phenotypes research which have not yielded fruit simply because of inadequate attention to the age-old query, 'What question am I trying to answer here?' In our experience the most common mistake in this respect occurs when a researcher comes across a genetic condition or other biologically discrete disorder which has not yet been reported to have a behavioural phenotype, and on that basis alone quickly proceeds to look for one. Although this phenomenon is to some extent a pleasing indication of the success and popularity of research in this area, it reflects poor technique. The result is predictable. In some cases, a behavioural phenotype is indeed suggested, despite the inherent limitations of working in this way. More often, the results obtained are equivocal. Research of this type is generally unhelpful, and it can also often be damaging, for any contact with research subjects necessarily has some effect upon them. At best, it might spoil or inhibit subsequent more rigorous and well thought out attempts to study a behavioural phenotype which may indeed be present. Certainly, any such work is very likely to miss a potential target, since unless a project is designed to test for the occurrence of an uncommon or otherwise unfamiliar behaviour in a given syndrome, then that

behaviour is unlikely to be identified. At worst, such sloppy research technique may have an adverse effect upon the subjects themselves. This can arise either from failure to look for suitable behaviours, or from looking for quite unsuitable ones. In either case, behaviours which are present or the perception of behaviours held by subjects and/or carers may be altered. This can be quite deleterious.

When researchers work with syndrome support societies there is no need for the scenario outlined above to happen. These groups have often supplied or at least suggested the direction of the initial research question for many studies of behavioural phenotypes. Indeed, one of the earliest and most productive of the current generation of such studies stemmed from discussions with parents of children affected by tuberous sclerosis. This group identified the occurrence of an idiosyncratic spectrum of behaviour which was not recognized as a consequence of that disorder by the clinicians who had seen their children, but was commonly encountered by most members of the parent network. In common with many other carer support societies, the Tuberous Sclerosis Association then initiated its own objective study of these behaviours. This survey in turn spawned the pivotal study of hyperactivity and autism in this disorder (Hunt and Dennis 1987). Their experience has since been shared by other syndrome-based parent/ carer support societies, who often begin by making their own observations, which are subsequently elaborated and clarified through the involvement of a scientific research team in a more systematic study.

There are, of course, other more conventional sources of the clinical observations which lead to the initial research questions that drive research in behavioural pheno-types. First and foremost, there is clinical experience. Many clinicians, however, particu-larly paediatricians, psychologists and psychiatrists who work with disabled children, are unlikely to see substantial numbers of subjects affected by any one rare condition. It is clearly essential therefore to establish close liaison with geneticists and genetic counsel-lors, whose objective clinical descriptions are invaluable in initiating the kind of detailed behavioural studies which are required in the delineation of behavioural phenotypes. The other principle source of suggested associations between syndrome and behaviour which indicate hypotheses for studies of this type is the myriad case reports which appear in the published literature. Indeed, although the psychiatric features of fragile X syndrome have now been subject to extensive detailed study (see Chapter 5), the case reports which indicated the directions for this line of enquiry appeared only comparatively recently (*e.g.* Gillberg *et al.* 1988).

Review articles and meta-analyses
Having decided to attempt to embark upon examining a question or research issue in behavioural phenotypes, the next step will be the literature review. To date, there is a surprising paucity of review articles in this field. With the notable exceptions of the relatively common Down and fragile X syndromes, on which there are several excellent authoritative reviews (Down—see Collacott 1993*a*; fragile X—see Turk 1992, 1995, and Chapter 5), there are few considered collations of findings in specific syndromes. Chapter 7 of this book goes some way to rectify this deficit, but the brief format there

does not allow the critical discussion which is required to further facilitate systematic rational enquiry. One of the greatest contributions an aspiring researcher can make in this field is to produce an updated review article on an important syndrome.

However, a note of caution must be sounded regarding the application of meta-analysis (*i.e.* analysis where the results of separate studies are brought together for consideration). The problem derives from the basic premise of this approach which assumes that either (i) the same raw data do not appear in the different studies, or (ii) where the same data do appear in different studies, then there is some means of detecting this. In some selected and highly specialized work on certain rare conditions the latter provision does apply. By convention, whenever neuropsychological studies of certain well-documented individuals with specific rare lesions are published, their coded initials are also published. Where this has been done carefully and deliberately, the precise extent of behaviours and deficits may be established, and their determinants studied. [For a good example of this method, consult the studies on corpus callosal agenesis in high functioning individuals (*e.g.* Jeeves and Temple 1987).] Unfortunately for the purpose of meta-analysis, such rigour is not the rule in most studies. Indeed, there are several rare genetic conditions on which multiple genomic behavioural phenotype studies have been carried out by different research teams who have employed the national or international sampling methods which are necessary in such rare conditions. Inevitably, there is repeat measurement of individual subjects, but there is no way of testing for this in the published reports of these studies. We therefore see limitations in applying meta-analysis to behavioural phenotypes.

Sample selection

The above issue highlights both the importance of care in selecting a sampling procedure and the need to consider the implications of the sample chosen. Parent support groups for a given syndrome are often approached for this purpose. Indeed, many such groups are sufficiently proactive and interested in behavioural research that they have either made the first approach to researchers themselves, or have even carried out their own studies or behavioural surveys. Some of the advantages of working in this way are clear from the above discussion on framing the research question. In addition, in our experience members of these groups are highly motivated to participate in behavioural research. This results in a high compliance rate in studies with which they become involved (*e.g.* Clarke *et al.* 1989).

However, there are also substantial limitations and disadvantages in proceeding in this way. Firstly, membership of a syndrome support society does not guarantee that an individual has the condition in question. For a variety of reasons, many of these organizations include children and adults who are not affected by the index syndrome. We refer here not to 'carriers' of disorders or to unaffected family members or carers, but to other individuals or families who wish to identify with certain disorders, or who mistakenly believe that they are affected by the relevant condition. Subsequent genetic investigation has revealed that most of these individuals represent phenocopies of the disorder on which the respective society is based. In carrying out research with such groups, independent validation of diagnosis is therefore necessary. This entails either carrying out or at least having sight of the results of relevant diagnostic investigations, including genetic analysis. Furthermore, where the diagnosis has been verified, it cannot be assumed that the members of such societies are necessarily representative of the general population of the disorder. It is often suggested that family or carer support groups attract more intelligent and vocal individuals. Also, it is unclear whether their affected children or relatives are at the more or less extreme end of the spectrum of severity of the condition. It is the impression of some that they tend to be at the more severe end. These children may therefore be more intellectually or developmentally delayed and behaviourally disturbed than is the norm for a given condition. Consequently, care must be taken in any extrapolation of the results derived from studies conducted along these lines. On the other hand, it is likely that the same selection biases operate in respect of different syndrome support societies. This is useful in planning cross-syndrome comparative research. (For further discussion of working with family and carer support societies, see O'Brien 1992*a,b*.)

There are several other options to choose from in sampling. The two most commonly employed are clinic samples and genetics registers. Both approaches have their advantages and disadvantages. In general, the more disabled subjects are more likely to be in contact with the relevant services, although by no means invariably (Richardson *et al.* 1986). This effect is relevant to both clinic populations and genetics registers. Clinic samples are often well-documented, locally available and amenable for detailed study. In addition, other selection biases operate, according to the nature and speciality orientation of the clinic in question. A Child Psychiatrist and a Developmental Paediatrician are both likely to see a child with a specific syndrome, but for different reasons. Their clinics therefore include quite contrasting populations of children. One attractive option is to carry out research through the medium of the Child Development Centre. These centres are a rich source of large populations of children with special needs, and they are in routine contact with other service networks. They also operate in a multidisciplinary fashion, which goes some way to avoid the selection bias problems of speciality clinics.

Another means of approaching and accessing children for the study of behavioural phenotypes is to work in liaison with school-based clinics. Of all options, this may require the greatest care and sensitivity, for there remains great concern over labelling and stigmatization in the field of education for special needs. This of itself is a challenge to any research endeavour which involves a diagnostic approach (Goacher *et al.* 1988). As discussed in Chapter 1, the issue can become most vexing when genetic study of the determinants of behaviour is proposed (Nelkin and Tancredi 1991). However, it is found that careful and thorough explanation of the nature and scope of this kind of research does facilitate cooperation. It seems that it is just as important to emphasize what one is not trying to investigate or establish, as it is to explain what is being studied. For example, the researcher must be careful not to create the impression that s/he is attempting to demonstrate that a host of cognitive, linguistic, social or motor characteristics of a group of children are the inevitable consequences of a given biological disorder. Moreover, it is crucial not to convey the impression that any behaviours identified will necessarily be refractory to educational efforts. This would not only be incorrect, but the collaboration of the relevant agencies would almost certainly not be forthcoming.

Genetics registers offer a unique resource for research into behavioural phenotypes (McGuffin *et al.* 1994). Although these registers are by no means comprehensive, they do allow the potential possibility of making contact with appreciable numbers of subjects with rare disorders spread over a given region. Also, through the development of national networks of such registers, large numbers of such children may be identifiable. This medium therefore offers an alternative to working with family support societies. The selection biases which operate in the two situations are different (Kaprio *et al.* 1990). On the one hand, many people continue to demonstrate a reluctance to engage in any activities associated with genetic testing, as recently experienced in respect of Huntington's disease (Tyler *et al.* 1992). It is possible that some such people may be more attracted toward contact with parent interest groups. On the other hand, the need to confirm diagnosis does not arise in genetics register based samples, or at least not in the same way as in family/carer support societies. Obviously it is possible to combine these two approaches to sample ascertainment in a study, as they are in many ways complementary.

Ideally, samples for research in this area should be derived from epidemiological surveys, whether screening for specific syndromes, behaviours or patterns of developmental delay. In practise, this is such a massive undertaking for research on any one condition that it is rarely done. A notable exception is Collacott's extensive programme of work on the psychopathology of adults with Down syndrome (Collacott 1993*b*). The most striking features of this cohort study were the extensive efforts made and different methods employed to identify the subjects for study. These were adults who were living in a variety of situations, and all of whom were subject to the same diagnostic procedure. Promisingly, the combination of the screening techniques for many conditions and the development of genetics registers should now facilitate further large-scale projects of this type.

Choice of syndrome for study
Much of the above discussion has assumed that a discrete biologically identifiable condition will be the focus for most research. In other words a *genomic* approach is proposed (see Chapter 1). This is true of most research into behavioural phenotypes. The choice of syndrome(s) for such work will be determined by the research questions framed. It is important to be aware that the issue of defining the syndrome for investigation can be more complicated than might at first be envisaged. The story of our emerging understanding of the molecular basis of fragile X syndrome (see Chapter 5) serves as a salutary reminder in this connection, since where there was previously a clear distinction made between 'carriers' and affected individuals, it is now understood that the situation is much more complex. The crucial issue, therefore, is to define clearly the nature of the group for study. For example, a project might aim to study all affected individuals with greater and lesser degrees of expression of a given genotype. Another study might focus only on the behavioural features of the full-blown condition, however that may be defined. In either case, many such genomic studies entail comparisons of behaviour

between different conditions. Special considerations which apply in this connection are outlined in the section on control and comparison groups which follows.

But what of the *phenomic* approach to research? As explained earlier (Chapter 1), the 'syndrome' for study by this strategy is delineated by observation, which in the present case comprises behavioural observation. Indeed, in the opinion of many workers in this field, the phenomic method holds great promise for further advance in the investigation of the genetic basis of behaviour, and is generally underused (Flint and Yule 1994). It is further proposed by Flint in Chapter 6 that this approach will come to even greater prominence in the future. We would suggest that when research proceeds in this way, the four behavioural domains contained in the definition of behavioural phenotype proposed in Chapter 1 might be usefully consulted. In this way, systematic description of cognitive, linguistic, motor and social dimensions of behaviour may be employed to delineate a behavioural phenotype, which can then be the subject for genetic and/or other biological investigation.

Control and comparison groups

This is one field where the adoption of 'normal controls' is contentious. The difficulty lies in deciding from which population a normal control group should be drawn. For example, if it is decided to employ a general population sample for this purpose, then any claims of an association between a biological disorder and a specific behavioural constellation will need to take into account any differences in intellect or other developmental capacity between the index and control groups. There will also be the issue of different environmental influences. These differences will be more pronounced with increasing severity of intellectual disability, because of the differences in life experience and general situation of people with severe intellectual or developmental disabilities. Another possibility when studying the behavioural phenotype of a condition causing mental retardation is to employ a representative sample of people with mental retardation. This is appealing at first sight, but demands careful consideration. Any such sample will include a wide variety of conditions, some of which will have their own behavioural features. In order to control for any chance effects of clustering of behaviours, a large control group would need to be employed. This in turn will have implications for index sample size. It has been suggested that a preferable control group would be drawn from a population for which no diagnosable disorder has been identified. This is even more problematic because such a control group would simply represent those for whom no causal diagnosis has *as yet* been demonstrated.

The factors considered most often in controlling include age, sex, general level of intelligence and immediate family and social environment (Einfeld and Hall 1994). There are well-documented difficulties in interpreting studies which have attempted to control for environmental influences, including the adopted-away twin studies discussed in Chapter 1. Other possible approaches which might be used include many of the conventional control methods employed in child psychology research, including non-affected siblings and school-based peers. The decision whether to control for other variables such as specific intellectual or cognitive delays will depend on the precise aim of the study in question. However, there have been few genomic studies of behavioural phenotypes to date which have reported on any control data as such (O'Brien 1992*a*).

One strategy which has found favour is to make comparisons of the behavioural characteristics of individuals affected by different, discrete and diagnosable biological conditions. This approach has much to commend it.

First, it is possible to select disorders which have similar impact in terms of general intellectual or developmental disability, and to carry out behavioural comparisons between them. Any behavioural comparisons carried out on a group of two or more such disorders are likely to be informative, since where certain behaviours are found to be common across all disorders, it is most likely that these behaviours are a reflection of the degree of intellectual or developmental disability in question. Moreover, where one condition is found to have a quite different set of behavioural concomitants, then there is evidence of a specific behavioural phenotype, which should be clarified through subsequent, more detailed study.

Second, where there is some preceding knowledge of specific cognitive deficits in a condition, then the relevance of those deficits to the behavioural phenotype of either the index condition or one studied in comparison may be more fully appreciated. For example, in studying the behavioural phenotype of a disorder which carries a mild degree of mental retardation, it would be quite conceivable to select fragile X subjects as a comparison group. Now, there is much known of the linguistic peculiarities of people affected by that disorder. Any similarities or differences in the linguistic domain which might then be found in the index group would be of great interest. The results would further clarify just how specific that language disorder is to fragile X syndrome, while exploring the role that any such linguistic factors might play in the behavioural phenotype of the disorder being studied. Similarly, where a set of biological disorders carry similar developmental impact yet arise by quite different aetiological mechanisms, detailed behavioural comparison may be most informative. This applies particularly to phenomic research. For example, a considerable body of evidence has indicated that autism is a feature of the behavioural phenotype of many biological disorders (Gillberg 1992). The studies from which this is derived can be difficult to interpret, not least because definitions and diagnostic criteria for autism continue to vary widely (Wing 1989). However, even when this is taken into account, the autism behavioural phenotype is associated with many such biological disorders. The first and natural conclusion to be drawn from this is that the occurrence of autism in these situations is largely developmentally determined. On more careful study, an additional effect is clear. Through the application of rigorous diagnostic criteria, 'secondary autism' can certainly be identified in many different genetic disorders. But it appears that the autism is not always of the same *nature*. In tuberous sclerosis, for example, there is admixture of hyperactivity and autism (Hunt and Dennis 1987). On the other hand, the fragile X behavioural phenotype certainly passes as autism on standard diagnostic measures, but is quite distinct (Turk 1995). Not only can such a research approach clarify the behaviours which are more common in a given disorder, but also the direction of further research into the biological basis of more discrete behaviours may be indicated.

Choice of behavioural measurement schedule

The chapter following concentrates on certain principals of behavioural measurement which apply to behavioural phenotypes research, and gives a critique of some of the more commonly employed measuring instruments. For the purpose of the present review, three points are to be noted. First, many instruments have now been used for research in this field. Indeed, a few have been developed specifically for this purpose (*e.g.* O'Brien 1994). Where possible, it is recommended that an established instrument should be used in any study (Singh *et al.* 1991). Second, where the focus of enquiry is a diagnosable psychiatric disorder, there remains a dearth of measurement schedules applicable to the more severely mentally retarded subjects (Reid 1994). Any attempts to develop new instruments for this purpose should concentrate on observable behaviour, as opposed to the measurement of cognition and emotion which are conventionally included in psychiatric diagnostic tools (Sturmey 1993). Third, recently there have been substantial developments in behavioural measurement. The use of new technology in recording and assessment techniques is of particular interest. Future studies of behavioural phenotypes will rely less on checklists and interview methods and more on these more sophisticated innovations in behavioural measurement.

Genetic model

This issue is examined in greater depth by Richards and Flint in Chapters 2 and 6 of this book. The development of techniques for the study of quantitative trait loci discussed there are of particular relevance to research on behavioural phenotypes. However, for the novice in behavioural genetics research, it should be noted that there are essentially two models of genetic investigation which are applicable to research into behavioural phenotypes. First, there are *linkage* studies. In this approach, family pedigrees are examined. The technique depends on the behaviour of genetic markers (points on the chromosome whose position and constituents are known) with reference to the disease gene in question, studied over successive generations. Linkage has been employed extensively in the study of familial transmission of major psychiatric disorders in the general population. However, some of the earlier claims of linkage have proven to have been over-zealous or even erroneous, and have subsequently been refuted (*e.g.* Kennedy *et al.* 1988).

The other approach is the study of *association*. In association studies, populations of people with a specific, diagnosable disorder are grouped together for study of the presence of a marker gene. Classical association studies rely on comparison with populations which do not possess that marker. Most behavioural phenotypes research is the study of association (for further reading see McGuffin *et al.* 1994).

Ethical issues

In Chapter 1 and at several other points in this text, we have described certain ethical concerns which are raised by research into behavioural phenotypes. Indeed, many commentators are concerned that policies which might amount to selective breeding on the basis of behaviour might yet emerge from this work. Faced with such a prospect, it is important that detailed consideration and rational ethical debate should be applied to these aspects of behavioural genetics. In all such discussions, the contributions of parents and parent advocate groups are clearly of crucial importance. For the present purpose the important issue concerns whether it is ethical to proceed with research into the behavioural phenotypes of developmentally disabling disorders. For such research may, however inadvertently, result in a revisitation of eugenics.

Three conventional approaches are employed in ethical thinking concerning medical practice. These are the Principles, Paradigms, and Perspectives approaches.

Four principles are generally recognized. These are: respect for autonomy; commitment to benefit; non-maleficence ('first do no harm'); and justice. Consideration of these is helpful in exploring the ethics of research in this area. We can ask such questions as:

• Is the work likely to promote the autonomy of the individuals being studied?

• Will the project be of benefit? (to whom?)

• Will the study harm anyone?

• Does the research proposed conform to ideas of justice, in that it will treat individuals fairly?

The paradigms approach is more often applied to considerations of issues in individual cases. Essentially, the usual procedure is to take a case in which there are difficulties in proceeding with logical discussion because of ethical and/or emotive issues, and to change it in some way which makes it easier to consider. This model may aid debate on ethical issues of research in behavioural phenotypes. For example, we might be rightly concerned regarding the labelling and stigmatizing consequences of any results which clearly demonstrate a pronounced behavioural phenotype for any one disorder. But if we shift the question toward study of the occurrence of some severe, dehumanizing or life-threatening physical medical condition in that same syndrome, our attitude may change. It may now seem that it is important to clarify the extent and nature of the problem, and to seek further means of alleviating it. If we now revisit the issue of studying a pronounced behavioural phenotype in some disorder, we might be clearer in our mind regarding the value of such a study.

The perspectives approach is really something of an *aide-mémoire*. It reminds us to consider the issue from the viewpoint of all involved parties, and to bear in mind the potential impact of the study upon them.

It is hoped that, through the application of these insights into contemporary ethical thought, rational debate might lead to fruitful research. For a further review of ethical thinking in this area see the ILSMH Issue Paper on bio-ethics (International League of Societies for Persons with Mental Handicap 1994).

ACKNOWLEDGEMENT

We are most indebted to Tony Hope for his contribution to the application of ethical thinking to behavioural phenotypes.

REFERENCES

Clarke, D.J., Waters, J., Corbett, J.A. (1989) 'Adults with Prader–Willi syndrome: abnormalities of sleep and behaviour.' *Journal of the Royal Society of Medicine*, **82**, 21–24.

Collacott, R.A. (1993*a*) 'Down's syndrome.' *Current Opinion in Psychiatry*, **6**, 650–654.

—— (1993*b*) 'Epilepsy, dementia and adaptive behaviour in Down's syndrome.' *Journal of Intellectual Disability Research*, **37**, 153–160.

Einfeld, S.L., Hall, W. (1994) 'When is a behavioural phenotype not a phenotype?' *Developmental Medicine and Child Neurology*, **36**, 467–470.

Flint, J., Yule, W. (1994) 'Behavioural phenotypes.' *In:* Rutter, M., Taylor, E., Hersov, L. (Eds.) *Child and Adolescent Psychiatry, 3rd Edn.* Oxford: Blackwell Scientific, pp. 666–687.

Gillberg, C.L. (1992) 'The Emanuel Miller Memorial Lecture 1991. Autism and autistic-like conditions: subclasses among disorders of empathy.' *Journal of Child Psychology and Psychiatry*, **33**, 813–842.

—— Ohlson, V-A., Wahlström, J., Steffenburg, S., Blix, K. (1988) 'Monozygotic female twins with autism and the fragile-X syndrome (AFRAX).' *Journal of Child Psychology and Psychiatry*, **29**, 447–451.

Goacher, B., Evans, J., Welton, J., Wedell, K. (1988) *Policy and Provision for Special Educational Needs.* London: Cassell.

Hunt, A., Dennis, J. (1987) 'Psychiatric disorder among children with tuberous sclerosis.' *Developmental Medicine and Child Neurology*, **29**, 190–198.

International League of Societies for Persons with Mental Handicap (1994) *Just Technology? From Principles to Practice in Bio-Ethical Issues. Issue Paper.* Brussels: ILSMH.

Jeeves, M.A, Temple, C.M. (1987) 'A further study of language function in callosal agenesis.' *Brain and Language*, **32**, 325–335.

Kaprio, J., Koskenvuo, M., Rose, R.J. (1990) 'Population-based twin registries: illustrative applications in genetic epidemiology and behavioral genetics from the Finnish Twin Cohort Study.' *Acta Geneticae Medicae et Gemellologiae*, **39**, 427–439.

Kennedy, J.L., Giuffra, L.A., Moises, H.W., Cavalli-Sforza, L.L, Pakstis, A.J., Kidd, J.R., Castiglione, C.M., Sjogren, B., Wetterberg, L., Kidd, K.K. (1988) 'Evidence against linkage of schizophrenia to markers on chromosome 5 in a northern Swedish pedigree.' *Nature*, **336**, 167–170.

McGuffin, P., Owen, M.J., O'Donovan, M.C., Thapar, A., Gottesman, I.I. (1994) 'Genetic counselling and ethical issues.' *In: Seminars in Psychiatric Genetics.* London: Gaskell, pp. 218–225.

Nelkin, D., Tancredi, L. (1991) 'Classify and control: genetic information in the schools.' *American Journal of Law and Medicine*, **17**, 51–53.

O'Brien, G. (1992*a*) 'Behavioural phenotypy in developmental psychiatry.' *European Child and Adolescent Psychiatry*, Suppl. 1, 1–61.

—— (1992*b*) 'Behavioural phenotypes and their measurement.' *Developmental Medicine and Child Neurology*, **34**, 365–367.

—— (1994) 'The developmental and behavioural consequences of corpus callosal agenesis and Aicardi syndrome.' *In:* Lassonde, M., Jeeves, M.A. (Eds.) *Callosal Agenesis—the Natural Split Brain.* New York: Plenum Press, pp. 235–246.

Reid, A.H. (1994) 'Psychiatry and learning disability.' *British Journal of Psychiatry*, **164**, 613–618.

Richardson, S.A., Koller, H., Katz, M. (1986) 'A longitudinal study of numbers of males and females in mental retardation services by age, IQ and placement.' *Journal of Mental Deficiency Research*, **30**, 291–300.

Rutter, M., Bolton, P., Harrington, R., Le Couteur, A., MacDonald, H., Simonoff, E. (1990) 'Genetic factors in child psychiatric disorders—I. A review of research strategies.' *Journal of Child Psychology and Psychiatry*, **31**, 3–37.

Singh, N.N., Sood, A., Sonenklar, N., Ellis, C.R. (1991) 'Assessment and diagnosis of mental illness in persons with mental retardation. Methods and measures.' *Behavior Modification*, **15**, 419–443.

Sturmey, P. (1993) 'The use of DSM and ICD diagnostic criteria in people with mental retardation. A review of empirical studies.' *Journal of Nervous and Mental Disease*, **181**, 38–41.

Turk, J. (1992) 'The fragile-X syndrome. On the way to a behavioural phenotype.' *British Journal of Psychiatry*, **160**, 24–35.

—— (1995) 'Fragile X syndrome.' *Archives of Disease in Childhood*, **72**, 3–5.

Tyler, A., Ball, D., Craufurd, D. (1992) 'Presymptomatic testing for Huntington's disease in the United Kingdom.' *British Medical Journal*, **304**, 1593–1596.

Wing, L. (1989) 'The diagnosis of autism.' *In:* Gillberg, C. (Ed.) *Diagnosis and Treatment of Autism.* New York: Plenum Press, pp. 5–22.

4
MEASUREMENT OF BEHAVIOUR

Gregory O'Brien

Any research endeavour in the field of behavioural phenotypes depends ultimately on two types of diagnostic measurement—investigation of the genotype and of the phenotype. As regards the genotype, there is general confidence in the reliability and validity of the procedures employed, and widespread interest in the ongoing development and elaboration of new approaches (see Chapters 2 and 6). Also, recent innovations in molecular biology continue to accelerate the pace of identification of genes implicated in behavioural phenotypes. Moreover, the techniques employed in genetic investigation are constantly being developed and further refined, resulting in increasing detail, precision and accuracy in the mapping of the human genome. That same degree of attention and sophistication in investigative method is required in our approach to the measurement of the phenotypes in question, the behaviours.

In this brief review of behavioural measurement, it is quite impossible to describe all of the instruments and techniques potentially available for the investigation of behavioural phenotypes. The aim is therefore to provide an overview of the types of tools which might be employed, with particular reference to those which have already proved to be of some value in studies of behavioural phenotypes. In keeping with research already carried out in this area, the majority of the measurement instruments reviewed in this chapter are questionnaires and interview schedules. There is also discussion of the use of direct behavioural observation techniques in behavioural phenotypes research. In addition, some examples of behavioural measurement methodologies which have not yet been employed extensively in research in this area (at least to our knowledge) are reviewed. These include techniques using electronic recording instruments and certain aspects of contemporary information technology. Again, there have been recent rapid developments in this area. Examples are given only of those devices and approaches which seem to be particularly appealing for the present purpose, based upon evidence of some experience of their use in behavioural phenotypes research and also from consideration of other related projects. The intention is to give an indication of the ways in which new innovations in behavioural measurement might be successfully employed in the investigation of behavioural phenotypes.

For further reading on measurement instruments for behaviour and psychiatric disorder in developmentally disabled subjects, the reader is directed to Lund (1989), Sturmey *et al.* (1991), O'Brien (1992), and particularly Aman (1991).

Behaviours, developmental attainments or psychiatric disorders?
Whatever type of measurement approach is to be employed—and as will be shown,

these range from simple questionnaires through to sophisticated electronic recording devices—it is necessary to decide in advance exactly what is to be measured. For example, in some cases it may be appropriate to concentrate on just a few behaviours, or even on one type of behaviour. This will generally be in those cases where there is already good evidence of specific behavioural anomalies occurring in some condition(s). Obvious examples include studies of eating behaviour or mood disorder in Prader–Willi syndrome, of self-injurious behaviour in Lesch–Nyhan syndrome, and of sleep-related behaviour disorder in tuberous sclerosis.

More often, a more general assessment of behaviour is required, as there are many biological disorders for which there is as yet little behavioural information. Where a study proceeds along these lines, it would seem logical to give some consideration to the four principal elements of behaviour we encounter in behavioural phenotypes—cognition, language, motor and social (see Chapter 1). Many such studies will require data on developmental attainments in addition to assessment of behaviour disorder. This is because any set of behaviours might be a reflection of the individual's general developmental level, or might be occurring in relation to some specific developmental delay, for example of language function. (For further discussion of the role of level of developmental and intellectual disability in the aetiology of behavioural phenotypes, see Chapters 1 and 3). Also, it is important to bear in mind the possibility that certain conditions might predispose to *superior* functioning in some areas of cognition. For example, in Williams syndrome preliminary evidence from 'Theory of Mind' experiments suggests that in tests of empathic perspective people affected by that condition may have unusually high capacities, amounting to over-empathizing (see Chapter 7). It is quite possible that this might be the basis of the long-standing observation of idiosyncratic 'adult-like' social manner in the Williams syndrome child.

Table 4.1 gives a summary of some behavioural measurement instruments that are suitable for studies which aim to make a general assessment of behaviour. The table also indicates whether each schedule also yields any data on developmental attainments, and shows the applicability of each instrument to child or adult samples. It does not include the many questionnaires which have been custom-designed for use in individual syndromes, often in conjunction with the relevant syndrome/carer support society—some examples of these instruments are included in Table 4.3 (see the section following, on informant questionnaires). Instruments which measure IQ and/or specific academic skills and/or cognitive abilities are not included, except where this is part of the overall assessment of behaviour disorder in a given instrument.

Other studies in the field of behavioural phenotypes seek to determine whether specific diagnosable psychiatric disorders occur in certain biological disorders. This approach often poses researchers with the greatest challenge, as it is notoriously difficult to diagnose psychiatric disorders in many of the potential study groups because of their associated intellectual and developmental levels. Nevertheless, substantial strides have recently been made in the development of psychiatric diagnostic schedules which might be applicable to this population. Some of these are summarized in Table 4.2. This table indicates the applicability of each schedule to children/adults, and provides a summary

TABLE 4.1
Measurement schedules for general behavioural assessment

Schedule* (Reference)	Child/adult**	Developmental assessment?	Interview required?
Adaptive Behavior Scale: ABS-RC:2 (Nihira *et al.* 1993)	Both	Yes	No
Aberrant Behavior Checklist (Aman *et al.* 1985)	Both	No	No
Additional Behavioural Inventory (Gath and Gumley 1986) (#)	Children	No	No
Behavioural Assessment Battery (Kiernan and Jones 1982)	Both	Yes	No
Behavioural Phenotypes Interview (Bax *et al.* 1995)	Children	Yes	Yes
Behaviour Disturbance Scale (Leudar *et al.* 1984) (#)	Adults	No	No
Child Behavior Checklist (McConachy and Achenbach 1988) (#)	Children	No	No
Developmentally Delayed Version of the Child Behaviour Checklist (Einfeld and Tonge 1991) (#)	Both	No	No
Handicap Behaviour and Skills Schedule (Wing 1980)	Both	Yes	Yes
Present Behaviour Examination—Mental Handicap Version (O'Brien and Whitehouse 1990)	Adults	No	Yes
Psychosocial Behaviour Scale (Espie *et al.* 1988)	Adults	No	No
Rett Syndrome Interview Schedules (Lindberg 1991)	Both	Yes	Yes
Reiss Screen for Maladaptive Behavior (Reiss 1988) (#)	Teenagers and adults	No	No
Rutter A and B Scales (Rutter *et al.* 1976) (#)	Both	No	No
SSBP Postal Questionnaire (O'Brien 1994, 1995)	Both	Yes (2 versions)	Yes

*This table lists some of the instruments for the measurement of behaviour in behavioural phenotypes research. Measurement schedules which either yield psychiatric diagnoses or measure psychiatric symptoms are summarized in Table 4.2. However, certain tools in this table do serve as screening instruments for psychiatric disorder, notably those labelled (#).

**Although many of these schedules were originally intended for children only, where studies have indicated applicability for adult use they are described as appropriate to both children and adults.

of the psychiatric diagnostic information yielded by each instrument. Note in particular that many of these instruments are limited to subgroups within the population of people with developmental disabilities. This is a reflection of the *pathoplastic* effect of level of retardation on psychiatric symptomatology (Fraser and Murti Rao 1991). The symptoms which suggest or indicate the presence of psychiatric disorder are different at differing

TABLE 4.2
Psychiatric diagnostic schedules of use in behavioural phenotypes research

Schedule (Reference)	Child/adult	Diagnoses	Notes	Interview required?
Autism Behavior Checklist (Krug *et al.* 1980)	Children	Autism	Useful screening instrument	No
Autism Diagnostic Interview (Le Couteur *et al.* 1989)	Both	Autism/ related disorders	Widely applicable	Yes
Beck Depression Inventory (Kazdin *et al.* 1983)	Adults	Depression	Suitable in mild retardation	No
Childhood Autism Rating Scale (Schopler *et al.* 1986)	Children	Autism	Recommended for studies of autism	No
Diagnostic Assessment for the Severely Handicapped (DASH) Scale (Matson *et al.* 1990)	Adults	DSM-III(R) diagnoses	Severe retardation only	Yes
Early Autistic Symptoms Questionnaire (Dahlgren and Gillberg 1989)	Children <2 years	Autism	Note age applicability	No
EAS Scale (Buss and Plomin 1984)	Children	Temperament	Short scale, widely used	No
Emotional Disorders Rating Scale— Developmental Disabilities (Feinstein *et al.* 1988)	Children/ teenagers	Mood and anxiety symptoms	Mild to moderate retardation	Yes
Goldberg Clinical Interview Schedule— Mental Handicap Version (Ballinger *et al.* 1975)	Adults	ICD-9 diagnoses	All levels retardation	Yes
Gillberg Interview for Mentally Retarded Teenagers (Gillberg *et al.* 1986)	Teenagers	ICD-9 diagnoses	Useful short interview	Yes
Hamilton Depression Scale—Mental Handicap Version (Sireling 1986)	Adults	Depression	Suitable in mild/moderate retardation	No
Kiddy-SADS-E5 (Orvaschel 1995)	Children	DSM-IV diagnoses	Applicable to mild retardation	Yes
Parental Account of Childhood Symptoms (Taylor *et al.* 1986)	Children	Hyperactivity	Widely applicable	No
Psychopathology Inventory for Mentally Retarded Adults (Senatore *et al.* 1985)	Adults	DSM-III diagnoses	Suitable in mild/moderate retardation	No
Zung Anxiety Scale: Adults Mental Handicap Version (Helsel and Matson 1988)	Adults	Anxiety symptoms	Self-report questionnaire requiring language use	No
Zung Depression Scale: Mental Handicap Version (Helsel and Matson 1988)	Adults	Depression	Self-report questionnaire requiring language use	No

levels of developmental disability. These symptoms are the diagnostic features on which the measurement schedules depend; therefore, an instrument which is suitable to diagnose, say, depression in mild to moderately mentally retarded individuals is likely to be unsuitable for use in more severely retarded subjects.

Informant questionnaires

The informant-based questionnaire has probably been the most widely used type of instrument for the investigation of behavioural phenotypes. As a research approach, the use of such a tool has many advantages. Firstly, and for practical purposes most importantly, there are the issues of ease of administration, and the possibility of accessing large samples. The latter issue refers to the use of questionnaires distributed through such forums as clinics with a special interest in certain disorders, and particularly family/syndrome support societies. There are various means by which these questionnaires can be used: by post; as an adjunct to an interview or clinical examination; and through distribution at large group meetings. It should be noted, incidentally, that the latter method seems to be favoured by many syndrome support societies. However, whichever mechanism is planned it is crucial to clarify whether the device was designed to be used in the manner and setting proposed by any one study. If the instrument was not designed with that intention, then its use will need to be subject to the appropriate reliability and/or validation procedures (see below).

Questionnaires have many limitations. Format, layout and language which may be entirely familiar to clinicians, scientists and professional researchers can be most off-putting to parents and other lay informants. Studies of questionnaire use and response have revealed that ambiguity is very common in questionnaires (Fallowfield 1995). Whereas in an interview this problem can be alleviated through sound technique and explanation, no such opportunity is afforded when using an informant-completed questionnaire. It is therefore particularly important to consider carefully the application of any questionnaire to behavioural phenotypes research. The instrument should first of all be self-explanatory, incorporating a rationale for the study and introducing the material to be explored. Items should be brief and to the point, with some clear relevance to the target group. Reliability—the capacity of the instrument to yield the same answers in different contexts, on separate occasions or with different informants—should be established by independent study. (Notes on reliability testing are included in the following section on interview schedules.) In fact, well-designed questionnaires often prove to be quite reliable. The greater problem with questionnaires is more often in connection with their validity. This is the capacity of an instrument to measure that which it is supposed to measure. In the case of behavioural measurement the ultimate test of validity is to compare results obtained through the application of an instrument with those derived from direct observation of behaviour. No other method can supply such robust data on the validity of any instrument. However, due to the difficulties and time investment inherent in direct observation of behaviour, other options are often employed. One technique commonly adopted involves taking some other instrument as a yardstick of known value in measurement, and comparing results of the two. Again, this method is

TABLE 4.3
Specific syndrome behavioural phenotype postal questionnaires

Schedule (Reference)	Child/adult	General comments
Mucopolysaccharidosis Questionnaire (Bax 1985)	Both; best for children	Incorporates Rutter A; behaviour and general health data
Noonan's Syndrome Association—Parent Questionnaire (Hill 1990)	Children	Developmental and family history, in addition to behaviour
Prader–Willi Association Teenage and Adult Questionnaire (Clarke *et al.* 1989)	Teenagers and adults	Fairly lengthy, 22 page questionnaire, including behaviour, health and family data
Rett Syndrome Association Questionnaire (Kerr 1992)	Children	Health and behaviour data, including epilepsy
Tuberous Sclerosis Association Questionnaire (Tuberous Sclerosis Association 1989)	Both	Health, behaviour, disability and social adjustment
Williams Syndrome Association Questionnaire (Udwin 1990)	Adults	Behaviour and service needs

far from foolproof: where the two agree, they may be in agreement regarding an error, unless the index tool has been validated against direct observation. Other useful indices of validity have been reviewed by Fallowfield (1990). In general, it is advisable to adopt an existing schedule where possible. However, if circumstances dictate that a new questionnaire must be developed, the reference guide by Streiner and Norman (1989) is recommended.

The questionnaires used in studies of behavioural phenotypes have included many which have been tailor-made for the purpose. In fact, most of these instruments are highly specialized in content, being designed for the study of an individual syndrome or biological disorder. Table 4.3 reviews a few examples of this kind of questionnaire. It is well worth while considering carefully the inclusion of such a schedule in a study protocol, where one exists for the condition in question. The nature and content of these questionnaires render them most 'informant friendly', which in turn tends to result in a high completion rate. More importantly, they are warmly welcomed by parents and carers because of their emphasis on the uniqueness of the subject's difficulties. However, we would recommend that some other schedule(s) should also be included, particularly one which might facilitate comparison with other conditions or some control group. Table 4.3 includes general comments on each of the syndrome-specific schedules listed, with notes of applicability to child/adult samples. All the questionnaires listed were designed for use in postal surveys.

Two informant questionnaires are worthy of special mention. These are the Developmentally Delayed Version of the Child Behaviour Checklist (DD-CBC) and the SSBP Postal Questionnaire. Of all those listed in Table 4.1, these two have been most widely employed in studies on behavioural phenotypes.

The DD-CBC has the advantage of being a derivative of one of the most successful tools used in child psychiatric diagnostic research, the original Achenbach CBC (McConachy and Achenbach 1988). Indeed, several studies on behavioural phenotypes have successfully employed the latter instrument, rather than its adaptation for developmentally delayed subjects (*e.g.* Wood *et al.* 1995). The DD-CBC was piloted on a very large population of developmentally delayed individuals (Einfeld and Tonge 1991). This is a particularly useful feature, in that there are therefore useful control data. The authors have proposed that this questionnaire might be of considerable value in behavioural phenotypes research.

The SSBP Postal Questionnaire was designed specifically to be sensitive to cross-syndrome differences in behavioural phenotypes. As summarized in Table 4.1 it includes developmental assessment, and it is primarily intended for use with children aged 2 to 18 years (O'Brien 1994). An adult version of the scale has now been piloted (O'Brien 1995).

Interview schedules

Interview schedules are particularly useful tools for the study of behavioural phenotypes. The adoption of any interview schedule in behavioural research is more likely to lead to greater validity than when a questionnaire is employed. This is most true where a skilled interviewer is able to use the interview situation to clarify and explain the meaning of the question items for the interviewee, and also to ensure that s/he has correctly understood and recorded the responses given by the informant. In short, it is the task of the interviewer to keep in tune with the interviewee. Furthermore, in the case of interviews concerning behaviour, examples of recent behaviours can be discussed in detail. In other words, the whole emphasis is to relate the interview, via the informant's observations of behaviour, as closely as possible to the subject's manifest behaviour. However, herein lies the *validity/reliability paradox*. For, just as highly reliable questionnaires do not necessarily carry high validity (see above), similarly the higher validity of the interview setting does not necessarily result in high scoring on certain tests of reliability. This depends to a great extent on the degree of structure of the schedule. The most highly structured interviews demand that question items be read verbatim, and not altered, and offer no opportunity to employ supplementary questioning. Many such highly structured instruments demand yes/no or other forced-choice answers. Clearly, this type of approach is more likely to yield the same answers on different occasions, and therefore to possess greater reliability. On the other hand, less structured interviews commonly incorporate probe questions with additional dependent items, while allowing the exploration of other material related to a particular question or domain of enquiry. The interview conducted in this fashion may well vary in content, depending on how much additional or supplementary material is explored by the interviewer.

In practise, these issues are examined in conventional tests of reliability, the most commonly used of which are: test–retest, done across time (28 days is usually an appropriate period); inter-rater, that is assessment of the same interview by separate raters, employing either direct observation or audio/video recording; and inter-informant, being the measure of agreement reached when different interviewees/informants are questioned concerning the behaviour of a given subject. As in all considerations of choice of measurement instrument in this field, it cannot be stressed too strongly that, where possible, an existing schedule should be employed. However, if this is deemed impossible or inappropriate—generally this will occur where no suitable schedule exists—then it is hoped that these comments will be of some guidance in design and development of a new instrument. Finally, it should be noted that in common with other research endeavours which entail interviewing on behaviour or psychopathology, the semi-structured interview schedule has proven to be the most popular type of interview instrument used in the study of behavioural phenotypes. Such instruments offer the maximal combination of reliability and validity.

Tables 4.1 and 4.2 indicate which instruments for general assessment of behaviour (Table 4.1) and psychiatric diagnosis (Table 4.2) are primarily interview schedules. These are measurement tools which are designed for use in an interview setting. As can be seen, many of the psychiatric diagnostic schedules fall into this category. In addition, some other instruments which appear in these tables—and some of the postal questionnaires described in Table 4.3—have been used in an interview context. Indeed there is considerable interest in certain quarters in the flexible use of highly structured questionnaires, employing them in this way (Aman 1991). However, it is of course generally not advisable to use behavioural measurement instruments in settings and contexts for which they were not designed. Moreover, while it may be possible to incorporate highly structured questionnaires into an interview methodology, the converse is much more problematic. Where an instrument is described as primarily intended for interview use in Tables 4.1 and 4.2, therefore, this should be taken as an indication that it cannot be assumed to be appropriate for use in any other manner. It should also be noted that most of these interviews require considerable clinical skills and expertise for proper use, and many also require special training. In all decisions regarding appropriateness of a measurement schedule for a given study, and especially where some novel or alternative method of administration is being considered, careful study of key published material on the development and use of the schedule, scrutiny of the instrument manual and possibly consultation with the instrument author will be required.

Certain interview schedules have already proved to be particularly promising for the study of behavioural phenotypes.

The Handicap Behaviour and Skills Schedule (Wing 1980) is a useful semi-structured informant-based interview, which takes between 50 and 90 minutes to complete by a trained interviewer, preferably one who is a qualified clinician. The informant should be a parent or carer who knows the subject well. In addition to interviewing such a reliable informant, it is also recommended that the subject should be at least briefly observed. Much of the material in the schedule is skills-based, including social skills. Approximately half of the items relate to autistic-type behaviours and related cognitive deficits. The instrument yields a single score, derived from the Vineland Scale. It has been used in individuals with all levels of intellectual and developmental disability; supplementary question items are available for testing very mildly retarded individuals.

The Present Behaviour Examination—Mental Handicap Version (O'Brien and Whitehouse 1990) is a precoded forced-choice informant-based interview, which takes around 90 minutes to complete. Informants should be any carer who can supply details of behaviour over a 24 hour period, including sleep-related behaviour. The approach taken in this interview has been the basis of a new instrument, the Behavioural Phenotypes Interview (Bax *et al.* 1995). This interview schedule has the advantage of having been designed and developed for the specific purpose of the study of behavioural phenotypes. Information on its use and on training in its administration are available from the author of the schedule.

The Autism Diagnostic Interview (Le Couteur *et al.* 1989) is a highly specialized interview schedule for the diagnostic assessment of autism and related pervasive developmental disorders. It is without doubt the one instrument for this purpose which is of the highest pedigree, with unrivalled sensitivity and specificity in measurement. A shorter version of the interview, taking around two hours to administer, has recently been developed. Researchers interested in using either version are advised to contact the authors and arrange to attend a special training course to learn techniques of its administration.

Direct behaviour observation schedules

There is no substitute for direct observation of behaviour. However, the novice researcher might ask, 'But what do I observe?' In order to bring structure and method to direct observation, many methodologies have been developed. Whichever direct observation schedule is adopted, certain basic tenets and principles apply. First and foremost, direct observation is the most naturalistic method of measuring manifest behaviour. No intervening confounding factors such as informants are involved. Also, in line with conventional ABC (Antecedent–Behaviour–Consequence, see Chapter 1) behavioural analysis, the behaviours under consideration can be studied properly within their context and in the presence of any causal or maintaining factors. Most direct observation schedules were originally devised for treatment purposes. The behavioural analysis data provided in this way form the basis of intervention programmes, particularly where environmental triggers or maintaining factors are identified, and/or where the behaviour is found to have some function for the individual within the setting in question. In order to supply such information, many of these schedules are lengthy, and take considerable time to implement. [For an account of the principles underlying any such behavioural analysis, see Yule (1987).]

Two examples of approaches to direct behavioural observation which are of potential interest to behavioural phenotypes researchers are reviewed. These are chosen to illustrate how such schedules may be fairly brief but effective and reliable, or more detailed, comprehensive and time-consuming.

One interesting approach is taken in the Balthazar Scales of Adaptive Behaviour (Balthazar 1973). This direct observation instrument is designed to assist in the measurement of a defined set of characteristic behaviour problems of severely and profoundly retarded subjects, both children and adults. By this method, six 10-minute observation sessions are carried out by a trained observer. Seven dimensions of behaviour are covered, of which stereotypy, repetitive verbalization, self-directed behaviour (*i.e.* self injury and other self stimulating behaviours) and aggressive withdrawal may be of particular relevance. It is therefore of potential value in the study of severely disabling conditions, in which many of the informant questionnaires and diagnostic interview schedules are of limited applicability. The regime of six 10-minute observation periods supplies multiple measurements at different times, and therefore more robust data than can be derived from single-period observations.

One of the most comprehensive schedules for direct observation is included in the Behavioural Assessment Battery (Kiernan and Jones 1982). This detailed and elaborate assessment guide is intended to be used in the behavioural analysis of refractory cases, and it is not really feasible for use in even moderate scale studies. However, it might well serve studies of behavioural phenotypes, either where used to validate other measures, or in detailed single case studies.

Electrophysiological behavioural recording and activity monitoring
There is a long tradition of the use of electrophysiological measurement and monitoring techniques in the study of behaviour in people with developmental disabilities. Some of the earliest applications focused on physiological correlates of sexual behaviour and aggression, with results which are considered by many reviewers to be at best equivocal (Travin *et al.* 1988). Currently, there is considerable contemporary interest in the application of electrophysiological measurement to other aspects of behaviour. Three examples which are of particular interest to behavioural phenotypes research include studies of sleep and epilepsy, and of general levels of activity.

Systematic study of sleep and sleep-related behaviour is of considerable importance. Not only does it clarify the extent of the burden imposed by disturbed sleep in respect of carers, there is also considerable theoretical interest in the pathogenesis of sleep disruption. Conditions in which pronounced sleep disorders have been reported include Down syndrome (Stores 1993), the mucopolysaccharidoses (reviewed by O'Brien 1992) and tuberous sclerosis (Hunt and Stores 1994). Probably the most useful approaches to this kind of sleep monitoring are those which entail 24 hour recording. Essentially there are three types of sleep problems which merit investigation, all of which are issues in behavioural phenotypes research. These are: sleeplessness, of whatever form; sleep-related behaviour disorders; and daytime hypersomnolence (Stores 1994). The monitoring devices in question incorporate electroencephalographic, electro-oculographic and electromyographic information, to monitor the onset, length and nature of the stages of sleep, in addition to other characteristics of the sleep–wake cycle. Recent innovations in these techniques have resulted in the advent of ambulatory polysomnography, which has largely removed the need for extensive laboratory-based investigations. Also of interest to behavioural phenotypes research are approaches which entail measurement of breathing disorders in sleep (Stradling 1992). There is considerable interest in the application of these measuring techniques to studies of breathing in Prader–Willi and Rett syndromes.

Many of the conditions for which behavioural phenotypes have been proposed feature epilepsy as part of their overall clinical phenotype. Aicardi syndrome, Angelman syndrome and tuberous sclerosis are good examples. Also, there is a wealth of evidence concerning the role played by epilepsy in behaviour disorders, particularly in people with developmental disabilities. Systematic study of behavioural phenotypes therefore includes consideration of epilepsy, and the means by which epilepsy might be a causal factor in behaviour problems, whether directly or indirectly (see discussion of the 'epileptic personality' idea in Chapter 1). As in sleep studies, the technology employed in epilepsy investigation is now such that continuous ambulatory recording is available quite widely (Stores 1994). Concomitant behavioural measurement can aid in clarification of the relationship between any epileptic activity and manifest behaviours. Some centres are equipped to use video recording for this purpose.

A recent innovation in behavioural measurement which holds out some promise for behavioural phenotypes research is the development of devices for activity monitoring. One such device, the Gaehwiler Electronic Z80 32K VI, incorporates a wrist-strap type monitor which records and stores data on the subject's movements. It has been proposed that this technique might be useful for studies of overactivity, sleep disorders, tics and other movement disorders including dystonias (Bramble, personal communication).

The advantages of all of these continuous recording approaches include the capacity to supply information concerning behaviours occurring at any time of day or night, and in any situation, while not relying on an individual acting as observer.

Use of recording media

A plethora of recording media are now available for potential application to behavioural phenotypes studies. These include audio and video recording, certain electrophysiological measurement techniques described above, and particularly new technology for computer-assisted recording of direct behavioural observation. One software system for the collection and analysis of observational data is of particular interest, and serves as an example of how contemporary technology can be applied to our research. This is the 'Observer' (Noldus 1991). 'Observer' effectively transforms any (IBM compatible) personal computer into an event recorder. The package requires the researcher to define the behaviours and other parameters to be recorded. It is mostly used in one of two ways: either on lap-top computer for real-time observation of behaviour, or for subsequent study of videotapes. 'Observer' was originally designed for use in animal and ethological studies, but has now been successfully applied in human behaviour studies. The system can supply sophisticated analysis of the timing, circumstances, extent and associations of behaviours.

Concluding comment

Some of the most exciting and revealing findings in studies of behavioural phenotypes come from studies employing neuropsychological investigation of specific cognitive deficits, for example the work on frontal functioning in fragile X syndrome (Mazzocco *et al.* 1992). It is not within the scope of this chapter to provide a review of the application of such refined neuropsychological testing procedures to research in behavioural phenotypes. Readers interested in exploring this specialist area may wish to consult De

Sonneville (1988), Dennis (1991), Levin *et al.* (1991), Mirsky *et al.* (1991), or Rourke and Fuerst (1991).

ACKNOWLEDGEMENT

The advice of Shaun Gravestock, Paul Smith and William Yule was invaluable in the preparation of this chapter.

REFERENCES

Aman, M.G. (1991) *Assessing Psychopathology and Behaviour Problems in Persons with Mental Retardation: a Review of Available Instruments.* Rockville, MD: US Department of Health and Human Services.
—— Singh, N.N., Stewart, A.W., Field, C.J. (1985) 'The Aberrant Behavior Checklist: a behavior rating scale for the assessment of treatment effects.' *American Journal of Mental Deficiency*, **89**, 485–491.
Ballinger, B.R., Armstrong, J., Presley, A.S., Reid, A.H. (1975) 'Use of a standardized psychiatric interview in mentally handicapped patients.' *British Journal of Psychiatry*, **127**, 540–544.
Balthazar, E.E. (1973) *Balthazar Scales of Adaptive Behaviour. II. Scales of Social Adaptation.* Palo Alto, CA:Consulting Psychologists Press.
Bax, M. (1985) *The Mucopolysaccharidosis Questionnaire.* London: Community Paediatric Research Unit, Chelsea and Westminster Hospital.
—— Dennis, J., MacKain, K., O'Brien, G., Udwin, O., Yule, W. (1995) *The Behavioural Phenotypes Interview.* London:Community Paediatric Research Unit, Chelsea and Westminster Hospital.
Buss, A.H., Plomin, R. (1984) *Temperament: Early Developing Personality Traits.* Hillsdale, NJ: Lawrence Erlbaum.
Clarke, D.J., Waters, J., Corbett, J.A. (1989) 'Adults with Prader–Willi syndrome: abnormalities of sleep and behaviour.' *Journal of the Royal Society of Medicine*, **82**, 21–24.
Dahlgren, S.O., Gillberg, C. (1989) 'Symptoms in the first two years of life. A preliminary population study of infantile autism.' *European Archives of Psychiatry and Neurological Sciences*, **238**, 169–174.
Dennis, M. (1991) 'Frontal lobe function in childhood and adolescence: a heuristic model for assessing attention, regulation, executive control, and the attentional states important for social discourse.' *Developmental Neuropsychology*, **7**, 327–358.
De Sonneville, L. (1988) *Paediatric Behavioural Neurology. Vol. 2. Aspects of Information Processing: a Computer-based Approach to Developmental Disorders.* Amsterdam: Suyi.
Einfeld, S.L., Tonge, B. (1991) 'Psychometric and clinical assessment of psychopathology in developmentally disabled children.' *Australian and New Zealand Journal of Developmental Disabilities*, **17**, 147–154.
Espie, C.A., Montgomery, J.M., Gillies, J.B. (1988) 'The development of a psychosocial behaviour scale for the assessment of mentally handicapped people.' *Journal of Mental Deficiency Research*, **32**, 395–403.
Fallowfield, L.J. (1990) *The Quality of Life. The Missing Instrument in Health Care.* London: Souvenir Press.
—— (1995) 'Questionnaire design.' *Archives of Disease in Childhood*, **72**, 76–79.
Feinstein, C., Kaminer, Y., Barrett, R.P., Tylenda, B. (1988) 'The assessment of mood and affect in developmentally disabled children and adolescents: the Emotional Disorders Rating Scale.' *Research in Developmental Disabilities*, **9**, 109–121.
Fraser, W.I., Murti Rao, J. (1991) 'Recent studies of mentally handicapped young people's behaviour.' *Journal of Child Psychology and Psychiatry*, **32**, 79–108.
Gath, A., Gumley, D. (1986) 'Behaviour problems in retarded children with special reference to Down's syndrome.' *British Journal of Psychiatry*, **149**, 156–161.
Gillberg, C., Persson, E., Grufman, M., Themner, U. (1986) 'Psychiatric disorders in mildly and severely retarded urban children and adolescents: epidemiological aspects.' *British Journal of Psychiatry*, **149**, 68–74.
Helsel, W.J., Matson, J.L. (1988) 'The relationship of depression to social skills and intellectual functioning in mentally retarded adults.' *Journal of Mental Deficiency Research*, **32**, 411–418.
Hill, P. (1990) *Noonan's Syndrome Association Parent Questionnaire.* London: Department of Child Psychiatry, St Georges Hospital Medical School.

Hunt, A., Stores, G. (1994) 'Sleep disorder and epilepsy in children with tuberous sclerosis: a questionnaire-based study.' *Developmental Medicine and Child Neurology*, **36**, 108–115.

Kazdin, A.E., Matson, J.L., Senatore, V. (1983) 'Assessment of depression in mentally retarded adults.' *American Journal of Psychiatry*, **140**, 1040–1043.

Kerr, A. (1992) 'Rett syndrome: British Longitudinal Study (1982–1990) and 1990 survey.' *In:* Roosenthal, J.J. (Ed.) *Mental Retardation and Medical Care.* Zeist: Uitgverij Kerckbosch.

Kiernan, C., Jones, N. (1982) *Behavioural Assessment Battery.* Windsor: NFER-Nelson.

Krug, D.A., Arick, J., Almond, P. (1980) 'Behavior checklist for identifying severely handicapped individuals with high levels of autistic behavior.' *Journal of Child Psychology and Psychiatry*, **21**, 221–229.

Le Couteur, A., Rutter, M., Lord, C., Rios, P., Robertson, S., Holdgrafer, M., McLennan, J. (1989) 'Autism Diagnostic Interview: a standardized investigator-based instrument.' *Journal of Autism and Developmental Disorders*, **19**, 363–387.

Leudar, I., Fraser, W.I., Jeeves, M.A. (1984) 'Behaviour disturbance and mental handicap: typology and longitudinal trends.' *Psychological Medicine*, **14**, 923–935.

Levin, H.S., Culahane, K.A., Hartman, J., Evankovich, K. (1991) 'Developmental changes in performance on tests of purported frontal lobe function.' *Developmental Neuropsychology*, **7**, 377–395.

Lindberg, B. (1991) *Understanding Rett Syndrome: a Practical Guide for Parents, Teachers, and Therapists.* Toronto: Hogrefe & Huber.

Lund, J. (1989) 'Measuring behaviour disorder in mental handicap.' *British Journal Of Psychiatry*, **155**, 379–383.

Matson, J.L., Coe, D.A., Gardner, W.I., Sovner, R. (1990) *Diagnostic Assessment for the Severely Handicapped (DASH) Scale (User Manual).* Baton Rouge, LA: Louisiana State University.

Mazzocco, M.M.M., Hagerman, R.J., Cronister-Silverman, A., Pennington, B.F. (1992) 'Specific frontal lobe deficits among women with the fragile X gene.' *Journal of the American Association of Child and Adolescent Psychiatry*, **31**, 1141–1148.

McConachy, S.H., Achenbach, T.M. (1988) *Practical Guide for the Child Behavior Checklist and Related Materials.* Burlington, VT: University of Vermont Department of Psychiatry.

Mirsky, A.F., Anthony, B.J., Duncan, C.C., Ahearn, M.B., Kellam, S.G. (1991) 'Analysis of the elements of attention: a neuropsychological approach.' *Neuropsychological Review*, **2**, 109–145.

Nihira, K., Leland, H., Lambert, N. (1993) *Adaptive Behaviour Scale – Residential and Community. 2nd Edn.* Texas: Pro-Ed.

Noldus LPJJ (1991) 'The Observer: a software system for collection and analysis of observational data.' *Behavioural Research Methods, Instruments, and Computers*, **23**, 415–429.

O'Brien, G. (1992) 'Behavioural phenotypy in developmental psychiatry.' *European Child and Adolescent Psychiatry*, Suppl. 1, 1–61.

—— (1994) 'The developmental and behavioural consequences of corpus callosal agenesis and Aicardi syndrome.' *In:* Lassonde, M., Jeeves, M.A. (Eds.) *Callosal Agenesis—The Natural Split Brain.* New York: Plenum Press, pp. 235–246.

——(1995) *SSBP Postal Questionnaire—Adult Version.* Northgate Hospital, Northumberland: Society for the Study of Behavioural Phenotypes.

—— Whitehouse, A.M. (1990) 'A psychiatric study of deviant eating behaviour among mentally handicapped adults.' *British Journal of Psychiatry*, **157**, 281–284.

Orvaschel, H. (1995) *Kiddy Schedule for Affective Disorders and Schizophrenia, Version 5.* Fort Lauderdale, FL: Center for Psychological Studies, Nova Southern University.

Reiss, S. (1988) *Test Manual for the Reiss Screen for Maladaptive Behaviour.* Orland Park, IL: International Diagnostic Systems.

Rourke, B.P., Fuerst, D.R. (1991) *Learning Disabilities and Psychosocial Functioning: a Neuropsychological Perspective.* New York: Guilford Press.

Rutter, M., Tizard, J., Yule, W., Graham, P., Whitmore, K. (1976) 'Isle of Wight Studies, 1964–1974.' *Psychological Medicine*, **6**, 313–332.

Schopler, E., Reichler, R.J., Renner, R. (1986) *The Childhood Autism Rating Scale (CARS) for Diagnostic Screening and Classification of Autism.* New York: Irvington.

Senatore, V., Matson, J.L., Kazdin, A.E. (1985) 'An inventory to assess psychopathology of mentally retarded adults.' *American Journal of Mental Deficiency*, **89**, 459–466.

Sireling, L. (1986) 'Depression in mentally handicapped patients: diagnostic and neuroendocrine evaluation.' *British Journal of Psychiatry*, **149**, 274–278.

57

Stores, G. (1994) 'Investigation of sleep disorders including home monitoring.' *Archives of Disease in Childhood*, **71**, 184–185.

Stores, R. (1993) 'Sleep problems in Down's syndrome: a summary report.' *Down's Syndrome: Research and Practice*, **1**, 72–74.

Stradling, J.R. (1992) 'Consensus report: sleep studies for sleep-related breathing disorders.' *Journal of Sleep Research*, **1**, 265–273

Streiner, D.L., Norman, G.R. (1989) *Health Measurement Scales. A Practical Guide to their Development and Use.* Oxford: Oxford University Press.

Sturmey, P., Reed, J., Corbett, J. (1991) 'Psychometric assessment of psychiatric disorders in people with learning difficulties (mental handicap): a review of measures.' *Psychological Medicine*, **21**, 143–155.

Taylor, E., Schachar, R., Thorley, G., Wieselberg, M. (1986) 'Conduct disorder and hyperactivity: 1. Separation of hyperactivity and antisocial conduct in British child psychiatric patients.' *British Journal of Psychiatry*, **149**, 760–767.

Travin, S., Cullen, K., Melella, J.T. (1988) 'The use and abuse of erection measurements: a forensic perspective.' *Bulletin of the American Academy of Psychiatry and the Law*, **16**, 235–250.

Tuberous Sclerosis Association (1989) *Questionnaire.* Park Hospital. Oxford: TSA.

Udwin, O. (1990) 'A survey of adults with Williams syndrome and idiopathic infantile hypercalcaemia.' *Developmental Medicine and Child Neurology*, **32**, 129–141.

Windle, M., Lerner, R.M. (1986) 'Reassessing the dimensions of temperamental individuality across the life span: the revised dimensions of temperament survey (DOTS–R).' *Journal of Adolescent Research*, **1**, 213–230.

Wing, L. (1980) 'The MRC Handicaps, Behaviour and Skills (HBS) Schedule.' *Acta Psychiatrica Scandinavica*, **62** (Suppl. 285), 241–248.

Wood, A., Massarano, A., Super, M., Harrington, R. (1995) 'Behavioural aspects and psychiatric findings in Noonan's syndrome.' *Archives of Disease in Childhood*, **72**, 153–155.

Yule, W. (1987) 'Identifying problems: functional analysis and observation and recording techniques.' *In:* Yule, W., Carr, J. (Eds.) *Behavioural Modification for People with Mental Handicaps. 2nd Edn.* London: Croom Helm, pp. 8–27.

5
LESSONS FROM FRAGILE X SYNDROME

Randi Hagerman

The fragile X syndrome was first reported in 1969 by Lubs, but it took almost 15 years before it was widely recognized as the most common inherited cause of mental retardation. It is caused by a mutation in the fragile X mental retardation–1 (*FMR-1*) gene, which is located at Xq27.3, the bottom end of the X chromosome. Recognition of this syndrome was dependent on advances in cytogenetics and the utilization of a tissue culture medium that was deficient in folic acid so that the fragile site or break in the chromosome at Xq27.3 was visible. When these techniques were consistently used, early reports emerged of large families demonstrating the fragile X chromosome.

The early phenotype
Although fragile X patients have always existed, the recognition of a cytogenetic marker allowed clinicians to separate fragile X patients from patients with other causes of mental retardation and assess commonalities. By 1980, Australian researchers, particularly Gillian Turner and her colleagues, had described the basic physical features including a long face, prominent ears and macro-orchidism. Remarkably consistent findings among fragile X males were noted in behavioral features. The similarities in their perseverative, litany-like speech, avoidance of eye contact, sensitivity to touch, hyperactivity, hand flapping and hand biting were notable, and they stimulated a plethora of descriptive papers in the early 1980s. Most of these reports did not utilize standardized assessments of behavior, *e.g.* Turner *et al.* (1980*b*) and Brondum Nielsen (1983), although others did (*e.g.* Brown *et al.* 1982, Levitas *et al.* 1983), with variable results.

At first only the most dramatically affected individuals were identified, and moderate to severe mental retardation was considered typical of the syndrome (Blomquist *et al.* 1982, Hagerman *et al.* 1983, Howard-Peebles and Finley 1983). Institutions for mentally retarded patients were screened, with a yield of approximately 2 to 10 per cent as fragile X positive, but again the focus was on the most severely affected (Carpenter *et al.* 1982, Froster-Iskenius *et al.* 1983, Primrose *et al.* 1986, Hagerman *et al.* 1988*a*). Each of the behavioral and physical features typical of fragile X were found at times in patients with other types of developmental delays, so they were not individually unique to fragile X. For instance, 13.5 per cent of adult males in our State institution had macro-orchidism but only 17 per cent of these individuals had fragile X syndrome. Hand biting was also common (13.5 per cent), but only 14 per cent of individuals with this behavior were fragile X positive (Hagerman *et al.* 1988*a*). Clinicians learned that the unique aspect of this syndrome was in seeing all of the features together in one individual, but it was difficult to package this overall gestalt in one measure. The instruments that focus on attention deficit hyperactivity disorder or autism did not seem effectively to delineate the unique features of fragile X. Attempts have been made to utilize typical fragile X features in screening checklists (Turner *et al.* 1986, Butler *et al.* 1991, Hagerman *et al.* 1991, Laing *et al.* 1991, Nolin *et al.* 1991) to identify high-risk individuals for subsequent diagnostic studies. This endeavor has been worthwhile, but these brief checklists are not robust enough for detailed behavioral studies between fragile X and other populations.

The association with autism

Brown *et al.* (1982) first reported the association between fragile X and autism when they noted that five of 27 patients fulfilled criteria for autism. Although previous reports had noted autism in isolated cases of fragile X (Turner *et al.* 1980a, Proops and Webb 1981, Meryash *et al.* 1982), it was Brown and his colleagues who noted a consistent pattern in several fragile X males utilizing standardized criteria. Subsequent reports confirmed this association (Levitas *et al.* 1983, August and Lockhart 1984, Kerbershian *et al.* 1984, Blomquist *et al.* 1985, Varley *et al.* 1985, Wahlström *et al.* 1986), and Gillberg *et al.* (1986) termed the subtype of autism with fragile X as 'AFRAX'.

In the mid- to late 1980s a variety of screening studies of autistic males demonstrated a low yield of fragile X patients, and several researchers became skeptical regarding the association between autism and fragile X (Venter *et al.* 1984, Goldfine *et al.* 1985, Payton *et al.* 1989). However, when all the screening studies were summarized, the overall frequency of fragile X in autistic males was 7 per cent (Brown *et al.* 1986, Hagerman 1990). This represents a significant subgroup of autism, and fragile X should be assessed in the work-up of the autistic individual.

The degree of autism within the fragile X population is variable, depending on how it is measured. Because autism is a behaviorally descriptive diagnosis, different instruments have different criteria regarding what constitutes autism. This problem was assessed in a study of various measures of autism, including DSM-III criteria, autism behavior checklist (ABC) criteria, and Rimland's E2 checklist criteria, in 50 fragile X males (Hagerman *et al.* 1986b). None of the subjects met Rimland's criteria, 30 per cent met ABC criteria and 15 per cent met DSM-III criteria. The most remarkable finding, however, was that 90 per cent of the males had poor eye contact, 88 per cent had hand stereotypies, including hand biting and hand flapping, and 96 per cent had perseverative or unusual speech. These autistic-like features affected the majority of fragile X patients and are perhaps the core features of fragile X because they are so consistent, even through all levels of intellectual ability. It has taken controlled studies, however, in the late 1980s and early 1990s, to further our understanding of the unique characteristics of fragile X.

Einfeld *et al.* (1989) compared the behavioral ratings of 44 males with fragile X and 45 mentally retarded males without fragile X matched on IQ. Since they found 4 per cent who were autistic in each group, they concluded that there was no association between fragile X and autism, beyond the deficits caused by mental retardation. However, they found a significantly higher frequency of gaze avoidance and hand flapping in the fragile X group compared to controls and they concluded that these features misled clinicians into thinking that fragile X and autism were associated. These features indeed are core features of fragile X and are caused by the underlying biochemical defect in this disorder which is also responsible for other autistic behaviors. In the future we will probably better understand the biochemical and neuroanatomical associations between fragile X and autism. For now, better controlled studies of more detailed assessments than Einfeld's behavior ratings have shed light on the association of fragile X and autism.

Cohen *et al.* (1988, 1989*b*) focused on the gaze avoidance characteristic in fragile X and found it to be unique in its pattern compared to that in non-fragile X autistic individuals and other mentally retarded controls. A fragile X male will look away more frequently when someone looks at him than controls do, suggesting a greater aversion to direct eye contact. In further controlled studies Sudhalter *et al.* (1990) found the speech of fragile X males to be more perseverative and dysfluent than that of non-fragile X autistic controls. More recently, Sudhalter (1992) performed a controlled study of the impulsive associative features of speech of fragile X patients. These appear to be unique and related to the disinhibition in fragile X which has neuropsychological and neurochemical underpinnings.

The study of Reiss and Freund (1990) most eloquently demonstrated the relationship between autism and fragile X. These authors utilized a semi-structured interview (Neuropsychiatric Developmental Interview) to assess DSM-III-R criteria in 34 fragile X boys and 32 IQ- and age-matched non-fragile X controls. The general and subcategories in the DSM-III-R criteria were compared, and fragile X patients showed statistically significantly increased dysfunction in peer social play, non-verbal communication (gaze aversion and gesturing), verbal communication (word/phrase perseveration and rate, volume) and repetitive motor behaviors (hand flapping and rocking). There was also a trend to show abnormal responsivity to sensory stimuli, as well as oversensitivity to sound and increased mouthing or smelling of objects compared to controls. The DSM-III-R criteria allow for delineation of the profile of features which characterizes autism, and this is critical in comparing autistic syndromes with different organic etiologies. In Reiss and Freund's study, the fragile X patients were found to be comparable to controls in their social interactions with caretakers. Indeed, they can be very sociable and friendly, which is one reason why controversy exists regarding the relationship with autism. If you believe that the primary deficit in autism consists of social interactional deficits, then very few fragile X patients meet this criterion alone unless they are severely retarded (Borghgraef *et al.* 1987). Social deficits are not the core deficits in fragile X. However, the subject's extreme sensitivity and over-responsiveness to many stimuli, perhaps related to disinhibition, is a core feature in fragile X and relatively consistent across IQ levels in males and in severely affected females.

Higher functioning fragile X males
As more individuals were identified with fragile X syndrome and as more detailed family studies took place, the spectrum of involvement expanded and higher functioning

fragile X males were described. Normal and borderline IQ fragile X males have been reported, but they show significant learning disabilities, particularly in mathematics, and attentional problems. They also consistently have social and emotional dysfunction, including shyness, social anxiety, avoidant behavior and poor eye contact (Hagerman *et al.* 1985, Goldfine *et al.* 1987). They have a milder version of fragile X syndrome both behaviorally and cognitively than that typically seen in moderately retarded males. Asperger syndrome, an autistic-like condition in high functioning individuals, has been described in two normal IQ fragile X males (Hagerman 1990, 1991*a*) who fulfilled Gillberg's (1985) criteria, including (i) inability to relate normally to other people, (ii) pedantic or perseverative speech, (iii) deviant non-verbal communication, (iv) repetitive activities and strong attachment to certain possessions, and (v) clumsy and poorly co-ordinated gross motor movements.

The non-retarded fragile X males are clearly affected by the syndrome and can be differentiated from non-penetrant carrier males, who are cytogenetically negative and unaffected by the syndrome. Non-penetrant males are often grandfathers of retarded male probands and they are difficult to study because when their grandchildren are identified they are often too old to test, uncooperative or dead. Loesch *et al.* (1987) carried out a unique study which carefully assessed three supposed non-penetrant grandfathers. She found cognitive deficits in all and significant emotional difficulties including nervous breakdowns and positive cytogenetic studies in two. This report suggested that perhaps not all male carriers are completely unaffected and stressed a broader continuum to fragile X syndrome involvement than previously considered. Further studies by Loesch *et al.* (1993, 1994) have carefully delineated this continuum in relation to the molecular factors described below.

Heterozygotes

Females were not the original focus in this field because males were more severely affected. In the first report of an X-linked pedigree (which was later shown to be fragile X positive), Martin and Bell (1943) described in detail several retarded males and only briefly mentioned two females who appeared to be 'slow'. Many early genetic studies were hampered by the lack of available cognitive testing, so it was hard to decipher who was significantly impaired and who was not. In a chapter regarding the history of the field, the Australian pioneer Gillian Turner (1983) described her surprise in the work-up of a fragile X family when 'a very normal looking, sweet little girl' turned out to be functioning in the moderately retarded range after cognitive testing. Turner subsequently screened a school for mildly retarded females and found that 5 per cent were cytogenetically positive for the fragile X chromosome (Turner *et al.* 1980*b*). This excited the interest of researchers, and subsequent broad surveys by Sherman *et al.* (1984, 1985) demonstrated that approximately one third of females with the fragile X gene were cognitively impaired with an IQ of less than 85.

The mid- to late 1980s experienced further work regarding the physical and behavioral phenotype in females, and indeed prominent ears, long face, poor eye contact, shyness and social anxiety turned out to be common in cytogenetically positive and affected females (Fryns 1986, Borghgraef *et al.* 1990, Cronister *et al.* 1991*a,b*). However, some normal IQ heterozygous females were also demonstrating emotional problems including chronic affective disorders, particularly depression (40 per cent), and schizotypal features, one third showing social isolation, inappropriate affect and odd communication patterns (Reiss *et al.* 1988, 1989). In addition, approximately one half of normal IQ girls who were cytogenetically positive were recognized as learning disabled by their schools (Hagerman *et al.* 1992). Many had attentional problems but often without hyperactivity, in addition to language deficits and difficulties in mathematics that required tutoring or individualized therapy (Hagerman *et al.* 1992). Freund *et al.* (1993) reported that 65 per cent of 17 fragile X positive girls compared to 12 per cent of age and IQ matched controls had an avoidant disorder or avoidant personality disorder, and 47 per cent had a mood disorder including major depression or dysthymia, compared to 6 per cent of controls. Moreover, 35 per cent had stereotypy/habit disorder including hand or nail biting, hand flapping and head banging, whereas no controls showed such behaviors. Although females with this syndrome are usually less severely affected than males, they are clearly having significant problems. Representing the severe end of the spectrum in females, autism has been reported in some cases (Hagerman *et al.* 1986*a*, Edwards *et al.* 1988, Gillberg *et al.* 1988, Le Couteur *et al.* 1988, Cohen *et al.* 1989*a*).

At the end of the 1980s the question uppermost in many researchers' minds was why some carriers were completely unaffected (both males and females) and why others ranged from mildly to severely affected.

The discovery of the *FMR-1* gene

In the spring of 1991 reports of hypermethylation of an expanded repetitive nucleotide sequence, CGG_n (Oberlé *et al.* 1991, Yu *et al.* 1991) led to the identification and sequencing of the *FMR-1* gene by a collaborative international effort (Verkerk *et al.* 1991). Subsequent reports demonstrated that greater than 200 CGG repeats (full mutation) at the *FMR-1* locus is associated with hypermethylation and lack of *FMR-1* protein production (Fu *et al.* 1991, Nakahori *et al.* 1991, Pieretti *et al.* 1991, Devys *et al.* 1993). In an affected male or female the CGG repeat number may be several hundred to 2000, whereas in unaffected carriers (male or female), the repeat number is approximately 52 to 200 (Fu *et al.* 1991, Yu *et al.* 1992). Normal individuals who are not carriers will have approximately five to 50 repeats, with an average of 29 to 30 (Fu *et al.* 1991, Snow *et al.* 1993). However, once the CGG repeat number is over 50 an instability occurs which can lead to expansion of the CGG mutation in subsequent offspring. Carriers with 52 to 200 CGG repeats are said to carry a premutation. The chance of expansion to a full mutation (>200 repeats) is low for carriers with 52 to 70 repeats but expansion almost always occurs in female carriers with >90 repeats who pass on the fragile X chromosome (Fu *et al.* 1991, Snow *et al.* 1993). The CGG repeat number will not expand significantly when passed on to the next generation through a male. Therefore, all daughters of non-penetrant males are carriers, but they are unaffected if they have a CGG repeat number in the premutation range. Usually the *FMR-1* region is not hypermethylated in unaffected carriers and the *FMR-1* protein is thought to be produced at normal levels. The full mutation in males causes the full fragile X syndrome in almost all cases. However, in females with the full mutation approximately half have cognitive deficits with a borderline IQ or mental retardation, and the rest have a normal IQ although specific learning disabilities are common (Rousseau *et al.* 1991*a*, 1994; Yu *et al.* 1991; Hagerman *et al.* 1992; Staley *et al.* 1993). For a review of molecular findings in fragile X syndrome, see Warren and Nelson (1994).

Cytogenetically positive but DNA negative individuals

With the advent of DNA testing for the CGG insert in the *FMR-1* gene (*FRAXA* locus), several subjects were reported who were cytogenetically positive with mental retardation but who did not have the CGG expansion (Rousseau *et al.* 1991*a*, Dennis *et al.* 1992, Knight *et al.* 1992). In a survey of 300 cytogenetically positive individuals, five females and three males were found without the CGG expansion (Hagerman 1992). Two of the boys had a normal IQ, one had a borderline IQ, and all had non-specific features in common with fragile X, such as hyperactivity, but none had the typical Martin–Bell phenotype of a long face and prominent ears.

Sutherland and Baker (1992) reported the presence of a distal mutation to the *FMR-1* gene in one cytogenetically positive family with mild mental retardation. They named this mutation *FRAXE*. Subsequently, Flynn *et al.* (1993) reported the *FRAXE* mutation in two additional families who were cytogenetically positive but again without the classical Martin–Bell phenotype. Knight *et al.* (1994) succeeded in sequencing the *FRAXE* mutation, which has a similar CGG amplification to that seen in *FRAXA*. Therefore, new cytogenetic and molecular techniques have allowed for a careful biologically based subdivision of families who are cytogenetically positive at Xq27.3. In differentiating these new families from those with the more common *FRAXA* mutation, the clinical characterization of physical, cognitive and behavioral characteristics has been invaluable. Yet another mutation, *FRAXF*, has recently been reported which is distal to *FRAXA* and *FRAXE* (Hirst *et al.* 1993). The cytogenetic fragility associated with *FRAXF* is unusual because it is folate insensitive, that is it will express when the tissue culture medium is not deficient in folate, unlike *FRAXA* and *FRAXE*. Parrish *et al.* (1994) have sequenced the *FRAXF* gene, which also contains a CGG repetitive sequence similar to *FRAXA* and *FRAXE*; however, it is inconsistently associated with mental retardation. It will take time to further characterize the behavioral phenotype in these new mutations because they are far less common than the *FRAXA* fragile X syndrome.

The phenomenon of a mutation caused by a triplet repeat expansion has been found in several other disorders which are associated with anticipation (an earlier onset or more severe disease in subsequent generations). At present the total number of triplet repeat expansions in the human genome is ten and they include Huntington's disease, myotonic dystrophy, Machado–Joseph disease and other degenerative disorders associated with anticipation (Willems 1994).

There appear to be additional rare mechanisms for developing the fragile X syndrome other than an expansion of the CGG repeat. Worhle *et al.* (1992) reported a micro-deletion of 250 kb across the *FMR-1* gene region in a 9-year-old boy with mild mental retardation and typical physical and behavioral features of fragile X syndrome. The CGG repeat and cytogenetic expression are absent but so is the *FMR-1* protein and therefore the patient has the classical features of fragile X syndrome. Numerous other deletions involving *FMR-1* have since been reported and all demonstrate physical and behavioral features which are typical of fragile X syndrome (Gedeon *et al.* 1992, Tarleton *et al.* 1993, Albright *et al.* 1994, Gu *et al.* 1994, Meijer *et al.* 1994, Hirst *et al.* 1995). Quan *et al.* (1995) reported a particularly large deletion which included the entire *FMR-1* gene and at least 9.0 megabases of flanking DNA mainly proximal to *FMR-1*. The patient had typical features of fragile X, in addition to other problems including anal atresia which were presumably related to the additional deleted material. One of two patients reported by Hirst *et al.* (1995) was an unusual mosaic with both normal cells and cells demonstrating a 660 base pair deletion in 40 per cent of lymphocytes. His phenotype was milder, presumably because of mosaicism, than that of the second patient they reported who had a similar sized deletion in all of his cells.

Lastly, DeBoulle *et al.* (1993) reported a severely retarded male with macro-orchidism who did not have the CGG expansion mutation but instead demonstrated a point mutation within the *FMR-1* gene which converted isoleucine to asparagine. This mutation occurs within a highly conserved region of *FMR-1* protein (FMRP) which is thought to be critical for its postulated function as an mRNA carrier or binding protein (Siomi *et al.* 1994). This patient has a more severe phenotype than that typically seen in fragile X syndrome. It is possible that the point mutation in FMRP caused a change in function of the protein which has a more severe deleterious effect than complete absence of the protein.

Molecular–clinical correlations

Males who have the full mutation are all considered to be affected by fragile X syndrome (Rousseau *et al.* 1991a, Snow *et al.* 1992, Yu *et al.* 1992). However, approximately 15 per cent of males have a mosaic pattern in DNA studies, meaning that both a full mutation and a premutation are seen. Rousseau *et al.* (1991a) and DeVries *et al.* (1993) found no significant cognitive difference between full mutation and mosaic males, but Staley *et al.* (1993) found that mosaic males had a higher mean IQ than full mutation males. Pieretti *et al.* (1991) found that four of 20 fragile X males produced mRNA for the *FMR-1* protein, and three of these four males were mosaics.

In a recent survey of 250 fragile X males, 13 per cent were found to have an IQ of ≥70 (Hagerman *et al.* 1994b). Although most experienced a subsequent IQ decline, five late-adolescent/adult males maintained an IQ above 70 and had a lower cytogenetic expression of the fragile X chromosome than the retarded fragile X males. Three of these males had a full mutation that was completely unmethylated, and one was mosaic. Methylation appears to play a critical role in turning off the gene to prevent protein production (Sutcliffe *et al.* 1992). Without complete methylation, three of these high functioning males have been shown to have limited FMRP production in the range of 10 to 35 per cent of normal levels in lymphoblastoid cell lines (Hagerman *et al.* 1994b, Merenstein *et al.* 1994). These initial data suggest that even minimal FMRP production is beneficial to the patient with fragile X syndrome and may be the causal factor for the high functioning (non-retarded) status in males. Future protein studies are critical to understanding the final outcome of molecular variations of the *FMR-1* gene.

In females the story is even more complex because there are two X chromosomes, one with the mutation and one normal. All females will randomly inactivate one of their X chromosomes and this process was thought to explain some of the phenotypic variability in fragile X females (Webb and Jacobs 1990). The molecular advances have helped to clarify the picture, and females with a premutation are usually cytogenetically negative and do not show neurocognitive or significant emotional problems compared to controls (Mazzocco *et al.* 1993, Reiss *et al.* 1993).

Only approximately 50 per cent of full mutation females show cognitive deficits, presumably because of the input of the normal X chromosome (Rousseau *et al.* 1991*a*). Preliminary data supported a significant correlation between IQ and the percentage of cells with the normal X as the active X chromosome in cytogenetic studies (McGavran *et al.* 1992) and in molecular studies (Rousseau *et al.* 1991*b*). However, a study by Taylor *et al.* (1994), utilizing Rousseau's molecular method to calculate the proportion of cells with the normal X as the active X, did not show a significant correlation between this activation ratio and IQ in full mutation females. At this point there are no clear methods to predict absolutely the degree of involvement in full mutation females. Although half will have significant cognitive impairment, many of those with a normal IQ will also have significant learning disabilities, including attentional and mathematics problems, in addition to shyness and avoidant personality disorder (Hagerman *et al.* 1992, Freund *et al.* 1993).

Neuropsychological deficits and emotional problems:
Recent work by Mazzocco *et al.* (1992*a,b*, 1993) has helped to develop an understanding of the interrelationship of emotional problems and cognitive deficits in fragile X females. The most subtle effect of the fragile X mutation can be characterized in studies of non-retarded heterozygotes in contrast to fully affected and retarded individuals. Significant frontal deficits were found in non-retarded but cytogenetically positive heterozygotes with a full mutation compared to controls and those with a premutation only. The frontal deficits included attentional and organizational problems, difficulties in shifting strategies in problem solving, significant perseveration, and problems in coordinating information in working memory, particularly the simultaneous consideration of information that is important in problem solving. These women often appear disorganized emotionally, with mood lability, tangential or perseverative speech and schizotypal features in addition to affective disorders (Reiss *et al.* 1988, 1989; Hagerman and Sobesky 1989). Sobesky *et al.* (1992) have also reported that affected females have a tendency to deny emotional difficulties as measured by a high lie scale on the Minnesota Multiphasic Personality Inventory compared to controls. They have difficulty in integrating past experiences with the present situation, and will often answer questions as if they were blindfolded, that is an 'out of sight, out of mind' approach to dealing with difficulties (Sobesky *et al.* 1992). A more accurate report of social or emotional problems can often be obtained

from a spouse or close family member so that treatment needs can be accurately assessed. We believe that the problems of denial and the 'blindfold effect' are caused or exacerbated by the frontal deficits in these females.

Additional neuropsychological deficits in affected females, including visuospatial organization deficits and dyscalculia, are reviewed by Baumgardner et al. (1992). The social and cognitive weaknesses described by Rourke (1987) in 'non-verbal learning disability' and by Weintraub and Mesulam (1983) in 'social learning disability' fit many of the characteristics of learning disabled fragile X females as reviewed by Miezejeski and Hinton (1992). The deficits in social learning involve right cerebral hemisphere dysfunction, and previous neuropsychological studies support a deficit in this region (Mazzocco et al. 1993).

It is also important to focus on areas of strength in fragile X patients, not only for treatment reasons but to better understand neuroanatomical and neurochemical correlations. Memory is a strength for affected males and females in addition verbal and visual learning and imitation (Dykens et al. 1987; Kemper et al. 1988; Pennington et al. 1991; Baumgardner et al. 1992; Mazzocco et al. 1992a, 1993).

Neuroanatomical and neurochemical correlations

Our task is to understand and improve the problems caused by an absent *FMR-1* protein. Studies by Reiss et al. (1991) have shown that a small posterior cerebellar vermis is present in affected males and females, and Murphy et al. (1991) have shown that the overall brain mass is larger in fragile X patients than in controls. More recent studies by Reiss et al. (1994) have shown an age-related decrease in the superior temporal gyrus which is greater in fragile X patients than in controls. In addition, the right and left hippocampal volumes were found to be greater in fragile X patients, and subsequently the caudate and thalamus have been shown to be larger in individuals affected by fragile X, compared to controls (Abrams and Reiss 1995). This suggests cellular over-proliferation, or a lack of the normal pruning process when FMRP is not present. Abitbol et al. (1993) studied expression of FMRP in normal human fetuses and found the highest expression in the nucleus basalis magnocellularis and in the hippocampus. The neuroanatomical and FMRP studies are consistent with the cognitive profiles described in fragile X patients, including strengths in memory but weaknesses in abstract reasoning and IQ decline, that have been previously reported (Lachiewicz et al. 1987, Hagerman et al. 1989, Freund and Reiss 1991). In addition, the behavioral problems in fragile X appear to be consistent with the neuroanatomical findings and studies of FMRP localization in the brain (for review, see Binstock 1995).

On a microscopic level Rudelli et al. (1985) and Wisniewski et al. (1991) have reported long and tortuous dendritic spines with a reduced synaptic contact area in fragile X patients. Berry-Kravis and Huttenlocher (1992) found significantly lower cAMP levels in the platelets of fragile X patients compared to controls including autistic subjects. Since cAMP is a central factor in influencing neurotransmitters, ion channels and even transcriptional processes important for neuronal structure, deficits in cAMP may be causal for many of the cognitive and behavioral problems including disinhibition seen in fragile X.

67

Treatment and future directions

Treatment for fragile X includes the use of medication to counteract some of the deficits described above. Stimulant medication has been shown to be helpful in fragile X males and females by improving attention and concentration and decreasing impulsive behavior (Hagerman *et al.* 1988*b*, Hagerman 1991*b*). Stimulation of the dopamine system improves frontal functioning (Aman *et al.* 1993) and that is of theoretical benefit in fragile X males and females with frontal deficits. Clonidine also appears to be beneficial in approximately 80 per cent of children with fragile X syndrome who have significant hyperactivity, tantrums or hyperarousal (Hagerman *et al.* 1995). Fluoxetine can be of benefit for affected males and females who suffer from mood lability, outburst behavior, anxiety or depression (Hagerman *et al.* 1994*a*). This serotonin re-uptake blocker can also enhance cAMP levels which is of theoretical benefit. As we gain insight into the structural and neurochemical problems in fragile X we can better define treatment programs that are beneficial. Eventually FMRP replacement may be possible, or gene therapy to turn on or replace a hypermethylated *FMR-1* mutation (Rattazzi 1995).

REFERENCES

Abitbol, M., Menini, C., Delezoide, A-L., Rhyner, T., Vekemans, M., Mallet, J. (1993) 'Nucleus basalis magnocellularis and hippocampus are the major sites of *FMR-1* expression in the human fetal brain.' *Nature Genetics*, **4**, 147–153.

Abrams, M.T., Reiss, A.L. (1995) 'Quantitative brain imaging studies of fragile X syndrome.' *Developmental Brain Dysfunction. (In press.)*

Albright, S.G., Lachiewicz, A.M., Tarleton, J.C., Rao, K.W., Schwartz, C.E., Richie, R., Tennison, M.B., Aylsworth, A.S. (1994) 'Fragile X phenotype in a patient with a large *de novo* deletion in Xq27–q28.' *American Journal of Medical Genetics*, **51**, 294–297.

Aman, C., Roberts, R., Pennington, B.F. (1993) 'The nature of the underlying deficit in ADHD: a neuropsychological examination of the frontal lobe and parietal lobe theories.' *Paper presented at the Annual Meeting of the Society for Research in Child Development, New Orleans, LA, March 1993.*

August, G.J., Lockhart, L.H. (1984) 'Familial autism and the fragile-X chromosome.' *Journal of Autism and Developmental Disorders*, **14**, 197–204.

Baumgardner, T.L., Freund, L., Hinton, V., Mazzocco, M.M.M. (1992) 'Workshop summary: neuropsychological deficits and learning strategies for fragile X females.' *In:* Hagerman, R.J., McKenzie, P. (Eds.) *1992 International Fragile X Conference Proceedings.* Denver, CO: Spectra/National Fragile X Foundation, pp. 79–83.

Berry-Kravis, E., Huttenlocher, P.R. (1992) 'Cyclic AMP metabolism in fragile X syndrome.' *American Neurology*, **31**, 22–26.

Binstock, T. (1995) 'Fragile X and the amygdala: cognitive, interpersonal, emotional and neuroendocrine considerations.' *Developmental Brain Dysfunction. (In press.)*

Blomquist, H.K., Gustavson, K-H., Holmgren, G., Nordenson, I., Sweins, A. (1982) 'Fragile site X chromosomes and X-linked mental retardation in severely retarded boys in a northern Swedish county: a prevalence study.' *Clinical Genetics*, **21**, 209–214.

—— Bohman, M., Edvinsson, S.O., Gillberg, C., Gustavson, K.H., Holmgren, G., Wahlström, J. (1985) 'Frequency of the fragile X syndrome in infantile autism. A Swedish multicenter study.' *Clinical Genetics*, **27**, 113–117.

Borghgraef, M., Fryns, J-P., Dielkens, A., Pyck, K., Van den Berghe, H. (1987) 'Fragile (X) syndrome: a study of the psychological profile in 23 prepubertal patients.' *Clinical Genetics*, **32**, 179–186.

—————— Van den Berghe, H. (1990) 'The female and the fragile X syndrome: data on clinical and psychological findings in 7 fra (X) carriers.' *Clinical Genetics*, **37**, 341–346.

Brondum Nielsen, K. (1983) 'Diagnosis of the fragile X syndrome (Martin–Bell syndrome): clinical findings in 27 males with the fragile site at Xq28.' *Journal of Mental Deficiency Research*, **27**, 211–226.

Brown, W.T., Jenkins, E.C., Friedman, E., Brooks, J., Wisniewski, K., Raguthu, S., French, J. (1982) 'Autism is associated with the fragile-X syndrome.' *Journal of Autism and Developmental Disorders*, **12**, 303–308.

—— —— Cohen, I.L., Fisch, G.S., Wolf-Schein, E.G., Gross, A., Waterhouse, L., Fein, D., Mason-Brothers, A., *et al.* (1986) 'Fragile X and autism: a multicenter survey.' *American Journal of Medical Genetics*, **23**, 341–352.

Butler, M.G., Mangrum, T., Gupta, R., Singh, D.N. (1991) 'A 15-item checklist for screening mentally retarded males for the fragile X syndrome.' *Clinical Genetics*, **39**, 347–354.

Carpenter, N.J., Leichtman, L.G., Say, B. (1982) 'Fragile X-linked mental retardation. A survey of 65 patients with mental retardation of unknown origin.' *American Journal of Diseases of Children*, **136**, 392–398.

Cohen, I L., Fisch, G.S., Sudhalter, V., Wolf-Schein, E.G., Hanson, D., Hagerman, R., Jenkins, E.C., Brown, W.T. (1988) 'Social gaze, social avoidance, and repetitive behavior in fragile X males: a controlled study.' *American Journal on Mental Retardation*, **92**, 436–446.

—— Brown, W.T., Jenkins, E.C., Krawczun, M.S., French, J.H., Raguthu, S., Wolf-Schein, E.G., Sudhalter, V., Fisch, G., Wisniewski, K. (1989*a*) 'Fragile X syndrome in females with autism.' *American Journal of Medical Genetics*, **34**, 302–303. *(Letter.)*

—— Vietze, P.M., Sudhalter, V., Jenkins, E.C., Brown, W.T. (1989*b*) 'Parent–child dyadic gaze patterns in fragile X males and in non-fragile X males with autistic disorder.' *Journal of Child Psychology and Psychiatry*, **30**, 845–856.

Cronister, A., Hagerman, R.J., Wittenberger, M., Amiri, K. (1991*a*) 'Mental impairment in cytogenetically positive fragile X females.' *American Journal of Medical Genetics*, **38**, 503–504.

—— Schreiner, R., Wittenberger, M., Amiri, K., Harris, K., Hagerman, R.J. (1991*b*) 'Heterozygous fragile X female: historical, physical, cognitive, and cytogenetic features.' *American Journal of Medical Genetics*, **38**, 269–274.

De Boulle, K., Verkerk, A.J.M.H., Reyniers, E., Vits, L., Hendrickx, J., Van Roy, B., Van Den Bos, F., de Graaff, E., Oostra, B.A., Willems, P.J. (1993) 'A point mutation in the *FMR-1* gene associated with fragile X mental retardation.' *Nature Genetics*, **3**, 31–35.

Dennis, N.R., Curtis, G., Macpherson, J.N., Jacobs, P.A. (1992) 'Two families with Xq27.3 fragility, no detectable insert in the *FMR-1* gene, mild mental impairment, and absence of the Martin–Bell phenotype.' *American Journal of Medical Genetics*, **43**, 232–236.

DeVries, B.A., Wiegers, A.M., deGraaff, E., Verkerk, A.J.M.H., van Hemel, J.O., Halley, D.J.J., Fryns, J-P., Curfs, L.M.G., Niermeijer, M.F., Oostra, B.A. (1993) 'Mental status and fragile X expression in relation to *FMR-1* gene mutation.' *European Journal of Human Genetics*, **1**, 72–79.

Devys, D., Lutz, Y., Rouyer, N., Bellocq, J-P., Mandel, J-L. (1993) 'The *FMR-1* protein is cytoplasmic, most abundant in neurons and appears normal in carriers of a fragile X premutation.' *Nature Genetics*, **4**, 335–340.

Dykens, E.M., Hodapp, R.M., Leckman, J.F. (1987) 'Strengths and weaknesses in the intellectual functioning of males with fragile X syndrome.' *American Journal of Mental Deficiency*, **92**, 234–236.

Edwards, D.R., Keppen, L.D., Ranells, J.D., Gollin, S.M. (1988) 'Autism in association with fragile X syndrome in females: implications for diagnosis and treatment in children.' *Neurotoxicology*, **9**, 359–365.

Einfeld, S., Molony, H., Hall, W. (1989) 'Autism is not associated with the fragile X syndrome.' *American Journal of Medical Genetics*, **34**, 187–193.

Flynn, G.A., Hirst, M.C., Knight, S.J.L., Macpherson, J.N., Barber, J.C.K., Flannery, A.V., Davies, K.E., Buckle, V.J. (1993) 'Identification of the *FRAXE* fragile site in two families ascertained for X linked mental retardation.' *Journal of Medical Genetics*, 30, 97–100.

Freund, L.S., Reiss, A.L. (1991) 'Cognitive profiles associated with the fra(X) syndrome in males and females.' *American Journal of Medical Genetics*, **38**, 542–547.

—— —— Abrams, M.T. (1993) 'Psychiatric disorders associated with fragile X in the young female.' *Pediatrics*, **91**, 321–329.

Froster-Iskenius, U., Felsch, G., Schirren, C., Schwinger, E. (1983) 'Screening for fra(X)(q) in a population of mentally retarded males.' *Human Genetics*, **63**, 153–157.

Fryns, J-P. (1986) 'The female and the fragile X. A study of 144 obligate female carriers.' *American Journal of Medical Genetics*, **23**, 157–169.

Fu, Y-H, Kuhl, D.P.A., Pizzuti, A., Pieretti M., Sutcliffe, J.S., Richards, S., Verkerk, A.J.M.H., Holden,

J.J.A., Fenwick, R.G., *et al.* (1991) 'Variation of the CGG repeat at the fragile X site results in genetic instability: resolution of the Sherman paradox.' *Cell,* **67**, 1047–1058.

Gedeon, A.K., Baker, E., Robinson, H., Partington, M.W., Gross, B., Manca, A., Korn, B., Poustka, A., Yu, S., *et al.* (1992) 'Fragile X syndrome without CCG amplification has an *FMR1* deletion.' *Nature Genetics,* **1**, 341–344.

Gillberg, C. (1985) 'Asperger's syndrome and recurrent psychosis—a case study.' *Journal of Autism and Developmental Disorders,* **15**, 389–397.

—— Persson, E., Wahlström, J. (1986) 'The autism–fragile-X syndrome (AFRAX): a population-based study of ten boys.' *Journal of Mental Deficiency Research,* **30**, 27–39.

—— Ohlson, V.A., Wahlström, J., Steffenburg, S., Blix, K. (1988) 'Monozygotic female twins with autism and the fragile-X syndrome (AFRAX).' *Journal of Child Psychology and Psychiatry,* **29**, 447–451.

Goldfine, P.E., McPherson, P.M., Heath, G.A., Hardesty, V.A., Beauregard, L.J., Gordon, B. (1985) 'Association of fragile X syndrome with autism.' *American Journal of Psychiatry,* **142**, 108–110.

—— —— Hardesty, V.A., Heath, G.A., Beauregard, L.J., Baker, A.A. (1987) 'Fragile-X chromosome associated with primary learning disability.' *Journal of the American Academy of Child and Adolescent Psychiatry,* **26**, 589–592.

Gu, Y., Lugenbeel, K.A., Vockley, J.G., Grody, W.W., Nelson, D.L. (1994) 'A *de novo* deletion in *FMR1* in a patient with a developmental delay.' *Human Molecular Genetics,* **3**, 1705–1706.

Hagerman, R.J. (1990) 'Chromosomes, genes, and autism.' *In:* Gillberg, C. (Ed.) *Autism—Diagnosis and Treatment: the State of the Art.* New York: Plenum Press, pp. 105–131.

—— (1991*a*) 'Physical and behavioral phenotype.' *In:* Hagerman, R.J., Silverman, A.C. (Eds.) *The Fragile X Syndrome: Diagnosis, Treatment and Research.* Baltimore, MD: Johns Hopkins University Press, pp. 3–68.

—— (1991*b*) 'Medical followup and pharmacotherapy.' *In:* Hagerman, R.J., Silverman, A.C. (Eds.) *The Fragile X Syndrome: Diagnosis, Treatment and Research.* Baltimore, MD: Johns Hopkins University Press, pp. 282–310.

—— (1992) 'Clinical conundrums in fragile X syndrome.' *Nature Genetics,* **1**, 157–158.

—— Sobesky, W.E. (1989) 'Psychopathology in fragile X syndrome.' *American Journal of Orthopsychiatry,* **59**, 142–152.

—— Smith, A.C.M., Mariner, R. (1983) 'Clinical features of the fragile X syndrome.' *In:* Hagerman, R.J., McBogg, P. (Eds.) *The Fragile X Syndrome—Diagnosis, Biochemistry, and Intervention.* Dillon, CO: Spectra, pp. 17–53.

—— Kemper, M., Hudson, M. (1985) 'Learning disabilities and attentional problems in boys with the fragile X syndrome.' *American Journal of Diseases of Children,* **139**, 674–678.

—— Chudley, A.E., Knoll, J.H., Jackson, A.W., Kemper, M., Ahmad, R. (1986*a*) 'Autism in fragile X females.' *American Journal of Medical Genetics,* **23**, 375–380.

—— Jackson, A.W., Levitas A., Rimland, B., Braden, M. (1986*b*) 'An analysis of autism in fifty males with the fragile X syndrome.' *American Journal of Medical Genetics,* **23**, 359–374.

—— Berry, R., Jackson, A.W., Campbell, J., Smith, A.C.M., McGavran, L. (1988*a*) 'Institutional screening for the fragile X syndrome.' *American Journal of Diseases of Children,* **142**, 1216–1221.

—— Murphy, M.A., Wittenberger, M.D. (1988*b*) 'A controlled trial of stimulant medication in children with the fragile X syndrome.' *American Journal of Medical Genetics,* **30**, 377–392.

—— Schreiner, R.A., Kemper, M.B., Wittenberger, M.D., Zahn, B., Habicht, K. (1989) 'Longitudinal IQ changes in fragile X males.' *American Journal of Medical Genetics,* **33**, 513–518.

—— Amiri, K., Cronister, A. (1991) 'Fragile X checklist.' *American Journal of Medical Genetics,* **38**, 283–287.

—— Jackson, C., Amiri, K., Silverman, A.C., O'Connor, R., Sobesky, W. (1992) 'Girls with fragile X syndrome: physical and neurocognitive status and outcome.' *Pediatrics,* **89**, 395–400.

—— Fulton, M.J., Leaman, A., Riddle, J., Hagerman, K., Sobesky, W. (1994*a*) 'Fluoxetine therapy in fragile X syndrome.' *Developmental Brain Dysfunction,* **7**, 155–164.

—— Hull, C.E., Safanda, J.F., Carpenter, I., Staley, L.W., O'Connor, R.A., Seydel, C., Mazzocco, M.M.M., Snow, K., *et al.* (1994*b*) 'High functioning fragile X males: demonstration of an unmethylated fully expanded *FMR-1* mutation associated with protein expression.' *American Journal of Medical Genetics,* **51**, 298–308.

—— Riddle, J.E., Robert, L.S., Brease, K., Fulton, M. (1995) 'A survey of the efficacy of clonidine in fragile X syndrome.' *Developmental Brain Dysfunction. (In press.)*

Hirst, M.C., Barnicoat, A., Flynn, G., Wang, Q., Daker, M., Buckle, V.J., Davies, K.E., Bobrow, M. (1993) 'The identification of a third fragile site, *FRAXF*, in Xq27–q28 distal to both *FRAXA* and *FRAXE*.' *Human Molecular Genetics*, **2**, 197–200.

—— Grewal, P., Flannery, A., Slatter, R., Maher, E., Barton, D., Fryns, J-P., Davies, K. (1995) 'Two new cases of *FMR1* deletion associated with mental impairment.' *American Journal of Human Genetics*, **56**, 67–74.

Howard-Peebles, P.N., Finley, W.H. (1983) 'Screening of mentally retarded males for macro-orchidism and the fragile X chromosome.' *American Journal of Medical Genetics*, **15**, 631–635.

Kemper, M.B., Hagerman, R.J., Altshul-Stark, D. (1988) 'Cognitive profiles of boys with the fragile X syndrome.' *American Journal of Medical Genetics*, **30**, 191–200.

Kerbeshian, J., Burd, L., Martsolf, J.T. (1984) 'Fragile X syndrome associated with Tourette symptomatology in a male with moderate mental retardation and autism.' *Journal of Developmental and Behavioral Pediatrics*, **5**, 201–203.

Knight, S.J.L., Hirst, M.C., Roche, A., Christodoulou, Z., Huson, S.M., Winter, R., Fitchett, M., McKinley, M.J., Lindenbaum, R.H., *et al.* (1992) 'Molecular studies of the fragile X syndrome.' *American Journal of Medical Genetics*, **43**, 217–223.

—— Voelckel, M.A., Hirst, M.C., Flannery, A.V., Moncla, A., Davies, K.E. (1994) 'Triplet repeat expansion at the *FRAXE* locus and X-linked mild mental handicap.' *American Journal of Human Genetics*, **55**, 81–86.

Lachiewicz, A.M., Gullion, C.M., Spiridigliozzi, G.A., Alysworth, A.S. (1987) 'Declining IQs of young males with the fragile X syndrome.' *American Journal on Mental Retardation*, **92**, 272–278.

Laing, S., Partington, M., Robinson, H., Turner, G. (1991) 'Clinical screening score for the fragile X (Martin–Bell) syndrome.' *American Journal of Medical Genetics*, **38**, 256–259.

Le Couteur, A., Rutter, M., Summers, D., Butler, L. (1988) 'Fragile X in female autistic twins.' *Journal of Autism and Developmental Disorders*, **18**, 458–460. *(Letter.)*

Levitas, A., Hagerman, R.J., Braden, M., Rimland, B., McBogg, P., Matus, I. (1983) 'Autism and the fragile X syndrome.' *Journal of Developmental and Behavioral Pediatrics*, **4**,151–158.

Loesch, D.Z., Hay, D.A., Sutherland, G.R., Halliday, J., Judge, C., Webb, G.C. (1987) 'Phenotypic variation in male-transmitted fragile X: genetic inferences.' *American Journal of Medical Genetics*, **27**, 401–417.

Loesch, D.Z., Huggins, R., Hay, D.A., Gedeon, A.K., Mulley, J.C., Sutherland, G.R. (1993) 'Genotype–phenotype relationships in fragile X syndrome: a family study.' *American Journal of Human Genetics*, **53**, 1064–1073.

—— Hay, D.A., Mulley, J. (1994) 'Transmitting males and carrier females in fragile X—revisited.' *American Journal of Medical Genetics*, **51**, 392–399.

Lubs, H.A. (1969) 'The marker X chromosome.' *American Journal of Human Genetics*, **21**, 231–244.

Martin, J.P., Bell, J. (1943) 'A pedigree of mental defect showing sex-linkage.' *Journal of Neurology and Psychiatry*, **6**, 154–157.

Mazzocco, M.M.M., Hagerman, R.J., Cronister-Silverman, A., Pennington B.F. (1992*a*) 'Specific frontal lobe deficits among women with the fragile X gene.' *Journal of the American Academy of Child and Adolescent Psychiatry*, **31**, 1141–1148.

—— —— Pennington, B.F. (1992*b*) 'Problem solving limitations among cytogenetically expressing fragile X women.' *American Journal of Medical Genetics*, **43**, 78–86.

—— Hagerman, R.J., Pennington, B.F. (1993) 'The neurocognitive phenotype of female carriers of fragile X: additional evidence for specificity.' *Journal of Developmental and Behavioral Pediatrics*, **14**, 328–335.

McGavran, L., Meltesen, L., Taylor, A., Hagerman, R.J. (1992) 'Preferential inactivation of the X chromosome bearing the *FMR-1* mutation inversely correlates with mental status in heterozygotes.' *American Journal of Human Genetics*, **51** (Suppl.), A84. *(Abstract.)*

Meijer, H., deGraff, E., Merckx, D.M.L., Jongbloed, J.E., deDie-Smulders, C.E.M., Engelen, J.J.M., Fryns, J-P., Curfs, P.M., Costra, B.A. (1994) 'A deletion of q1.6Kb proximal to the CGG repeat of the *FMR1* gene causes the clinical phenotype of the fragile X syndrome.' *Human Molecular Genetics*, **3**, 615–620.

Merenstein, S.A., Shyu, V., Sobesky, W.E., Staley, L., Berry-Kravis, E., Nelson, D.L., Lugenbeel, K.A., Taylor, A.K., Pennington, B.F., Hagerman, R.J. (1994) 'Fragile X syndrome in a normal IQ male with learning and emotional problems.' *Journal of the American Academy of Child and Adolescent Psychiatry*, **33**, 1316–1321.

71

Meryash, D.L., Szymanski, L.S., Gerald, P.S. (1982) 'Infantile autism associated with the fragile-X syndrome.' *Journal of Autism and Developmental Disorders*, **12**, 295–301.

Miezejeski, C.M., Hinton, V.J. (1992) 'Fragile X learning disability: neurobehavioral research, diagnostic models and treatment options.' *In:* Hagerman, R.J., McKenzie, P. (Eds.) *1992 International Fragile X Conference Proceedings.* Denver, CO: Spectra/National Fragile X Foundation, pp. 85–98.

Murphy, D., Shapiro, M.B., Haxby, J., Hagerman, R.J., Rappaport, S.I. (1991) 'Fragile X adults: neuropsychology, brain metabolism and anatomy.' *Paper presented at the Annual Meeting of the American Psychiatric Association, New York.*

Nakahori, Y., Knight, S.J.L., Holland, J., Schwartz, C., Roche, A., Tarleton, J., Wong, S., Flint, T.J., Froster-Iskenius, U., *et al.* (1991) 'Molecular heterogeneity of the fragile X syndrome.' *Nucleic Acids Research*, **19**, 4355–4359.

Nolin, S.L., Snider, D.A., Jenkins, E.C., Brown, W.T., Krawczun, M., Stetka, D., Houck, G., Dobkin, C.S., Strong, G., *et al.* (1991) 'Fragile X screening program in New York State.' *American Journal of Medical Genetics*, **38**, 251–255.

Oberlé, I., Rousseau, F., Heitz, D., Kretz, C., Devys, D., Hanauer, A., Boué, J., Bertheas, M.F., Mandel, J.L. (1991) 'Instability of a 550-base pair DNA segment and abnormal methylation in fragile X syndrome.' *Science*, **252**, 1097–1102.

Parrish, J.E., Oostra, B.A., Verkerk, A.J.M.H., Richards, C.S., Reynolds, J., Spikes, A., Shaffer, L.G., Nelson, D.L. (1994) 'Isolation of a CGG repeat showing expansion in *FRAXF*, a fragile site distal to *FRAXA* and *FRAXE*.' *Nature Genetics*, **8**, 229–235.

Payton, J.B., Steele, M.W., Wenger, S.L., Minshew, N.J. (1989) 'The fragile X marker and autism in perspective.' *Journal of the American Academy of Child and Adolescent Psychiatry*, **28**, 417–421.

Pennington, B., O'Connor, R., Sudhalter, V. (1991) 'Toward a neuropsychological understanding of fragile X syndrome.' *In:* Hagerman, R.J., Silverman, A.C. (Eds.) *The Fragile X Syndrome—Diagnosis, Treatment and Research.* Baltimore, MD: Johns Hopkins University Press, pp. 173–201.

Pieretti, M., Zhang, F., Fu Y-H, Warren, S.T., Oostra, B.A., Caskey, C.T., Nelson, D.L. (1991) 'Absence of expression of the *FMR-1* gene in fragile X syndrome.' *Cell*, **66**, 817–822.

Primrose, D.A., El-Matmati, R., Boyd, E., Gosden, C., Newton, M. (1986) 'Prevalence of the fragile X syndrome in an institution for the mentally handicapped.' *British Journal of Psychiatry*, **148**, 655–657.

Proops, R., Webb, T. (1981) 'The 'fragile' X chromosome in the Martin–Bell–Renpenning syndrome and in males with other forms of familial mental retardation.' *Journal of Medical Genetics*, **18**, 366–373.

Quan, F., Zonana, J., Gunter, K., Peterson, K.L., Magenis, R.E., Popovich, B.W. (1995) 'An atypical case of fragile X syndrome caused by a deletion that includes the *FMR-1* gene.' *American Journal of Human Genetics*, **56**, 1042–1051.

Rattazzi, M. (1995) 'Protein therapy in fragile X syndrome.' *Developmental Brain Dysfunction. (In press.)*

Reiss, A.L., Freund, L. (1990) 'Fragile X syndrome, DSM-III-R, and autism.' *Journal of the American Academy of Child and Adolescent Psychiatry*, **29**, 885–891.

—— Hagerman, R.J., Vinogradov, S., Abrams, M., King, R.J. (1988) 'Psychiatric disability in female carriers of the fragile X chromosome.' *Archives of General Psychiatry*, **45**, 25–30.

—— Freund, L., Vinogradov, S., Hagerman, R.J., Cronister, A. (1989) 'Parental inheritance and psychological disability in fragile X females.' *American Journal of Human Genetics*, **45**, 697–705.

—— Aylward, E., Freund, L. S., Joshi, P.K., Bryan, R.N. (1991) 'Neuroanatomy of fragile X syndrome: the posterior fossa.' *Annals of Neurology*, **29**, 26–32.

—— Freund, L., Abrams, M.T., Boehm, C., Kazazian, H. (1993) 'Neurobehavioral effects of the fragile X premutation in adult women: a controlled study.' *American Journal of Human Genetics*, **52**, 884–894.

—— Lee, J., Freund, L. (1994) 'Neuroanatomy of fragile X syndrome: the temporal lobe.' *Neurology*, **44**, 1317–1324.

Rourke, B.P. (1987) 'Syndrome of non-verbal learning disabilities. The final common pathway of white-matter disease/dysfunction?' *Clinical Neuropsychologist*, **1**, 209–234.

Rousseau, F., Heitz, D., Biancalana, V., Blumenfeld, S., Kretz, C., Boué, J., Tommerup, N., Van Der Hagen, C., DeLozier-Blanchet, C., *et al.* (1991*a*) 'Direct diagnosis by DNA analysis of the fragile X syndrome of mental retardation.' *New England Journal of Medicine*, **325**, 1673–1681.

—— —— Oberlé, I., Mandel, J-L. (1991*b*) 'Selection in blood cells from female carriers of the fragile X syndrome: inverse correlation between age and proportion of active X chromosomes carrying the full mutation.' *Journal of Medical Genetics*, **28**, 830–836.

—— —— Tarleton, J., MacPherson, J., Malmgren, H., Dahl, N., Barnicoat, A., Mathew, C., Mornet, E., *et al.* (1994) 'A multicenter study on genotype–phenotype correlations in the fragile X syndrome, using direct diagnosis with probe StB12.3: the first 2,253 cases.' *American Journal of Human Genetics*, **55**, 225–237.

Rudelli, R.D., Brown, W.T., Wisniewski, K., Jenkins, E.C., Laure-Kamionowska, M., Connell, F., Wisniewski, H.M. (1985) 'Adult fragile X syndrome. Clinico-neuropathologic findings.' *Acta Neuropathologica*, **67**, 289–295.

Sherman, S.L., Morton, N.E., Jacobs, P.A., Turner, G. (1984) 'The marker (X) syndrome: a cytogenetic and genetic analysis.' *Annals of Human Genetics*, **48**, 21–37.

—— Jacobs, P.A., Morton, N.E., Froster-Iskenius, U., Howard-Peebles, P.N., Nielsen, K.B., Partington, M.W., Sutherland, G.R., Turner, G., Watson, M. (1985) 'Further segregation analysis of the fragile X syndrome with special reference to transmitting males.' *Human Genetics*, **69**, 289–299.

Siomi, H., Choi, M., Siomi, M.C., Nussbaum, R.L., Dreyfuss, G. (1994) 'Essential role for KH domains in RNA binding: impaired RNA binding by a mutation in the KH domain of *FMR1* that causes fragile X syndrome.' *Cell*, **77**, 33–39.

Snow, K., Doud, L., Hagerman, R., Hull, C., Hirst, M.C., Davies, K.E., Thibodeau, S.L. (1992) 'Analysis of mutations at the fragile X locus using the DNA probe Ox1.9.' *American Journal of Medical Genetics*, **43**, 244–254.

Sobesky, W.E., Hull, C.E., Hagerman, R.J. (1992) 'The emotional phenotype in mildly affected carriers.' *In:* Hagerman, R.J., McKenzie, P. (Eds.) *1992 International Fragile X Conference Proceedings.* Denver, CO: Spectra/National Fragile X Foundation, pp. 99–106.

Staley, L.W., Hull, C.E., Mazzocco, M.M.M., Thibodeau, S.N., Snow, K., Wilson, V.L., Taylor, A., McGavran, L., Weiner, D., *et al.* (1993) 'Molecular–clinical correlations in children and adults with fragile X syndrome.' *American Journal of Diseases of Children*, **147**, 723–726.

Sudhalter, V. (1992) 'The language system of males with fragile X syndrome.' *In:* Hagerman, R.J., McKenzie, P. (Eds.) *1992 International Fragile X Conference Proceedings.* Denver, CO: Spectra/National Fragile X Foundation, pp. 107–120.

—— Cohen, I.L., Silverman, W., Wolf-Schein, E.G. (1990) 'Conversational analyses of males with fragile X, Down syndrome and autism: comparison of the emergence of deviant language.' *American Journal on Mental Retardation*, **94**, 431–441.

Sutcliffe, J.S., Nelson, D.L., Zhang, F., Pieretti, M., Caskey, C.T., Saxe, D., Warren, S.T. (1992) 'DNA methylation represses FMR-1 transcription in fragile X syndrome.' *Human Molecular Genetics*, **1**, 397–400.

Sutherland, G.R. (1979) 'Heritable fragile sites on human chromosomes. I. Factors affecting expression in lymphocyte culture.' *American Journal of Human Genetics*, **31**, 125–135.

—— Baker, E. (1992) 'Characterisation of a new rare fragile site easily confused with the fragile X.' *Human Molecular Genetics*, **1**, 111–113.

Tarleton, J., Richie, R., Schwartz, C., Rao, K., Aylsworth, A.S., Lachiewicz, A. (1993) 'An extensive *de novo* deletion removing *FMR1* in a patient with mental retardation and the fragile X syndrome phenotype.' *Human Molecular Genetics*, **2**, 1973–1974.

Taylor, A.K., Safanda, J.F., Fall, M.Z., Quince, C., Lang, K.A., Hull, C.E., Carpenter, I., Staley, L.W., Hagerman, R.J. (1994) 'Molecular predictors of cognitive involvement in female carriers of the fragile X syndrome.' *Journal of the American Medical Association*, **271**, 507–514.

Turner, G. (1983) 'Historical overview of X-linked mental retardation.' *In:* Hagerman, R.J., McBogg, P.M. (Eds.) *The Fragile X Syndrome—Diagnosis, Biochemistry, and Intervention.* Dillon, CO, Spectra, pp. 1–16.

—— Brookwell, R., Daniel, A., Selikowitz, M., Zilibowitz, M. (1980*a*) 'Heterozygous expression of X-linked mental retardation and X chromosome marker fra (X) (q27)'. *New England Journal of Medicine*, **303**, 662–664.

—— Daniel, A., Frost, M. (1980*b*) 'X-linked mental retardation, macro-orchidism, and the Xq27 fragile site.' *Journal of Pediatrics*, **96**, 837–841.

—— Robinson, H., Laing, S., Purvis-Smith, S. (1986) 'Preventive screening for the fragile X syndrome.' *New England Journal of Medicine*, **315**, 607–609.

Varley, C.K., Holm, V.A., Eren, M.O. (1985) 'Cognitive and psychiatric variability in three brothers with fragile X syndrome.' *Journal of Developmental and Behavioral Pediatrics*, **6**, 87–90.

Venter, P.A., Op't Hof, J., Coetzee, D.J., Van der Walt, C., Retief, A.E. (1984) 'No marker (X) syndrome in autistic children.' *Human Genetics*, **67**, 107.

Verkerk, A.J.M., Pieretti, M., Sutcliffe, J.S., Fu, Y-H., Kuhl, D.P.A., Pizzuti, A., Reiner, O., Richards, S., Victoria, M. F., *et al.* (1991) 'Identification of a gene (*FMR-1*) containing a CGG repeat coincident with a breakpoint cluster region exhibiting length variation in fragile X syndrome.' *Cell,* **65**, 905–914.

Wahlström, J., Gillberg, C., Gustavson, K-H., Holmgren, G. (1986) 'Infantile autism and the fragile X. A Swedish multicenter study.' *American Journal of Medical Genetics,* **23**, 403–408.

Warren, S.T., Nelson, D.L. (1994) 'Advances in molecular analysis of fragile X syndrome.' *Journal of the American Medical Association,* **271**, 536–542.

Webb, T., Jacobs, P.A. (1990) 'Fragile Xq27.3 in female heterozygotes for the Martin–Bell syndrome.' *Journal of Medical Genetics,* **27**, 627–631.

Weintraub, S., Mesulam, M-M. (1983) 'Developmental learning disabilities of the right hemisphere. Emotional, interpersonal and cognitive components.' *Archives of Neurology,* **40**, 463–468.

Willems, P.J. (1994) 'Dynamic mutations hit double figures.' *Nature Genetics,* **8**, 213–215.

Wisniewski, K.E., Segan, S.M., Miezejeski, C.M., Sersen, E.A. Rudelli, R.D. (1991) 'The fra (X) syndrome: neurological, electrophysiological, and neuropathological abnormalities.' *American Journal of Medical Genetics,* **38**, 476–480.

Wöhrle, D., Kotzot, D., Hirst, M.C., Manca, A., Korn, B., Schmidt, A., Barbi, G., Rott, H-D., Poustka, A., *et al.* (1992) 'A microdeletion of less than 250 kb, including the proximal part of the *FMR-1* gene and the fragile-X site, in a male with the clincal phenotype of fragile-X syndrome.' *American Journal of Human Genetics,* **51**, 299–306.

Yu, S., Pritchard, M., Kremer, E., Lynch, M., Nancarrow, J., Baker, E., Holman, K., Mulley, J. C., Warren, S. T., *et al.* (1991) 'Fragile X genotype characterized by an unstable region of DNA.' *Science,* **252**, 1179–1181.

—— Mulley, J., Loesch, D., Turner, G., Donnelly, A., Gedeon, A., Hillen, D., Kremer, E., Lynch, M., *et al.* (1992) 'Fragile X syndrome: unique genetics of the heritable unstable element.' *American Journal of Human Genetics,* **50**, 968–980.

6
PATHWAYS FROM GENOTYPE TO PHENOTYPE

Jonathon Flint

Genetic approaches to the analysis of behaviour have had very mixed success up to the present. Although quantitative genetic analysis has now established that variations in intelligence, personality and psychiatric illness have a genetic contribution, progress in delineating more precisely how these traits are genetically determined has not been smooth. With the availability of a large number of DNA polymorphisms, the most promising strategy appeared to be the use of linkage analysis to localize genes determining behavioural traits. Over the last few years linkage methods have indeed been employed to justify claims that possessing a variant of just one gene is enough to confer susceptibility to psychiatric illness. Thus a genetic variant on chromosome 5 was thought to be a major susceptibility locus for schizophrenia (Sherrington *et al.* 1988), and one on chromosome 11 a locus for manic depressive psychosis (Egeland *et al.* 1987). Despite the molecular methodology, none of these claims have been replicated, and some have been withdrawn (Pauls 1993).

This chapter argues that an understanding of the molecular basis of dysmorphic syndromes with well characterized behavioural phenotypes offers an alternative approach: molecular dissection of a behavioural phenotype may be an effective way of following the pathway from genotype to phenotype. I should stress at the outset that there are currently no fully fledged examples from the behavioural phenotype literature to show how this hope can be realized. All I can do at present is demonstrate the potential, and to do so my argument has to draw inferences from work on physiological rather than behavioural traits, and from animal rather than human genetics. I shall start with the main advantage that behavioural phenotype analysis has over conventional analyses of behavioural traits.

If we confine the investigation of behavioural phenotypes to clinical syndromes where there is either a known genetic basis or a strong suspicion of one, then the investigation can be considered analogous to a mutagenesis screen for behavioural variants. In effect, the investigator is asking whether there are any genetic alterations that result in behavioural abnormalities, and if any are found will proceed to characterize the mutations, seeking to determine how the genetic aberration determines the behavioural phenotype. This approach contrasts with the linkage and association studies that have been used to localize susceptibility genes for psychiatric disorders because it does not rely on normal allelic variation. The advantage thus gained is perhaps best explained with an example.

Suppose that we were trying to identify the genetic basis of sleep patterns in humans. We could justifiably collect a sample of families with members showing various degrees of variation in their requirements for sleep, and attempt to find whether some chromosomal regions were shared by people with similar sleep behaviour, indicating the presence of a genetic determinant in that region. However, it could be that ten or more genes were involved in sleep behaviour, but only one of these had allelic variants. Thus, although the analysis might find an association between the genetic variant and variations in sleep, it would not identify any of the other nine genes because they were monomorphic. Furthermore, it could be the case that, for physiological reasons, variation could only occur in the least important parts of the genetic pathway, so the linkage analysis would find only a relatively trivial genetic determinant.

In contrast, an investigator who looks for sleep disturbances in people with genetic abnormalities could uncover a mutation which affects a crucial determinant of sleep behaviour. We can reasonably expect that many more of the genes in the pathway are liable to mutations with relatively extreme effects (with a phenotype regarded as pathological rather than a normal variant) than are liable to have allelic variants with small effects. Indeed this has been the experience of workers looking for genes that determine circadian behaviour in the mouse. Where investigation of natural variants had only suggested the presence of genetic control, a mutagenesis screen provided evidence of a gene on chromosome 5 that was involved in the control of circadian rhythmicity (Vitaterna *et al.* 1994). So molecular dissection of genetically abnormal patients with a behavioural phenotype that includes sleep disorder could lead to the discovery of biochemical pathways involved in sleep that would not be readily detectable by other approaches.

Of course the patients who would be surveyed for sleep abnormalities are not the result of a mutagenesis experiment. Their genetic abnormalities will be much more heterogeneous, and sleep abnormalities are very unlikely to be their sole or even their major problem. This book describes the clinical groups in whom behavioural phenotypes are sought, and in general they are characterized by developmental delay (or mental retardation) and congenital abnormalities. (I shall refer to these conditions as dysmorphic syndromes.) The behavioural abnormalities could be secondary phenomena, possibly learnt as a way of coping with the characteristic physical features of the condition, or occurring in response to treatment regimens. Thus any investigator must have some way of deciding whether the behavioural phenotype is genetically determined. For the purposes of this argument, let us assume that an experiment can be designed to test this hypothesis, and that there are grounds for believing the behaviour to be genetically controlled.

We have now to consider two other assumptions that sustain the hopes of investigation into behavioural phenotypes. The first is that the behavioural abnormalities found in dysmorphic syndrome patients are relevant either to normal behaviour or to other psychiatric disorders. It is sometimes assumed that a psychiatric condition found in association with a dysmorphic syndrome must be of the same nature as that found in the general population. Indeed, the discovery of psychosis segregating with a dysmorphic syndrome due to a rearrangement of chromosome 5 prompted the search for genetic markers on this chromosome linked to schizophrenia (Sherrington *et al.* 1988). Yet psychosis has been found in association with genetic and non-genetic insults (Mirsky and Duncan 1986); indeed it could be argued that the psychosis is a non-specific consequence of injury to a developing brain, whether that injury is biochemical, infectious, traumatic or genetic. So the behavioural phenotype may only be a phenotypic copy of a behaviour, or of a behavioural disorder found in the general population, without also being a genetic copy.

The second assumption is that the pathway from genotype to phenotype is sufficiently close so that knowing the genotype would tell us something useful about how the phenotype arose. Unfortunately, however specific and characteristic a behaviour may be of a dysmorphic syndrome, indeed even where a behaviour is pathognomonic of a syndrome, that is no guarantee that the relationship between the two is direct. Let us suppose that we are interested in the cognitive differences between the sexes, but know nothing about the chromosomal or genetic basis of sex differences (this makes the example analogous to an investigation of a dysmorphic syndrome of unknown aetiology which happens to show a distinctive cognitive profile, similar perhaps to Turner's syndrome). There is a consistent but small difference in the way that males and females perform on sub-tests of adult intelligence tests, and for argument's sake we may consider this difference a behavioural phenotype. However, what we know from the molecular characterization of sex determination suggests that there will be no easy way of correlating genotype and phenotype.

The genetic description of sexual development in mammals is briefly as follows: first, the Y chromosome acts as a dominant male determinant (XY, XXY and XXXY individuals are all male); second, sexual characteristics are regulated by sex hormones produced by the gonads (a female phenotype develops in the absence of hormones produced in males); third, there is a single genetic determinant that distinguishes the sexes, and this is located on the Y chromosome.

During our supposed investigations into the cognitive profile associated with this genetic 'abnormality' we might hope that molecular characterization of the gene would inform us about the behavioural phenotype. The gene was recently cloned and is referred to as *SRY* (Berta *et al.* 1990, Koopman *et al.* 1991); our knowledge of the nature of sexual differentiation should alert us to the fact that this gene is likely to be so high up in a hierarchy of developmental switches that it can give us very few clues as to the origins of behavioural differences. Indeed, the molecular evidence bears this out: the *SRY* protein has the characteristics of a DNA binding protein, indicating that its role is in the regulation of a series of other genes. We will have to trace the action of *SRY* down many pathways before it informs us about the cognitive differences between the sexes.

Thus, even where a complex behavioural phenotype has a relatively simple genetic origin (in this case a single gene on the Y chromosome), and is specifically associated with and characteristic of that genetic variant (either presence or absence of the *SRY* gene product), that is no reason to expect there to be a specific relationship between gene and phenotype.

What then can be said in defence of the view that behavioural phenotypes will tell us something useful about the genetic basis of behaviour, normal as well as abnormal? There is now some evidence that supports the first assumption and I will outline this next; however, defence of the second assumption requires us to review the lessons for human behavioural genetics that accrue from the study of behaviour in other species, a review that concludes this chapter.

Are behavioural phenotypes merely phenocopies?

The genetic contribution to most behaviour and most behavioural disorders is very likely to be polygenic. Until recently this was assumed to mean that the action of a large number of genes, each with small effect, gave rise to the genetically determined component of the phenotypic variance. In other words, there were no major genes, no loci of particular importance. A number of discoveries have served to blur the distinction between polygenic and single gene disorders. On the one hand there have been the first reports of how many loci actually make up a polygenic trait, and how much each locus contributes to the phenotype. An essentially complete genome analysis of a diabetic mouse (Ghosh *et al.* 1993, Risch *et al.* 1993) shows that 23 susceptibility loci account for virtually all the genetic variation. These loci however are not of equal effect; some have more than twice the effect of others. Moreover, more than half of the genetic variation is due to interactive effects; this means that it is not so much the number of susceptibility loci present that determines the phenotype as the combination of loci. Work on rat models of hypertension show a similar picture. Again, a relatively small number of loci contribute to most of the genetic variants (indeed almost a quarter of systolic blood pressure readings after sodium chloride loading could be explained by a single locus on chromosome 10), and interactive effects are important (Hilbert *et al.* 1991).

On the other hand we have a series of reports of the complex effects exerted by single gene abnormalities. These show that complex phenotypes thought to have a polygenic basis can have a relatively simple genetic origin. Thus Hirschsprung's disease, characterized by congenital megacolon with absence of intramural intestinal ganglion cells, was long considered to be an example of sex modified polygenic inheritance. It is now known to arise, at least in some cases, from a mutation in the *RET* oncogene (Romeo *et al.* 1994), or a mutation in the endothelin-B receptor gene (Puffenberger *et al.* 1994).

Could the same observations be true for behaviour? If so, then it is likely that genetic analysis of behavioural phenotypes will be of value for an understanding of normal behaviour and psychiatric disorders. Let us consider each point in turn.

The genetic architecture of behaviour

Analysis of a polygenically determined trait in humans requires a large number of highly polymorphic markers, and a system that can use them to genotype hundreds of individuals within a reasonably short period of time. It is only within the last year that these requirements have been met and a full genome search has been completed in a search for the genetic basis of diabetes (Davies *et al.* 1994). No similar study has been reported for a behavioural trait in humans.

For technical reasons a genome search is easier in animals. There are difficulties with extrapolating the results of animal experiments to humans, but while we can argue about the relevance of a particular animal model to human behaviour, the genetic architecture is likely to be similar. Just as the way genes determine diabetes and hypertension in rodents is a good guide to how genes determine these physiological traits in humans, so too the genetic basis of behaviour in animals is likely to tell us about the genetic basis of behaviour in humans.

To date there is only one study that has completely mapped an animal genome for genes determining behaviour, and that is an analysis of morphine preference in inbred mouse strains (Berrettini *et al.* 1994). Nearly 85 per cent of the genetic variance could be explained by allelic variation at just three loci. This picture of major loci contributing substantially to the genetic variance is in agreement with analyses of polygenically determined physiological traits. However, the latter work would predict that a large number of genes will account for the remaining genetic variance; indeed, work on alcohol preference in mice has implicated over 100 loci affecting drug responses in mice (Crabbe *et al.* 1994, Phillips *et al.* 1994). Nevertheless, the presence of a few major genetic determinants of behaviour is likely.

'Polygenically determined' behaviour arising from mutation in a single gene

This paradoxical heading indicates that a single gene abnormality can give rise to a complex phenotype which appears to be indistinguishable from the type of behavioural abnormalities commonly seen in psychiatric clinics. The best example of this is undoubtedly the behavioural phenotype associated with a deficiency of the mono-aminoxidase A (*MAOA*) gene (Brunner *et al.* 1993*a,b*).

A few years ago in a hospital in Holland a woman sought advice about a behavioural abnormality that turned up again and again in her family. One of her relatives had attempted to rape his sister, another had tried to run over his employer when told that his work was not good enough, and two more were arsonists. This woman's case might have received no more than the usual admonition that such problems do tend to run in families were it not for the fact that the clinician noticed an intriguing genetic feature about this Dutch kindred. All members who exhibited violent behaviour were male and were either mildly mentally retarded or had borderline intelligence. In contrast, no-one else in the family showed signs of cognitive impairment or psychiatric disorders. The consistent association between abnormal behaviour, mild mental retardation and being male, raised the suspicion that there might be an X-linked gene determining the phenotype. The value of molecular genetics is that it allows such suspicion to be put to the test by looking for the co-segregation of polymorphisms on the X chromosome with the condition.

The geneticists involved with the family discovered that the region of DNA containing the *MAOA* gene was linked to the disorder. That is to say, in this kindred affected individuals have inherited the same length of DNA around Xp11.4–11.3, while unaffected individuals have not. Of course this might be a chance association, and it is possible to work out how often chance could produce such a result (the probability is about 1 in 25). The fact that the *MAOA* gene was in the region of DNA did not necessarily indicate an abnormality of mono-amine metabolism as the cause for the condition. Many other genes genetically linked to the *MAOA* gene (and therefore in the same stretch of DNA common to all affected members) might be responsible. But here researchers had a stroke of luck. They measured the concentration of *MAOA* in the urine and found it to be elevated. Again this did not conclusively demonstrate an *MAOA* abnormality but it made it worthwhile trying to find one.

One way to do this is to see if there is anything wrong with the DNA that codes for the *MAOA* enzyme. If the normal DNA sequence is known, as it was in this case, the experiment is relatively straightforward. It turned out that all affected individuals had a mutation in the *MAOA* gene that introduced a termination codon into the messenger RNA. The mutation therefore resulted in a truncated and non-functional enzyme, as could be confirmed by assaying *MAOA* activity in cultured fibroblasts (Brunner *et al.* 1993a).

It is important to be clear that this result still does not unequivocally implicate *MAOA* deficiency in the pathogenesis of the behavioural disorder, as the finding is still an association, though a very striking one, which could have arisen by chance. We do not know whether every case of *MAOA* deficiency occurs with mental retardation and aggressive behaviour, and we do not know if other genes linked to *MAOA* are abnormal in this family and are responsible for the phenotype. However, on balance it is likely that the *MAOA* deficiency has a role to play in the aetiology of the abnormal behaviour.

The behavioural abnormality has not been characterized in detail but there is as yet no evidence to suggest that it is qualitatively different from other cases of aggressive behaviour. It appears, on the face of it at least, that an increased tendency to extremely antisocial behaviour arises from a defect in *MAOA*.

This finding has excited a lot of interest because it suggests a direct route to understanding the biological basis of aggression. Researchers interested in the genetic basis of complex physical phenotypes with a supposed polygenic basis, such as the pathological elevation of blood pressure, have become interested in so-called 'intermediate phenotypes', which are traits directly related to single genes that determine the overall phenotype (for example blood pressure). The *MAOA* deficiency is a good example of such an intermediate phenotype. We might expect, for instance, to find in a quantitative genetic analysis of aggression that a locus including the *MAOA* gene contributes substantially to the genetic variance of aggressive behaviour. Characterization of other behavioural phenotypes associated with single gene disorders may help in the quantitative analysis of psychiatric disorders.

In summary, there is evidence that variation in normal and pathological behaviour is determined by relatively few genes. Furthermore, we find that mutations in a single gene can affect behaviour which is considered to have a polygenic basis. These findings imply that behavioural phenotypes occurring in dysmorphic syndromes could indeed be more than mere phenocopies of behavioural traits found in the general population, though only investigation will demonstrate how true this is in each case. What has next to be established is whether knowing the genetic basis will tell us anything about the pathway from gene to behaviour.

The relationship between genotype and phenotype

I now turn to the second assumption discussed above: that the relationship between gene and behaviour will be direct enough so that knowing molecular dissection can tell us something about the path from genotype to phenotype. Our understanding of the relationship between genotypes and phenotypes has accumulated from the study of many single gene disorders, and it is worth briefly reviewing this work. Perhaps the most relevant discovery is that the correlation between genotype and phenotype becomes less predictable as a path between the two becomes longer.

A good example comes from the study of sickle cell disease, which is due to a mutation in the gene that codes for haemoglobin. We know with almost absolute certainty that a homozygote with a DNA mutation in the sixth codon of the β-globin component of the haemoglobin molecule will have no normal adult β-globin protein. But we know with far less certainty how much of the haemoglobin present will be functional. There may be a mutation present that increases the amount of fetal haemoglobin, thus providing a protein that can substitute for some of the functions of the damaged β-globin chain. Further along the pathway we find that the β-globin gene mutation does not predict the occurrence and severity of various clinical phenomena, which are determined by the genetic and environmental determinants of numerous other physiological processes, each of which has its own complex genotype–phenotype interaction (Noguchi et al.1993, Serjeant 1993).

A second relevant discovery is that mutations in the same gene can produce a remarkable variety of phenotypes or, more technically, phenotypic diversity is the result of an allelic series (Suthers and Davies 1992, Romeo and McKusick 1994). This has been suspected for over 20 years, but definitive evidence has only emerged with the ability to sequence the DNA of different alleles at a locus. Thus it has now emerged that different forms of craniosynostosis (conditions involving premature fusion of skull sutures) result from mutations in the same gene (Jabs *et al.* 1994). Perhaps the most remarkable example is that different mutations in one gene (the *RET* oncogene) give rise to different forms of cancer (multiple endocrine neoplasia 2A or 2B, medullary thyroid carcinoma) and to Hirschsprung's disease (Edery *et al.* 1994, Hofstra *et al.* 1994, Romeo *et al.* 1994).

In the context of behavioural phenotypes these two points are very discouraging. *A priori*, it is unlikely that any behavioural trait is as closely related to a genotype as sickle cell disease is to mutations in the β-globin gene, so the degree to which modifying genetic loci, let alone other influences, determine the phenotype will be very marked, and almost certainly explain the variety within behavioural phenotypes described elsewhere in this volume. Furthermore, if different mutations in the same gene can give rise to such different phenotypes as Hirschsprung's disease and thyroid carcinoma, can we possibly expect the pathways from gene to behaviour to be any less surprising and unpredictable?

These considerations should alert us to the fact that genetic analysis will only be a very preliminary step in biological investigations of behaviour. The route may well be very arduous, but is it likely to be too arduous? Unfortunately there is no way to know except by trying, and here we have very little evidence to help us choose the right path. Indeed, available evidence is not encouraging: the molecular basis of Lesch–Nyhan syndrome has been known for many years, without this materially advancing knowledge of why sufferers harm themselves.

An even more apposite example is fragile X syndrome. The behavioural phenotype of this condition is one of the better characterized (see chapter 5), and the surprisingly complicated genetics of the disorder are now yielding to molecular analysis. Thus we have a good example as to how a gene may be related to a behavioural phenotype. In brief, we find that molecular analysis reveals a lot about the molecular processes that go on and little about anything else.

Inactivation of the gene *FMR-1* produces the syndrome, which occurs most frequently because of amplification of a trinucleotide repeat in the 5′ untranslated region of the gene (Verkerk *et al.* 1991) but also by a deletion or nucleotide mutation (Gedeon *et al.* 1992, De Boulle *et al.* 1993). There has been a lot of interest in trinucleotide repeats, aggravated by the discovery that repeat expansion at other loci was associated with other motor and mental disorders (Willems 1994), including Huntington's disease. The novelty of the finding and the suggestion that triplicate repeat expansion characterizes neuropsychiatric disorders has inspired some researchers to look at correlations between behavioural disorders in fragile X and the number of repeats, presumably in the belief that a direct link between genotype and phenotype might exist. Moreover, other researchers have tried to look in other psychiatric conditions for features of the genetics of fragile X which might indicate the action of trinucleotide repeat expansion.

It is now fairly well established that if such a correlation exists then it plays a relatively small part in determining the phenotype of the fragile X syndrome. We know a good deal about the behaviour of the repeat size; we know how repeat size expansion accounts for departures from mendelian inheritance, that repeat expansion can be pre-zygotic and post-zygotic (monozygotic twins show similar repeat lengths in Huntington's disease but not in fragile X syndrome), and that this difference is reflected in the contrast between somatic instability of repeats in fragile X and myotonic dystrophy but in somatic stability in Huntington's disease (Reyniers *et al.* 1993, Kruyer *et al.* 1994, Telenius *et al.* 1994). However, intriguing as these findings are, they do not tell us much about the relationship between genotype and phenotype in the fragile X syndrome. It is clear that further progress requires an understanding of what the *FMR-1* gene does.

The gene almost certainly has a non-specific effect on behaviour, probably by controlling some fundamental processes of cell biology. All the available evidence suggests that the gene encodes a protein with such a function. First, the gene is conserved across species (Verkerk *et al.* 1991). Second, the gene is widely expressed, although at very low levels in some tissues (Verkerk *et al.* 1991, Devys *et al.* 1993, Hinds *et al.* 1993). It is most abundant in neurons in both peripheral and central nervous systems (Devys *et al.* 1993), and there is no evidence for anatomical localization to explain the behavioural phenotype. Third, the gene produces a protein that binds RNA *in vitro* and may well do so *in vivo* (Siomi *et al.* 1993, 1994). If so, the gene probably acts by regulating expression of other genes, in other words it acts indirectly.

The fragile X story has not revealed more about gene behaviour relationships than the cloning of the *SRY* gene has done in exposing the biological basis of cognitive differences between the sexes. The only difference is that while nobody expected the *SRY* discovery to do anything of the kind, there had been hopes that the fragile X gene would tell us something about the origins of the behavioural phenotype.

Animal models for investigating behaviour

The fragile X example is only one of many syndromes with a behavioural phenotype, and need not be typical. In the absence of molecular information about other syndromes, is there evidence from other sources that points to the likely ways that genetic abnormalities determine behaviour? For this, I now turn to experiments on animal behaviour.

From a genetic point of view there is only 1.6 per cent difference between chimpanzees and humans, that is to say 98.4 per cent of our DNA sequence is the same as that of the chimpanzee. The possibility that the 1.6 per cent sequence divergence might represent those genes responsible for the behavioural differences between the species is extremely unlikely. Indeed, it is the extent of sequence similarity between species that must be stressed: this similarity is both a handicap to the behavioural geneticist, because it implies a long and complex path between genotype and phenotype, and also the strength of the geneticist's approach to characterizing properties of genes, because it allows their manipulation in different species.

To those whose working lives are spent in molecular biology laboratories, the idea of similarity between diverse cellular processes and also between the same process in different species is now so familiar they take it for granted. But it is not so obvious to those whose interests are less molecular, particularly if they have a knowledge of neuropharmacology and neurophysiology. Given the diverse behavioural reactions to the same compound exhibited by different species, it might seem impossible that the same genetic mechanisms could be operating in the two. Yet, geneticists have shown again and again that what works in a yeast cell often works well in a human cell. However, while it may be expected that general principles of organization are maintained through evolution, it is not so clear that the same should apply to features unique to man, which are primarily behavioural.

We can address this problem in two ways. First, we can look at animal models of human genetic disease with a behavioural phenotype and ask if the DNA homology can become a behavioural homology. Currently there are only two examples, mouse models of Lesch–Nyhan syndrome (Hooper *et al.* 1987, Kuehn *et al.* 1987) and of fragile X syndrome (Dutch–Belgian Fragile X Consortium 1994). These cases do give qualified support to the view that animal models are relevant, and, in the case of Lesch–Nyhan syndrome, they show how a combination of molecular and biochemical techniques can make progress along the path from gene to behaviour. The example of Lesch-Nyhan syndrome is given below.

Second, animal experiments are possible that can give general answers about the specificity of the relationship between behavioural traits and DNA rearrangements; the evidence here is that the link can be much more direct than many people expected.

A mouse model of Lesch–Nyhan syndrome

Lesch–Nyhan syndrome arises from a lack, or very low levels, of hypoxanthine phosphoribosyltransferase (HPRT). HPRT is involved in pathways that re-synthesize the components of nucleic acids from their breakdown products. Details of this become important later so I will outline them now. Polymers of purine and pyrimidine bases constitute nucleic acids. Free purines can be degraded to urate for excretion or phosphorylated ready for further use in the assembly of nucleic acids or in one of many second messenger or energy transfer systems. There are three purine bases involved (adenine, guanine and hypoxanthine), and the enzymes that salvage them are different: adenine phosphoribosyltransferase (APRT) works on adenine, while HPRT works on hypoxanthine and guanine.

Following the discovery of the metabolic basis of Lesch–Nyhan syndrome there were numerous investigations into the purine pathway of the nervous system. It emerged that basal ganglia cells produce HPRT with high specific activity, and *de novo* synthesis of purines is low, making these cells peculiarly dependent on the salvage pathway. Dopamine levels in the basal ganglia were less than 30 per cent of normal in Lesch–Nyhan patients (Lloyd *et al.* 1981), so it was suggested that there may be a connection between purine concentrations and the establishment of dopaminergic transmission during the morphogenesis of the basal ganglia.

The creation of the mouse model of Lesch–Nyhan syndrome promised to advance the study of the pathogenesis of this condition substantially. By introducing cells deficient in HPRT into a mouse embryo, and then breeding from the resulting chimera, research has produced the first genetically manipulated model of human disease. But the HPRT-deficient mice showed no abnormal neurological function, and no inclination to self-mutilate. Indeed, when first examined, there appeared to be nothing wrong with these mice (Hooper *et al.* 1987, Kuehn *et al.* 1987).

One possible explanation for the discrepancy between mouse and human responses to HPRT deficiency could lie in a different regulation of the nucleotide pool. The relative activities of the two salvage enzymes HPRT and APRT are different in mice and humans, so could this indicate that APRT took on a larger share of the work processing purines in mice than it did in humans? We now know that it does. Wu and Melton (1993) developed a pharmacological method for specifically inactivating APRT in mice, and discovered that APRT inhibitors produced self-mutilation in HPRT-deficient mice. The failure of the HPRT-deficient mice to display the behavioural phenotype turns out to be due to the ability of APRT to take over most (if not all) of the function of HPRT.

This result tells us that purine metabolism is very likely to be directly related to self-injurious behaviour (and probably to stereotypic behaviour). The effect of HPRT deficiency could have been mediated by its action on a developmental process (for instance, lack of the enzyme in the fetus could alter brain development and architecture, which would in turn predispose the organism to stereotypic behaviour in adulthood), but this explanation, although not excluded, is made much less plausible by the new work on the HPRT-deficient mouse. Thus the animal model has begun to delineate the biochemical pathways underlying self-injurious behaviour.

The construction of behavioural phenotypes in animals

HPRT and the fragile X gene are only two of many whose function has been investigated by the process of transgenesis. The basis of this technique is the propensity of cells to accept DNA that is injected into their cytoplasm and incorporate it into their own chromosomes. This can happen in a random fashion (the foreign DNA is included anywhere and in many copies), or it can be more specifically targeted to a single gene. In the latter case a mutant copy of the gene can replace the functional gene (the replacement occurs by means of homologous recombination), and if this occurs in embryonic stem cells then a complete animal can be grown that carries the genetically altered material. The final result is the creation of an animal that is either heterozygous, or homozygous for the mutant. Thus an experimenter can delete any gene of interest and see what effect that has on the animal.

The relevance to behavioural phenotypes is that this technique creates animals with behavioural phenotypes, but, in contrast to the situation in humans, the genetic lesion is known. Furthermore, when something is also known about the physiological and biochemical nature of the phenotype, then we can use the genetic analysis to work out how genes affect the trait. An experiment along these lines can determine whether behavioural phenotypes are always at a great remove from the underlying genetic abnormality. The example I give below is taken as representative of a growing number of investigations in this field, most of which fortunately demonstrate that the pathway from phenotype to genotype is not always impossibly tortuous.

One way to study a complex phenomenon is to break it down into increasingly simple components which are more amenable to experimental manipulation. In this way memory functions can be dissected, and, at the simplest level, they can be regarded as alterations in synaptic signalling. In one such simple system, analysis of mollusc synaptic modulation indicates that after serotonin has activated adenylyl cyclase, thus generating an increase in the second messenger cAMP, the amount of neurotransmitter released from a neuron following an action potential is increased. Experimentally induced alterations in cAMP levels confirm that concentrations of this molecule are critical for alterations in synaptic transmission. Furthermore, two types of alteration can be produced: in the first, a single stimulus leads to an enhanced response for a brief period of time (considered to be the equivalent of short-term memory); in the second, a series of stimuli produces a similar effect, but for a prolonged time (the equivalent of long-term memory). The latter alteration involves the synthesis of new proteins, and is induced by a cAMP-responsive element-binding protein (*CREB*).

There is a parallel to these findings in the mammalian brain. In the hippocampus there is a well known electrophysiological phenomenon called long-term potentiation (LTP), in which the strength of excitatory synaptic connections can be enhanced for prolonged periods after a short burst of high frequency synaptic activity (Bliss and Collingridge 1993). However, what this phenomenon has to do with memory, if anything, was not clear before the advent of molecular dissection by transgenesis. Until then, the main support for the role of LTP in memory was the effect of pharmacological agents that blocked hippocampal glutamate receptors of the *N*-methyl-D-aspartate class:

these compounds prevented the induction of LTP and impaired spatial learning in rodents. However, there were many possible explanations for this association, not all of which required LTP to be involved in memory. The new molecular approach made it possible to inactivate genes that were believed to determine LTP.

In the first series of experiments, phosphorylating enzymes (kinases) that were thought to control LTP were disrupted. This was achieved by replacing in a mouse the functional gene for the enzyme with a mutated, non-functional copy. Mice without a calmodulin kinase or a *fyn* tyrosine kinase produced in this way were then tested for memory defects (Grant *et al.* 1992; Silva *et al.* 1992a,b). In both cases LTP was reduced; furthermore, there was impaired spatial learning, indicating that selective inactivation of a gene could produce a specific alteration in behaviour. In the second set of experiments, the role of cAMP was directly investigated by disrupting the *CREB* gene (Bourtchuladze *et al.* 1994). Again mice were constructed which lacked the gene, and tested for LTP and learning impairment. Remarkably, it was found that loss of *CREB* function disrupted long-term memory for conditioning, without affecting initial memory. *CREB*-deficient and control mice were exposed to a conditioned stimulus (a tone) followed by an un-conditioned stimulus (foot shock). Thirty minutes and one hour after training, both control and mutant mice showed a fear response when exposed to the conditioned stimulus; two hours after training only the control mice exhibited this behaviour. The fact that initial memory was unchanged makes it very difficult to explain these results as the effect of motor, sensory, motivational or attentional abnormalities.

The transgenic mice can be compared to humans with dysmorphic syndromes and behavioural phenotypes. In a sense, the mice have been designed to have a behavioural phenotype, and the success of the strategy is encouraging for the analysis of human behavioural phenotypes. It shows that a phenomenon as complex as memory can be investigated by analysis of genetic mutations. Moreover, it is not only memory that is determined in this way.

Low concentrations of serotonin have been associated with impulsive violence in humans, without clear evidence for a causal link. Activation of one serotonin receptor (5-HT$_{1B}$) has been seen to lead to a decrease in aggressive behaviour, but without specific antagonists it has not been possible to investigate the association further. Gene disruption again provides an alternative method of analysis, and in an experiment akin to those described above, mice were constructed that lack the 5-HT$_{1B}$ receptor (Saudou *et al.* 1994). After a month of isolation and in the presence of an intruder, the mutant mice were found to be more aggressive than controls: mutants attacked intruders faster and more frequently.

These experiments demonstrate that molecular dissection of behaviour is possible, and that the effect of a mutation on a behaviour is not so removed that it is meaningless. The hope is that behavioural phenotypes in human dysmorphic syndromes will be similar to those observed in these mouse mutants, and indeed the parallels with the *MAOA* gene mutation in humans is striking. Whether other cases will live up to this promise is not clear. However, these experiments must not give the view that the relationship between gene and behaviour is turning out to be simple. It may be more direct than expected, but it is certainly complex.

The *CREB* gene is part of a signalling pathway used by many different cell types widely distributed throughout the body; similarly, expression of the genes for calmodulin kinase and the 5-HT$_{1B}$ receptor is not restricted to the central nervous system. Why therefore should disruption of genes involved in many different pathways have such specific effects? The answer is probably that specificity arises from interaction of numerous different components, each of which has a certain degree of redundancy. Thus there are known to be a number of isoforms of *CREB*, which may be able to substitute for the mutated *CREB* in some tissues, but not all. There is therefore a degree of redundancy in the actions of these genes. Redundancy has been noted in other behavioural mutants, for example in work on the genetic basis of the capacity of *Drosophila* to distinguish between an odour that has been paired with an electric shock and one that has not (Davis and Dauwalder 1991, Hoffmann 1991, Levin *et al.* 1992).

It should also be noted that other behavioural abnormalities have turned up in the engineered mutant mice. Calmodulin kinase deficient mice show abnormal fear responses and aggressive behaviour (Chen *et al.* 1994), and *fyn* kinase deficient mice have been found to have impaired suckling behaviour (Yagi *et al.* 1993). There is a parallel here again with human behavioural phenotypes: we find a number of specific behavioural abnormalities in a genetic mutant that cannot be easily related by known mechanisms. The examples of the mutant mice described here indicate that those specific abnormalities can be the result of mutations in a single gene.

The animal work is very encouraging for behavioural phenotype studies. It confirms that behaviour can be the result of mutations in a single gene; it shows that molecular dissection is a useful tool for analysing the biology of behaviour; and it demonstrates that the path from genotype to phenotype need not be so long that starting at a genetic level is just too far from the phenotype (though as we have seen this may be true in some disorders). The next challenge is to show that the results culled from work on insects, molluscs and mice are true for humans as well. The study of behavioural phenotypes has a good chance of helping in this endeavour.

REFERENCES

Berrettini, W.H., Ferraro, T.N., Alexander, R.C., Buchberg, A.M., Vogel, W.H. (1994) 'Quantitative trait loci mapping of three loci controlling morphine preference using inbred mouse strains.' *Nature Genetics*, **7**, 54–58.

Berta, P., Hawkins, J.R., Sinclair, A.H., Taylor, A., Griffiths, B.L., Goodfellow, P.N., Fellous, M. (1990) 'Genetic evidence equating *SRY* and the testis-determining factor.' *Nature*, **348**, 448–450.

Bliss, T.V.P., Collingridge, G.L. (1993) 'A synaptic model of memory: long-term potentiation in the hippocampus.' *Nature*, **361**, 31–39.

Bourtchuladze, R., Frenguelli, B., Blendy, J., Cioffi, D., Schutz, G., Silva, A.J. (1994) 'Deficient long-term memory in mice with a targeted mutation of the cAMP-responsive element-binding protein.' *Cell*, **79**, 59–68.

Brunner, H.G., Nelen, M., Breakefield, X.O., Ropers, H.H., van Oost, B.A. (1993*a*) 'Abnormal behavior associated with a point mutation in the structural gene for monoamine oxidase A.' *Science*, **262**, 578–580.

——— —— van Zandvoort, P., Abeling, N.G.G.M., van Gennip, A.H., Wolters, E.C., Kuiper, M.A., Ropers, H.H., van Oost, B.A. (1993*b*) 'X-linked borderline mental retardation with prominent behavioral disturbance: phenotype, genetic localization, and evidence for disturbed monoamine metabolism.' *American Journal of Human Genetics*, **52**, 1032–1039.

Chen, C., Rainnie, D.G., Greene, R.W., Tonegawa, S. (1994) 'Abnormal fear response and aggressive behavior in mutant mice deficient for α-calcium-calmodulin kinase II.' *Science*, **266**, 291–294.

Crabbe, J.C., Belknap, J.K., Buck, K.J. (1994) 'Genetic animal models of alcohol and drug abuse.' *Science*, **264**, 1715–1723.

Davies, J.L., Kawaguchi, Y., Bennett, S.T., Copeman, J.B., Cordell, H.J., Pritchard, L.E., Reed, P.W., Gough, S.C.L., Jenkins, S.C., et al. (1994) 'A genome-wide search for human type 1 diabetes susceptibility genes.' *Nature*, **371**, 130–136.

Davis, R.L., Dauwalder, B. (1991) 'The *Drosophila dunce* locus: learning and memory genes in the fly.' *Trends in Genetics*, **7**, 224–229.

De Boulle, K., Verkerk, A.J.M.H., Reyniers, E., Vits, L., Hendrickx, J., Van Roy, B., Van Den Bos, F., de Graaff, E., Oostra, B.A., Willems, P.J. (1993) 'A point mutation in the *FMR-1* gene associated with fragile X mental retardation.' *Nature Genetics*, **3**, 31–35.

Devys, D., Lutz, Y., Rouyer, N., Bellocq, J-P., Mandel, J-L. (1993) 'The FMR-1 protein is cytoplasmic, most abundant in neurons and appears normal in carriers of fragile X premutation.' *Nature Genetics*, **4**, 335–340.

Dutch–Belgian Fragile X Consortium (1994) '*Fmr1* knockout mice: a model to study fragile X mental retardation.' *Cell*, **78**, 23–33.

Edery, P., Lyonnet, S., Mulligan, L.M., Pelet, A., Dow, E., Abel, L., Holder, S., Nihoul-Fékété, C., Ponder, B.A.J., Munnich, A. (1994) 'Mutations of the *RET* proto-oncogene in Hirschsprung's disease.' *Nature*, **367**, 378–380.

Egeland, J.A., Gerhard, D.S., Pauls, D.L., Sussex, J.N., Kidd, K.K., Allen, C.R., Hostetter, A.M., Housman, D.E. (1987) 'Bipolar affective disorders linked to DNA markers on chromosome 11.' *Nature*, **325**, 783–787.

Gedeon, A.K., Baker, E., Robinson, H., Partington, M.W., Gross, B., Manca, A., Korn, B., Poustka, A., Yu, S., et al. (1992) 'Fragile X syndrome without CCG amplification has an *FMR1* deletion.' *Nature Genetics*, **1**, 341–344.

Ghosh, S., Palmer, S.M., Rodrigues, N.R., Cordell, H.J., Hearne, C.M., Cornall, R.J., Prins, J.-B., McShane, P., Lathrop, G.M., et al. (1993) 'Polygenic control of autoimmune diabetes in nonobese diabetic mice.' *Nature Genetics*, **4**, 404–409.

Grant, S.G.N., O'Dell, T.J., Karl, K.A., Stein, P.L., Soriano, P., Kandel, E.R. (1992) 'Impaired long-term potentiation, spatial learning, and hippocampal development in *fyn* mutant mice.' *Science*, **258**, 1903–1910.

Hilbert, P., Lindpaintner, K., Beckmann, J.S., Serikawa, T., Soubrier, F., Dubay, C., Cartwright, P., De Gouyon, B., Julier, C., et al. (1991) 'Chromosomal mapping of two genetic loci associated with blood-pressure regulation in hereditary hypertensive rats.' *Nature*, **353**, 521–529.

Hinds, H.L., Ashley, C.T., Sutcliffe, J.S., Nelson, D.L., Warren, S.T., Housman, D.E., Schalling, M. (1993) 'Tissue specific expression of *FMR-1* provides evidence for a functional role in fragile X syndrome.' *Nature Genetics*, **3**, 36–43.

Hoffmann, F.M. (1991) '*Drosophila abl* and genetic redundancy in signal transduction.' *Trends in Genetics*, **7**, 351–355.

Hofstra, R.M.W., Landsvater, R.M., Ceccherini, I., Stulp, R.P., Stelwagen, T., Luo, Y., Pasini, B., Höppener, J.W.M., Ploos van Amstel, H.K., et al. (1994) 'A mutation in the *RET* proto-oncogene associated with multiple endocrine neoplasia type 2B and sporadic medullary thyroid carcinoma.' *Nature*, **367**, 375–376.

Hooper, M., Hardy, K., Handyside, A., Hunter, S., Monk, M. (1987) 'HPRT-deficient (Lesch–Nyhan) mouse embryos derived from germline colonization by cultured cells.' *Nature*, **326**, 292–295.

Jabs, W.E., Li, X., Scott, A.F., Meyers, G., Chen, W., Eccles, M., Mao, J-i., Charnas, L.R., Jackson, C.E., Jaye, M. (1994) 'Jackson–Weiss and Crouzon syndromes are allelic with mutations in fibroblast growth factor receptor 2.' *Nature Genetics*, **8**, 275–279.

Koopman, P., Gubbay, J., Vivian, N., Goodfellow, P., Lovell-Badge, R. (1991) 'Male development of chromosomally female mice transgenic for *Sry*.' *Nature*, **351**, 117–121.

Kruyer, H., Milà, M., Glover, G., Carbonell, P., Ballesta, F., Estivill, X. (1994) 'Fragile X syndrome and the (CGG)ₙ mutation: two families with discordant MZ twins.' *American Journal of Human Genetics*, **54**, 437–442.

Kuehn, M.R., Bradley, A., Robertson, E.J., Evans, M.J. (1987) 'A potential animal model for Lesch–Nyhan syndrome through introduction of HPRT mutations into mice.' *Nature*, **326**, 295–298.

Levin, L.R., Han, P.-L., Hwang, P.M., Feinstein, P.G., Davis, R.L., Reed, R.R. (1992) 'The Drosophila learning and memory gene *rutabaga* encodes a Ca^{2+}/calmodulin-responsive adenylyl cyclase.' *Cell*, **68**, 479–489.

Lloyd, K.G., Hornykiewicz, O., Davidson, L., Shannak, K., Farley, I., Goldstein, M., Shibuya, M., Kelley, W.N., Fox, I.H. (1981) 'Biochemical evidence of dysfunction of brain neurotransmitters in the Lesch–Nyhan syndrome.' *New England Journal of Medicine*, **305**, 1106–1111.

Mirsky, A.F., Duncan, C.C. (1986) 'Etiology and expression of schizophrenia: neurobiological and psychosocial factors.' *Annual Review of Psychology*, **37**, 291–319.

Noguchi, C.T., Schechter, A.N., Rodgers, G.P. (1993) 'Sickle cell disease pathophysiology.' *Baillière's Clinical Haematology*, **6**, 57–91.

Pauls, D.L. (1993) 'Behavioural disorders: lessons in linkage.' *Nature Genetics*, **3**, 4–5.

Phillips, T.J., Crabbe, J.C., Metten, P., Belknap, J.K. (1994) 'Localization of genes affecting alcohol drinking in mice.' *Alcoholism: Clinical and Experimental Research*, **18**, 931–941.

Puffenberger, E.G., Hosoda, K., Washington, S.S., Nakao, K., deWit, D., Yanagisawa, M., Chakravarti, A. (1994) 'A missense mutation of the endothelin-B receptor gene in multigenic Hirschsprung's disease.' *Cell*, **79**, 1257–1266.

Reyniers, E., Vits, L., De Boulle, K., Van Roy, B., Van Velzen, D., de Graaff, E., Verkerk, A.J.M.H., Jorens, H.Z.J., Darby, J.K., *et al.* (1993) 'The full mutation in the FMR-1 gene of male fragile X patients is absent in their sperm.' *Nature Genetics*, **4**, 143–146.

Risch, N., Ghosh, S., Todd, J.A. (1993) 'Statistical evaluation of multiple-locus linkage data in experimental species and its relevance to human studies: application to nonobese diabetic (NOD) mouse and human insulin-dependent diabetes mellitus (IDDM).' *American Journal of Human Genetics*, **53**, 702–714.

Romeo, G., McKusick, V.A. (1994) 'Phenotypic diversity, allelic series and modifier genes.' *Nature Genetics*, **7**, 451–453.

—— Ronchetto, P., Luo, Y., Barone, V., Seri, M., Ceccherini, I., Pasini, B., Bocciardi, R., Lerone, M., *et al.* (1994) 'Point mutations affecting the tyrosine kinase domain of the *RET* proto-oncogene in Hirschsprung's disease.' *Nature*, **367**, 377–378.

Saudou, F., Amara, D.A., Dierich, A., LeMeur, M., Ramboz, S., Segu, L., Buhot, M-C., Hen, R. (1994) 'Enhanced aggressive behavior in mice lacking 5-HT$_{1B}$ receptor.' *Science*, **265**, 1875–1878.

Serjeant, G.R. (1993) 'The clinical features of sickle cell disease.' *Baillière's Clinical Haematology*, **6**, 93–115.

Sherrington, R., Brynjolfsson, J., Petursson, H., Potter, M., Dudleston, K., Barraclough, B., Wasmuth, J., Dobbs, M., Gurling, H. (1988) 'Localization of a susceptibility locus for schizophrenia on chromosome 5.' *Nature*, **336**, 164–167.

Silva, A.J., Paylor, R., Wehner, J.M., Tonegawa, S. (1992*a*) 'Impaired spatial learning in α-calcium-calmodulin kinase II mutant mice.' *Science*, **257**, 206–211.

—— Stevens, C.F., Tonegawa, S., Wang, Y. (1992*b*) 'Deficient hippocampal long-term potentiation in α-calcium-calmodulin kinase II mutant mice.' *Science*, **257**, 201–206.

Siomi, H., Siomi, M.C., Nussbaum, R.L., Dreyfuss, G. (1993) 'The protein product of the fragile X gene, FMR1, has characteristics of an RNA-binding protein.' *Cell*, **74**, 291–298.

—— Choi, M., Siomi, M.C., Nussbaum, R.L., Dreyfuss, G. (1994) 'Essential role for KH domains in RNA binding: impaired RNA binding by a mutation in the KH domain of FMR1 that causes fragile X syndrome.' *Cell*, **77**, 33–39.

Suthers, G.K., Davies, K.E. (1992) 'Phenotypic heterogeneity and the single gene.' *American Journal of Human Genetics*, **50**, 887–891. *(Editorial.)*

Telenius, H., Kremer, B., Goldberg, Y.P., Theilmann, J., Andrew, S.E., Zeisler, J., Adam, S., Greenberg, C., Ives, E.J., *et al.* (1994) 'Somatic and gonadal mosaicism of the Huntington disease gene CAG repeat in brain and sperm.' *Nature Genetics*, **6**, 409–414.

Verkerk, A.J.M.H., Pieretti, M., Sutcliffe, J.S., Fu, Y-H., Kuhl, D.P.A., Pizzuti, A., Reiner, O., Richards, S., Victoria, M.F., *et al.* (1991) 'Identification of a gene (*FMR-1*) containing a CGG repeat coincident with a breakpoint cluster region exhibiting length variation in fragile X syndrome.' *Cell*, **65**, 905–914.

Vitaterna, M.H., King, D.P., Chang, A-M., Kornhauser, J.M., Lowrey, P.L., McDonald, J.D., Dove, W.F., Pinto, L.H., Turek, F.W., Takahashi, J.S. (1994) 'Mutagenesis and mapping of a mouse gene, *Clock*, essential for circadian behavior.' *Science*, **264**, 719–725.

Willems, P.J. (1994) 'Dynamic mutations hit double figures.' *Nature Genetics*, **8**, 213–215.

Wu, C-L., Melton, D.W. (1993) 'Production of a model for Lesch–Nyhan syndrome in hypoxanthine phosphoribosyltransferase-deficient mice.' *Nature Genetics*, **3**, 235–240.

Yagi, T., Aizawa, S., Tokunaga, T., Shigetani, Y., Takeda, N., Ikawa, Y. (1993) 'A role for Fyn tyrosine kinase in the suckling behaviour of neonatal mice.' *Nature*, **366**, 742–745.

7
PSYCHOLOGICAL AND BEHAVIOURAL PHENOTYPES IN GENETICALLY DETERMINED SYNDROMES: A REVIEW OF RESEARCH FINDINGS

Orlee Udwin and Jennifer Dennis*

Introduction

This chapter reviews the psychological and behavioural phenotypes that are associated with a number of genetically determined disorders. Most of these conditions came to be recognized as syndromes through the identification of distinct patterns of physical and neurological features, often including a characteristic facial appearance. More recently, as psychologists, paediatricians and psychiatrists have become involved in supporting and advising parent self-help groups for these different conditions, they have become aware of distinct behavioural and personality characteristics and particular cognitive profiles and patterns of learning difficulties that are also associated with each syndrome. In other cases, such as Lesch–Nyhan and cri du chat syndromes, it was the distinctive behaviours which led to a demarcation of the syndromes, and these in turn now have biological markers.

It is not suggested that particular behaviours or cognitive patterns are necessarily unique to a given syndrome. Rather, it is the *combination* of particular cognitive and behavioural characteristics that is unique and that differentiates each syndrome from others. It is important to stress that not all individuals with a given syndrome will show *all* of the features that characterize that syndrome. There is variation within syndromes in the number and severity of features (both physical and psychological) that are shown, and the extent of variability itself varies from syndrome to syndrome.

In the following pages the genetic underpinnings, physical features and natural history of some 30+ syndromes are briefly reviewed, in so far as these are known, followed by descriptions of the cognitive profiles, learning difficulties and behavioural characteristics that are associated with each syndrome. At the end of each section there is

---

*Orlee Udwin is responsible for the major part of this chapter, with the exception of the sections on Down syndrome, Lowe syndrome, the sex chromosome aneuploidies, Smith–Magenis syndrome and tuberous sclerosis complex, which were written by Jennifer Dennis.

Editorial note: In line with emerging practice, eponymous syndrome names are given in the non-possessive form (*e.g.* Lowe syndrome rather than Lowe's), although it is recognized that the reverse still holds currency in many circles (most notably with 'Down's syndrome').

a list of key references which contain overviews of the syndromes and further details on syndrome characteristics.

For many of the syndromes, research into their cognitive and behavioural phenotypes is still in its infancy. In these cases descriptions are still largely anecdotal, and confirmation of, and elaboration on the information must await further research. However, findings on psychological and behavioural phenotypes are already proving valuable for parents, teachers and clinicians in informing intervention efforts and facilitating the sharing of information about appropriate educational and behaviour management approaches.

ACKNOWLEDGEMENTS

I am grateful to the following colleagues, who reviewed sections of this chapter and helped to ensure the accuracy of the material: Martin Bax (London), Martine Borghgraef (Leuven), David Clarke (Birmingham), Michael Clarke (Manchester), Gillian Clayton-Smith (Manchester), Trevor Cole (Birmingham), John Corbett (Birmingham), Judith Dawkins (London), Dian Donnai (Manchester), Eleanor Feldman (Nottingham), Rosalie Ferner (London), Richard Gibbons (Oxford), Peter Hill (London), Tony Holland (Cambridge), Susan Huson (Oxford), Maggie Ireland (Newcastle upon Tyne), Alison Kerr (Scotland), Julie McGaughran (Manchester), Neil Martin (Canterbury), Gregory O'Brien (Morpeth), David Sansom (Birmingham), Isobel Smith (London), Jeremy Turk (London), Jonathan Waters (Birmingham) and Michele Zappella (Italy).

Orlee Udwin

AICARDI SYNDROME

First description
The condition was first described by Aicardi *et al.* (1965).

Incidence/prevalence
The syndrome is found only in girls and is very rare, with something over 200 cases identified to date. However, under-reporting is likely in view of the variable expression of the phenotype.

Genetics/aetiology
Aicardi syndrome is an X-linked dominant disorder affecting only girls and individuals with two X chromosomes; it is lethal in males. All cases have been sporadic. Familial transmission has not been reported: affected females are severely disabled and therefore less likely to become pregnant. Cytogenetic abnormalities involving the Xp22–Xpter region have been described in a number of cases. Current gene mapping suggests that the syndrome is probably allelic or contiguous with Goltz syndrome and microphthalmia with linear skin defects, in which these cytogenetic abnormalities have also been described, and which show considerable overlap in phenotype (Ballabio and Andria 1992).

Physical phenotype, natural history and life expectancy
The three defining features of Aicardi syndrome are the presence of agenesis of the corpus callosum, infantile spasms, and eye lesions or choroidoretinal lacunae, often accompanied by severe visual deficits. The spasms are mostly asymmetrical or unilateral, and frequently become apparent between 3 and 6 months of age, or even earlier, with multiple episodes commonly occurring daily. Electroencephalograph (EEG) tracings typically consist of complex paroxysmal bursts separated by intervals of low voltage, almost inactive record (Aicardi 1982). The paroxysmal bursts are often unilateral or completely asynchronous over both hemispheres. Infantile spasms often cease before 2 years of age. Other types of seizures, mostly partial, unilateral or atypical, are frequently associated with the spasms and may precede them. The seizures tend to persist.

It is now suggested that the original definition of the syndrome, as described above, may be too narrow, and that there needs to be acknowledgment of some variability in the phenotype. Other features that have been described in affected children include spinal and rib abnormalities in about 40 per cent of cases (*e.g.* hemivertebrae, fused ribs) which often result in a marked scoliosis, muscular hypotonia, microphthalmia (in about one third of cases), and retinal colobomas, facial asymmetry and plagiocephaly. Microcephaly is not present initially, but develops over time in about one-fifth of cases. Hypertelorism, an upturned nose and low-set ears have been described in some children, but there is no characteristic facial appearance. Sexual development appears to be normal.

Only some affected individuals achieve independent walking. Hemiplegia or spastic diplegia is evident in many cases. Death in infancy is common, usually as a result of pulmonary infection, which may be aggravated by kyphoscoliosis. A few individuals survive into childhood, but survival into adolescence or early adulthood is rare (Carney *et al.* 1993).

CT and MRI scans reveal multiple central nervous system malformations involving the midline structures and cerebral hemispheres, for example an irregular ventricular contour with heterotopic nodules projecting into the lateral ventricles, variable degrees of cortical atrophy, cystic formations and localized ventricular dilations. Neuropathological findings suggest the presence of a neuronal migration defect involving several areas of the brain.

Psychological and behavioural phenotype

Nearly all affected children have severe learning difficulties. Most demonstrate a developmental level below 12 months of age, with no expressive language. The majority are uncommunicative and lethargic, show little spontaneous activity, and remain totally dependent on adults for their self care (O'Brien 1994). However, Talens *et al.* (1987) present a brief description of a programme of early stimulation for two affected girls who were subsequently reported to have some comprehension of language, to walk with support, and to be fairly responsive to the environment. Self-injurious behaviours have been reported in over half of affected children, and aggression towards people and objects in about one-quarter. Frequent night waking is also common (O'Brien 1994).

KEY REFERENCES

Aicardi, J. (1982) 'The syndrome of callosal agenesis, choroidal lacunae and infantile spasms. Aicardi syndrome.' *In:* Wise, G.B., Blaw, M.E., Procopis, P.G. (Eds.) *Topics in Child Neurology, 17.* New York: S.P. Medical and Scientific, pp. 205–214.
Carney, S.H., Brodsky, M.C., Good, W.V., Glasier, C.M., Greibel, M.L., Cunniff, C. (1993) 'Aicardi syndrome: more than meets the eye.' *Survey of Ophthalmology*, **37**, 419–424.
O'Brien, G. (1994) 'The behavioural and developmental consequences of corpus callosal agenesis and Aicardi syndrome.' *In:* Lassonde, M., Jeeves, M.A. (Eds.) *Callosal Agenesis.* New York: Plenum Press, pp. 235–246.
Talens, C., Andres, M., Rebagliato, M. (1987) 'Early stimulation: psychomotor development of two girls with Aicardi syndrome.' *Child: Care, Health and Development*, **13**, 101–109.

ADDITIONAL REFERENCES

Aicardi, J., Lefebvre, J., Lerique-Koechlin, A. (1965) 'A new syndrome: spasm in flexion, callosal agenesis, ocular abnormalities.' *Electroencephalography and Clinical Neurophysiology*, **19**, 609P–610P.
Ballabio, A., Andria, G. (1992) 'Deletions and translocations involving the distal short arm of the human X chromosome: review and hypotheses.' *Human Molecular Genetics*, **1**, 221–227.

ANGELMAN SYNDROME

Alternative name
'Happy puppet' syndrome (no longer used because of its pejorative connotations).

First description
Angelman (1965) was the first to describe a disorder characterized by severe learning difficulties, inappropriate bouts of laughter, jerky ataxic limb movements and similar facial appearance in affected individuals.

Incidence/prevalence
The incidence is unknown but is thought to be in the region of 1:20,000 to 1:30,000. The syndrome occurs across all ethnic and racial groups and males and females are equally affected.

Genetics/aetiology
Most cases are sporadic. A deletion of the proximal long arm of chromosome 15 (15q11–q13) has been detected in 60–75 per cent of cases, similar to the deletion seen in Prader–Willi syndrome but always occurring on the maternally derived chromosome (Knoll *et al.* 1989). In a few of these cases the deletion arises as a result of a maternal chromosome 15 rearrangement, for example a translocation or inversion. Uniparental disomy of chromosome 15 has been reported in a few cases, but the remaining cases do not show detectable deletions or uniparental disomy. These may be accounted for by submicroscopic deletions or mutations at the Angelman locus. Abnormalities of this type may be transmitted in an autosomal dominant fashion (Wagstaff *et al.* 1992) and they explain most familial occurrences of the disorder. It has further been suggested that Angelman syndrome may be a contiguous gene syndrome where the loss or silencing of multiple imprinted genes is responsible for the syndrome phenotype.

Physical phenotype, natural history and life expectancy
The syndrome is characterized by ataxic movements, epilepsy and/or an abnormal EEG, delayed psychomotor development and lack of speech, and inappropriate bouts of laughter. The typical facial appearance consists of a long face and prominent jaw, a wide mouth with wide-spaced teeth, thin upper lip, mid-face hypoplasia and deep-set eyes, and a flat occiput. Microcephaly is a common finding, reflecting the abnormality in underlying brain development which affects the growth of the skull and facial bones. Affected individuals habitually keep their mouths open, with varying degrees of tongue protrusion. Prognathism and deformation of the primary dentition are probably caused by the behaviour of constant tongue thrusting (Clayton-Smith 1993). Blue eyes and blonde hair are described in two thirds of cases.

Early feeding problems due to difficulties with sucking and swallowing or persistent regurgitation of feeds are reported in about 70 per cent of cases, and severe gastro-oesophageal reflux in 40 per cent. Behaviours such as pica, rumination and repeated placing of objects or hands into the mouth are fairly common (Penner *et al.* 1993).

Motor development is delayed. An ataxic gait and jerky voluntary movements with associated tremulousness are present in all cases. Most children learn to walk, though the age at which walking commences ranges from 18 months to 7 years. Truncal hypotonia and limb hypertonia with brisk reflexes are found on examination, resulting in the tendency to walk with a stiff-legged, wide-based gait. In addition, there is a character-istic posture of the arms which are upheld with flexion at the wrists and elbows. Hand flapping occurs especially when walking or with excitement. Scoliosis is found in up to 10 per cent of cases. It is apparent at birth or during early childhood, and tends to worsen in adolescence.

Upper respiratory tract infections and otitis media are common after infancy, but otherwise general health is usually good. There is a tendency to obesity with age, especially in adult females.

Epilepsy is found in 86 per cent of cases. The seizures commence at variable ages up to 6 years, typically between 18 and 24 months, and are often difficult to control. The first seizure is often precipitated by a febrile illness or by teething. Clayton-Smith (1993) has identified a characteristic pattern to the seizures, with severe bouts of uncontrollable seizures lasting up to several weeks, interspersed with seizure-free periods of several months. Seizures are worst at around 4 years of age, then decrease in frequency and severity, often with complete cessation by age 10.

A characteristic EEG pattern is found in all cases, comprising large amplitude slow wave activity which persists during sleep, very large amplitude slow activity occurring in runs and more prominent anteriorly, and spikes or sharp waves mixed with large amplitude components seen posteriorly which are facilitated by or only seen with eye closure. These features are a strong diagnostic marker for the syndrome, although they become less apparent after age 10 when some alpha rhythm tends to appear. Neuro-imaging studies show some cortical atrophy, ventricular enlargement or dysmyelination in a few cases.

Life expectancy is probably normal, but as yet little is known about adults with the syndrome.

Psychological and behavioural phenotype

Information about the cognitive and behavioural characteristics associated with Angel-man syndrome is still largely anecdotal. The syndrome is characterized by severe or profound learning difficulties and lack of speech. Development of pre-speech skills such as babbling and vocal play is also deficient, and individuals typically acquire no more than three words. Many children have no speech at all. Penner *et al.* (1993) evaluated the function of the speech mechanism and motor imitation in a small sample and found sig-nificant difficulties in the execution of motor acts, which may reflect an underlying oral motor dyspraxia. They also noted poor social interaction and communication skills more generally. By contrast, Zori *et al.* (1992) and Clayton-Smith (1993) have found that a significant number of affected individuals want to communicate and use non-verbal means of communication, including gestures, signs and picture boards. They suggest that comprehension of speech is significantly better than expression, and that affected individuals have a good memory, especially for people's faces and for directions.

Many children become toilet trained and can feed themselves, and as adults they are capable of performing basic household tasks such as dusting and setting the table under supervision (Clayton-Smith 1993).

Affected children are typically described as sociable and affectionate, liking physical contact and with a cheerful and happy affect. Smiling is usually very frequent, but is not necessarily in response to social overtures. Individuals display frequent definite attacks of giggling and easily provoked bouts of laughter, which may be inappropriate to the circumstances and do not necessarily indicate happiness or enjoyment (Clayton-Smith 1993). The children are said to love music and water, and there are anecdotal accounts of children jumping into the bath fully clothed and attempting to get into lakes and swimming pools at any opportunity. They are also said to be fascinated by mirrors, reflections and plastic. Hand clapping and hand flapping are common, the latter especially when walking or with excitement. Chewing and mouthing of objects are frequently described. Claims that two-thirds of affected children have autism or pervasive developmental disorder require more extensive investigation.

Overexcitability, overactivity and limited attention span are characteristic in childhood, but become less apparent with age, and concentration appears to improve. There are some accounts of aggressive behaviour and temper tantrums in affected individuals, but these have not been confirmed in other reports. Difficulties initiating and maintaining sleep are commonly reported (in about 90 per cent of cases) (Clayton-Smith 1993). Affected children appear to need less sleep than other children, often napping only for short intervals, and sleeping on average five to six hours a night. A period of particularly poor sleep sometimes precipitates a bout of seizures. Parents frequently report destruction of bedroom furniture during the night, and severely disrupted nights are typical. Summers *et al.* (1992) reported some success in treating sleep problems using a combined behavioural and pharmacological approach. Fortunately, length of sleep seems to increase with age.

KEY REFERENCES

Clayton-Smith, J. (1993) 'Clinical research on Angelman syndrome in the United Kingdom: observations on 82 affected individuals.' *American Journal of Medical Genetics*, **46**, 12–15.

—— Pembrey, M.E. (1992) 'Angelman syndrome.' *Journal of Medical Genetics*, **29**, 412–415.

Zori, R.T., Hendrickson, J., Woolven, S., Whidden, E.M., Gray, B., Williams, C.A. (1992) 'Angelman syndrome: clinical profile.' *Journal of Child Neurology*, **7**, 270–280.

ADDITIONAL REFERENCES

Angelman, H. (1965) '"Puppet children": a report on three cases.' *Developmental Medicine and Child Neurology*, **7**, 681–683.

Knoll, J.H.M., Nicholls, R.D., Magenis, R.E., Graham, J.M., Lalande, M., Latt, S.A. (1989) 'Angelman and Prader–Willi syndromes share a common chromosome 15 deletion but differ in parental origin of the deletion.' *American Journal of Medical Genetics*, **32**, 285–290.

Penner, K.A., Johnston, J., Faircloth, B.H., Irish, P., Williams, C.A. (1993) 'Communication, cognition, and social interaction in the Angelman syndrome.' *American Journal of Medical Genetics*, **46**, 34–39.

Summers, J.A., Lynch, P.S., Harris, J.C., Burke, J.C., Allison, D.B., Sandler, L. (1992) 'A combined behavioural/pharmacological treatment of sleep–wake schedule disorder in Angelman syndrome.' *Journal of Developmental and Behavioral Pediatrics*, **13**, 284–287.

Wagstaff, J., Knoll, J.H.M., Glatt, K.A., Shugart, Y.Y., Sommer, A., Lalande, M. (1992) 'Maternal but not paternal transmission of 15q11–13-linked nondeletion Angelman sydrome leads to phenotypic expression.' *Nature Genetics*, **1**, 291–294.

CORNELIA DE LANGE SYNDROME

Alternative names
Brachmann–de Lange syndrome; Amsterdam dwarfism.

First description
The first published case was by Brachmann (1916), but de Lange (1933) was the first to suggest that the manifestations comprised a new syndrome.

Incidence/prevalence
The syndrome is relatively rare, with an incidence of 1:40,000 to 1:100,000 live births. However, some writers consider it to be much more common, and quote an incidence of 1:10,000 (Opitz 1985). Males and females are equally affected.

Genetics/aetiology
The aetiology is unclear. Most cases are sporadic, but a few affected sibling pairs, a three-generation family, and some mildly affected parents have been reported, suggesting an autosomal dominant mode of inheritance with germline mosaicism to explain the recurrence in siblings. Vertical transmission appears to be largely maternal, but this may be due to the greater likelihood of girls with mild to moderate learning difficulties becoming pregnant, when compared with the likelihood of males of similar ability levels fathering children. There are as yet no biochemical or chromosomal markers for the syndrome. Chromosomal abnormalities have been found in some cases, and Ireland *et al.* (1991) have made a preliminary assignment of the gene responsible to the long arm of chromosome 3 (at 3q26.3), but as yet findings are inconsistent. There is phenotypic overlap with duplication of chromosome 3q (25–29).

Physical phenotype, natural history and life expectancy
Cornelia de Lange syndrome is characterized by low birthweight, severe growth retardation, small stature, developmental delay, limb abnormalities and distinct facial anomalies. Clinical findings demonstrate wide variation. Ireland *et al.* (1993) have argued for a clear phenotypic dichotomy, with severe cases and mildly affected cases forming two distinct groups. Those in the mildly affected group have a much better prognosis.

Facial characteristics found in up to 80–90 per cent of affected individuals include a small upturned nose, anteverted nostrils, neat well-defined arched eyebrows which often fan out laterally as well as meeting in the middle, long curly eyelashes, thin lips and a crescent-shaped mouth, a long philtrum, high arched palate and micrognathia. The facial features may change with age, especially in affected males, with the eyebrows becoming bushy, the nostrils normally placed, the philtrum of normal length, and the nose and lips well-developed.

Typical limb abnormalities include miniaturization, short forearms and short hands and feet. Shortening of the preaxial and postaxial digits is common in post-pubertal individuals. Other digital abnormalities include partial syndactyly of the second and third toes and absence of the second or third or both interdigital triradii on the hands. Dental abnormalities (late eruption of widely spaced teeth) are found in up to 90 per cent of cases, and hearing abnormalities (including sensorineural deafness) in at least 60 per cent. Lower birthweight has been found to correlate with a more severe phenotype, specifically including severe upper limb malformations and greater psychomotor retardation (Hawley *et al.* 1985).

Anomalies that occur less often include myopia, microcornea, astigmatism, optic atrophy, coloboma of the optic nerve, strabismus, cleft palate, congenital heart defects (most commonly ventricular septal defect), hiatus hernia, pyloric stenosis, brachyoesophagus, undescended testes and other genital abnormalities in males (Hawley *et al.* 1985).

In infancy, failure to thrive and feeding difficulties (regurgitation, vomiting, chewing and swallowing difficulties) have been documented in 70–100 per cent of cases and are potentially life-threatening. Feeding difficulties remain a problem in about 70 per cent of children, and recurrent respiratory infections are also common. Aspiration pneumonia is a frequent problem with a high early mortality. Increased muscle tone is not uncommon in early infancy, although spasticity has been noted in some children in later years. Nearly half of one sample were ambulatory, with the average age of independent walking being 3 years (Hawley *et al.* 1985). Sexual development appears to be normal, and there are increasing numbers of reports of affected individuals who have reached adulthood.

Psychological and behavioural phenotype
Most affected individuals have moderate or severe learning difficulties, although cognitive abilities in the low-average and borderline range have been reported in some cases (Kline *et al.* 1993). Perceptual organization, visuospatial memory and fine motor skills are particular strengths, while verbal communication is an area of deficit. Kline *et al.* therefore suggest that teaching approaches which emphasize visuospatial skills and visual memory (*e.g.* using computers) would be preferable to standard methods of verbal instruction. There are many reports of limited speech development or absence of speech in affected individuals, even in some who are more cognitively able. In one report of 64 children, about half were able to obey simple commands and only 12 per cent were able to combine words expressively (Hawley *et al.* 1985). In another study, half of those aged over 4 years were able to combine two or more words into sentences, while one third had fewer than three words. Only 4 per cent were judged to have language skills within normal limits (Goodban 1993). Overall, language expression is inferior to comprehension, and syntactic skills are particularly poor, even in children with well developed vocabularies (Kline *et al.* 1993). An unusual phenomenon reported in this population is the utterance of a clear, meaningful word or phrase once only, which is never used again. Articulation errors are common. Many children have a guttural vocal quality, which is low in pitch and quality. Crying and other sounds are often described as low-pitched, growling, deep and raucous (Goodban 1993). Many affected individuals are able to cope with their everyday needs and continue to acquire new skills even into their late teens.

However, in one sample fewer than half the cases attained any self-help skills (Hawley *et al.* 1985).

A behavioural phenotype can be identified, although affected children also show great variability in their behaviour. In general, the children are not very talkative, even when they have well developed vocabularies. Autistic features have been described, including a lack of social relatedness and impassivity, rejection of physical contact, little reaction to sounds or to pain, and stereotypic self-stimulatory movements such as moving round and round (twirling) (Johnson *et al.* 1976). More mildly affected individuals are reported to show rigidity and inflexibility to change, and a preference for a structured environment. Affected individuals react with pleasure to vestibular stimulation, for example bouncing or spinning in a chair. However, tactile defensiveness has also been described (Hawley *et al.* 1985, Goodban 1993).

Some children with Cornelia de Lange syndrome are placid and good-natured, but many others are said to be restless, overactive, distractible and irritable. Self-injurious behaviour and aggression are striking characteristics of the syndrome. Over half of one sample of affected individuals manifested behaviour difficulties, including screaming, tantrums, biting and hitting self or others. The self-injurious behaviour and other repetitive behaviours tend to be stereotypical and performed repeatedly, but they are different in each individual. In many cases the self-injury is relatively mild; in other cases it may result in scarring and tissue loss. However, in contrast to the self-injury characteristic of Lesch–Nyhan syndrome, the self-mutilation in Cornelia de Lange syndrome does not have a compulsive quality to it and shows a good response to behaviour modification (Schroeder *et al.* 1990). The high levels of aggression may be related to low serotonin levels in whole blood (Greenberg and Coleman 1976). It has also been suggested that the aggressive outbursts may be evoked by feelings of discomfort or frustration or by some painful physical condition. For example, in a few cases temperament was reported to improve significantly after treatment for reflux vomiting.

KEY REFERENCES

Goodban, M.T. (1993) 'Survey of speech and language skills with prognostic indicators in 116 patients with Cornelia de Lange syndrome.' *American Journal of Medical Genetics*, **47**, 1059–1063.

Hawley, P.P., Jackson, L.G., Kurnit, D.M. (1985) 'Sixty-four patients with Brachmann–de Lange syndrome: a survey.' *American Journal of Medical Genetics*, **20**, 453–459.

Ireland, M., Donnai, D., Burn, J. (1993) 'Brachmann–de Lange syndrome. Delineation of the clinical phenotype.' *American Journal of Medical Genetics*, **47**, 959–964.

Kline, A.D., Stanley, C., Belevich, J., Brodsky, K., Barr, M., Jackson, L.G. (1993) 'Developmental data on individuals with the Brachmann–de Lange syndrome.' *American Journal of Medical Genetics*, **47**, 1053–1058.

ADDITIONAL REFERENCES

Brachmann, W. (1916) 'Ein Fall von symmetrischer Monodaktylie durch Ulnadefekt, mit symmetrischer Flughautbildung in den Ellenbogen sowie anderen Abnormalitäten.' *Jahrbuch für Kinderheilkunde und Physische Erziehung*, **84**, 225–235.

de Die-Smulders, C., Theunissen, P., Schrander-Stumpel, C., Fryns, J-P. (1992) 'On the variable expression of the Brachmann–de Lange syndrome.' *Clinical Genetics*, **41**, 42–45.

de Lange, C. (1933) 'Sur un type nouveau de dégénération (typus Amstelodamensis).' *Archives de Médecine des Enfants*, **36**, 713–719.

Greenberg, A., Coleman, M. (1976) 'Depressed 5-hydroxyindole levels associated with hyperactive and aggressive behaviour. Relationship to drug response.' *Archives of General Psychiatry*, **33**, 331–336.

Ireland, M., English, C., Cross, I., Houlsby, W.T, Burn, J. (1991) 'A *de novo* translocation t(3;17)(q26.3; q23.1) in a child with Cornelia de Lange syndrome.' *Journal of Medical Genetics*, **28**, 639–640.

Johnson, H.G., Ekman, P., Friesen, W. (1976) 'A behavioral phenotype in the de Lange syndrome.' *Pediatric Research*, **10**, 843–850.

Opitz, J.M. (1985) 'The Brachmann–de Lange syndrome.' *American Journal of Medical Genetics*, **22**, 89–102. *(Editorial.)*

Schroeder, S.R., Rojahn, J., Mulick, J.A., Schroeder, C.S. (1990) 'Self-injurious behavior.' *In:* Matson, J.L. (Ed.) *Handbook of Behavior Modification with the Mentally Retarded. 2nd Edn.* New York: Plenum Press, pp. 141–180.

CRI DU CHAT SYNDROME

Alternative names
Deletion 5p– syndrome; chromosome 5 short arm deletion.

First description
The syndrome was first described by Lejeune *et al.* (1963).

Incidence/prevalence
Cri du chat syndrome has an incidence of approximately 1:50,000 live births, with a female:male ratio of 4:3 (Niebuhr 1978*a*).

Genetics/aetiology
The syndrome results from a partial deletion of the short arm of chromosome 5. There is a great degree of cytogenetic heterogeneity, including simple terminal deletions of varying sizes, interstitial deletions and a variety of structural rearrangements. The majority of cases (85 per cent) are due to *de novo* deletions, mostly paternal in origin. Most of the remaining cases result from unbalanced translocations, which may be maternally or paternally derived. The critical region for the development of the syndrome is thought to be 5p15.2 (Niebuhr 1978*b*), but to date no genes have been mapped to this region.

Individuals with familial and *de novo* translocations manifest more severe physical anomalies and lower cognitive abilities than individuals with isolated deletions. In the latter group, the size of the missing chromosome segment has been found to correlate negatively with the physical phenotype and with IQ (Wilkins *et al.* 1983).

Physical phenotype, natural history and life expectancy
Affected individuals have a striking facial appearance. In infancy the face is round with hypertelorism, epicanthal folds, slanting palpebral fissures, posteriorly rotated low-set ears with preauricular tags, a broad flat nose and microretrognathia. The facial features show a consistent progression with age: the face lengthens and loses much of its infantile fullness, although the epicanthal folds and oblique palpebral fissures remain. In adolescence the facial features appear to coarsen, and prominent supraorbital ridges, deep-set eyes, a hypoplastic nasal bridge and severe dental malocclusion are typical. A relatively large mouth and a full lower lip are also common in older individuals. A minority of cases have a cleft lip and palate, and there may be clinodactyly.

Affected children demonstrate prenatal growth retardation, with low birthweight and microcephaly. The infants are often hypotonic, and common neonatal complications include poor sucking, vomiting, failure to thrive, respiratory distress and jaundice. These gradually improve with age. Although there is a significant mortality in the first few months of life, in recent years life expectancy has significantly improved. Marked growth retardation continues in childhood and into adulthood, with decreased height, poor weight gain and significant microcephaly.

Developmental milestones are significantly delayed in many cases. Some affected individuals never learn to walk; those who do tend to have an unsteady broad-based stooping gait with bent knees. Coordination difficulties are common.

Respiratory and ear infections occur frequently. Cardiac abnormalities are common, and include septal defects and patent ductus arteriosus. Gastrointestinal anomalies, such as intestinal malrotation and Hirschsprung disease, are found occasionally. Severe constipation is a chronic problem in approximately half the cases, and otitis media persists in about one third. In males, undescended testes are frequently found in the younger age groups, and in adults the testes are sometimes small. Inguinal hernia, diastasis recti and scoliosis are fairly common, especially in older individuals. Small hands and feet, poor muscular development and prematurely greying hair have also been noted in some cases.

Psychological and behavioural phenotype

Many affected children have severe learning difficulties and develop minimal or no speech and very limited self-care skills, for example in toileting and dressing. Others, however, show only mild or moderate learning difficulties, and achieve a moderate degree of independence in self-care skills (Wilkins *et al.* 1980, Carlin 1990).

In most cases there is a marked discrepancy between verbal and non-verbal abilities, with language development being particularly delayed. Just under half of one series of cases did not develop speech, though some of the children were able to use basic sign or gestural language for communication (Carlin 1990).

The most striking feature in affected infants is an unusual cry, variously described as high-pitched, plaintive, weak, monotonous or shrill, similar to the mewing of a cat. This feature is ascribed to abnormal laryngeal development. It is not seen in all cases, and one third of infants with this characteristic cry are said to lose it by 2 years of age. Alternatively, it may be that crying simply becomes less frequent after that age. Individuals who develop speech display a characteristic, relatively high-pitched, monochromatic voice timbre.

Affected individuals tend to be amiable and placid. However, hyperactivity, restlessness, irritability, destructiveness and self-stimulatory behaviours can be major problems in at least 50 per cent of cases (Wilkins *et al.* 1980, 1983). Affected children with severe learning difficulties commonly exhibit behaviours such as head banging, hand waving and hand sucking, and they often display withdrawn behaviour, with roving eye movements and apparently decreased awareness of their surroundings.

KEY REFERENCES

Carlin, M.E. (1990) 'The improved prognosis in cri-du-chat (5p–) syndrome.' *In:* Fraser, W.I. (Ed.) *Key Issues in Mental Retardation Research.* London: Routledge, pp. 64–73.
Niebuhr, E. (1978a) 'The cri du chat syndrome: epidemiology, cytogenetics and clinical features.' *Human Genetics*, **44**, 227–275.
Wilkins, L.E., Brown, J.A., Wolf, B. (1980) 'Psychomotor development in 65 home- reared children with cri-du-chat syndrome.' *Journal of Pediatrics*, **97**, 401–405.

—— —— Nance, W.E., Wolf, B. (1983) 'Clinical heterogeneity in 80 home-reared children with cri du chat syndrome.' *Journal of Pediatrics*, **102**, 528–533.

ADDITIONAL REFERENCES

Lejeune, J., Lafourcade, J., Berger, R., Vialette, J., Bowswillwald, M., Serginge, P., Turpin, R. (1963) 'Trois cas de deletion partielle du bras court d'un chromosome 5.' *Comptes Rendus de l'Académie des Sciences*, **257**, 3098–3102.

Niebuhr, E., (1978*b*) 'Cytologic observations in 35 individuals with a 5p– karyotype.' *Human Genetics*, **42**, 143–156.

DOWN SYNDROME

Alternative names
Trisomy 21.

First description
The syndrome which now bears his name was first described by John Langdon Down in 1866. Due to the characteristic facies he termed the condition 'mongolism', but this title is no longer deemed acceptable.

Incidence/prevalence
The natural incidence averages approximately 1:600 live births and increases with increasing maternal age, rising from 1:2500 below age 30 to 1:80 at age 40 and 1:32 at age 45. There is very significant early fetal loss.

Genetics/aetiology
The underlying cytogenetic abnormality (trisomy 21) was identified by Lejeune *et al.* in 1959. Three main genotypes are now recognized:
(1) Non-disjunction (~95 per cent) 47,XX (or 47,XY) +21. Non-familial; non-specific recurrence risk around 1:200.
(2) Translocations (1–5 per cent). Unbalanced Robertsonian translocation, usually between chromosomes 14 and 21, *e.g.* 46,XX, –14, +t (14q21q). Often occurs as a *de novo* mutation but one parent may carry balanced translocation, hence recurrence risk 1:4, sometimes higher.
(3) Mosaic forms (traditionally said to be 1–2 per cent but probably many undiagnosed); two cell lines, one trisomic, one normal; proportions vary from child to child. Usually associated with less severe impairment.

The mechanism whereby increased gene dosage produces profound phenotypic change in trisomic disorders is not understood. Shapiro (1994) argues in terms of amplified developmental instability—those features which are most unstable in the general population are those most affected by the presence of extra genetic material, the larger the additional chromosome the greater the effect. This argument does not look for explanations in terms of genes specifically encoded on chromosome 21. With regard to the latter, a small region encompassing the distal part of the long arm of chromosome 21 (distal part of band 21q22.1–22.3) would appear to be sufficient for the generation of many of the associated phenotypic features. Increased dosage of loci outside this region is also required for the full expression of the phenotype. The almost universal finding of Alzheimer-type neuropathology, with or without clinically expressed dementia, among older people with Down syndrome has been ascribed to overexpression of the β–amyloid precursor protein gene encoded on 21q21.1. Genetic variation in the *ApoE* gene appears to be an important factor in determining lifespan and the extent to which dementia is clinically expressed in this population (Royston *et al.* 1994).

Physical phenotype, natural history and life expectancy

The most common features of Down syndrome are: upward-, outward-slanting eyes; epicanthus; wide nasal bridge; Brushfield spots; large posterior fontanelle; brachycephaly; low nuchal hair line; single transverse palmar crease; large cleft between first and second toe; and short stature with relatively short upper arms. Neonatal hypotonia is usually present but some improvement usually occurs over time. There is often generalized joint laxity. Thyroid dysfunction is overrepresented at all ages. 15 per cent of adolescents are hypothyroid, and thyroid function declines further in adult life. 50 per cent have congenital heart disease, around 15 per cent with full atrioventricular septal defect (AVSD). 7 per cent have congenital upper intestinal obstruction of varying degree.

Glue ear affects around 80 per cent of children at some time and this may continue into adult life. Sensorineural deafness may develop in adolescence. There is a higher than average incidence of myopia and hypermetropia. Nasal catarrh and partial upper airway obstruction are relatively common. The incidence of leukaemia is 1 per cent.

Many adults with otherwise uncomplicated Down syndrome develop Alzheimer-type dementia with onset from age 35. Others survive fit and well into their seventies. Recent figures (Baird and Sadovnick 1989) suggest that 44 per cent of people with the syndrome now survive beyond age 60 and 14 per cent beyond age 68. Those with untreated AVSD progress to Eisenmenger syndrome and die in respiratory and cardiac failure any time from late teens to late twenties. Antibiotics have dramatically reduced deaths in the early years but propensity to infections increases the morbidity among those with leukaemia.

Psychological and behavioural phenotype

Cognitive aspects

The IQ distribution among 6-year-olds with Down syndrome is shifted about 50 points downward, with a mean of 55 and with the top 10 per cent falling within the lower end of the normal range. As the children get older, mean IQ appears to fall. By age 8, Gath and Gumley (1984) found a mean IQ of 45 with a range of 20–80. There is often further decline in adult life. All studies show that as a group, boys have lower IQ than girls. Testing at all ages is influenced by the grave specific difficulties with speech and language which are almost universal among those with the syndrome. Permeating all aspects of functioning is a general slowing of central processing time. This has been documented for motor processing times (Kerr and Blais 1985).

For most teenagers some aspects of expressive language are at around a 3-year level. While vocabulary may progress quite well, the syntactic element of language is severely retarded (Fowler 1990). Short sentence length and key-word speech are characteristic. Speech production difficulties complicate the picture. For most of those with the syndrome their level of general sophistication, social awareness and desire to communicate far exceeds their ability to do so. This deficit constitutes the single gravest disadvantage for these people. Some of the factors which underpin these difficulties have to do with phonological processing and short-term auditory memory deficits.

Many adults with the syndrome have mild/moderate hearing impairment. The influence of this on speech and language development is somewhat conflicting. Some studies find a threshold effect, others a graduated one.

In the last ten years the work of Buckley and colleagues at the Sarah Duffen Centre in Portsmouth has shown that many children with the syndrome appear to have enhanced ability to recognize written words in the preschool years. When this skill is present it can be harnessed both to increase syntactic and phonological awareness and to give the children advantage on school entry. S. Buckley (personal communication) estimates that around 75 per cent of children with the syndrome can learn to read, though at varied levels of competence.

Behavioural aspects

It was the recognition of the behavioural as well as the physical aspects of different mentally handicapping disorders which in 1866 led Langdon Down to propose his 'ethnic classification of idiots'. He later wrote, 'by a recognition of type we are able to determine the physical as well as mental and moral characteristics of the child in a way which astonishes the mother, who finds one is able to anticipate all she has to relate' (Down 1887). He went on to describe: power of imitation and mimicry; a strong sense of the ridiculous; humorous remarks and laughter; obstinacy ('they can only be guided by consummate tact'); solitary rehearsal of real or imagined conversations; and general amiability.

This stereotyped view continues to be widely held, and it is only recently that within-syndrome variability has been acknowledged and investigated. Green *et al.* (1989) showed that among very young children there was a distinct subgroup, around 25 per cent, who were chaotic and/or difficult to engage and who rated significantly for conduct-type disorder and attention deficit.

Berger (1990) in an excellent chapter on parent–child interactions, reviews evidence for considerable deviations in attentional development in the early years. Krakow and Kopp (1983) present data about deficits in social referencing in children with Down syndrome, and Sinson and Wetherick (1982) have made some classical observations about aberrations of mutual gaze which lead to social isolation.

Jennifer Wishart's ongoing elegant studies highlight the problems many of these children face in 'learning to learn' (Wishart 1988). The majority, despite reasonable underlying cognitive skills, seem to lack the motivation necessary to carry forward their own learning. They evade, with every social strategy available, actually getting down to a task, or remaining on a task which has become challenging, or continuing with a task if they feel even a hint of external pressure.

There is now a considerable body of evidence which shows a significant incidence of conduct disorder, some of it severe, not only among older children with the syndrome but also in those of pre-school age. Gath and Gumley (1984) draw attention to a central problem which has bedevilled behavioural research among people with learning disabilities—that instruments devised and standardized for the ordinary population are inappropriate for those with learning disability, in particular in their failure to tap specific behaviours which may pose major management problems for parents and carers. In the decade since Gath and Gumley's comments the situation has been to some extent redressed. It is a particular focus of interest for the Society for the Study of Behavioural Phenotypes. Gath (personal communication) compared children with Down syndrome with others with learning disability from other causes and found that, for some, 'sitting down' (in the middle of the road, in supermarkets, etc.) and 'escaping' were significant problems. Escaping behaviours are particularly difficult to deal with. In some cases it is necessary to lock these children into their own homes and erect high boundary fences in an attempt to ensure their safety. They show considerable ingenuity in evading these restrictions, but the basic 'escaping' impulse seems triggered by wide open spaces, open doors, gaps in hedges, etc. These behaviours, if consistently handled, do seem to ease off for many children during adolescence. Similarly, 'sitting down' and refusing to budge is a scenario familiar to most parents and carers of those of all ages.

This contemporary work echoes right back to Langdon Down's observation that 'they can only be guided by consummate tact'. The work of Berger and Cunningham (1981) on the facilitation of early smiling may also tap into this same area. He observed that smiling was most quickly elicited when parents were asked only to imitate their baby's own facial movements rather than try specifically to elicit smiling.

Psychiatric disorder

There is a body of literature concerning associations between Down syndrome and autism (see Howlin *et al.* 1995). Definitions vary, but the core behavioural deviations are specified in Gillberg's paper (Gillberg 1992). A standardized approach is much needed. There is no doubt that this population is more at risk than the general population for behaviours which fall within the autistic spectrum, but often empathic functioning seems little impaired. A minority show notable avoidant and oppositional behaviours and motor stereotypies.

As always, psychiatric disorder among older children and adults may be under-diagnosed where learning disability coexists. Teenagers and young adults are at risk for depressive illness. It is critically important to keep this possibility in mind when performance and general competence unexpectedly decline, particularly in those who are relatively able. Alzheimer-type dementia is clinically apparent in 40–50 per cent of over-45s. The biological basis and impact of this has been excellently reviewed by Berg *et al.* (1993). Early warning signs are loss of self-care skills and excessive tearfulness. Here again these classical hallmarks of dementia may be missed and falsely attributed to environmental factors in the presence of preexisting learning disability.

KEY REFERENCES

Berg, J.M., Karlinsky, H., Holland, A.J. (1993) *Alzheimer Disease, Down Syndrome and their Relationship.* Oxford: Oxford University Press.

Cicchetti, D., Beeghly, M. (Eds.) (1990) *Children with Down Syndrome: a Developmental Perspective.* Cambridge: Cambridge University Press.

Down, J.L. (1887) *Mental Affections of Childhood and Youth.* (Reprinted as *Classics in Developmental Medicine No. 5.* by Mac Keith Press, London, 1990.)

ADDITIONAL REFERENCES

Baird, P.A., Sadovnick, A.D. (1989) 'Life tables for Down syndrome.' *Human Genetics*, **82**, 291–292.

Berger, J. (1990) 'Interactions between parents and their infants with Down syndrome.' *In:* Cicchetti, D., Beeghly, M. (Eds.) *Children with Down Syndrome: a Developmental Perspective.* Cambridge: Cambridge University Press, pp. 101–146.

—— Cunningham, C.C. (1981) 'Early development of social interactions in Down's syndrome and non-handicapped infants.' *In: Finland Speaks: The Report of EASE 80 Conference, Helsinki, August 1981.*

Down, J.L. (1866) 'Observations on an ethnic classification of idiots.' *London Hospital Reports*, **3**, 259–262. (Reprinted in Down, J.L. *Mental Affections of Childhood and Youth. Classics in Developmental Medicine No. 5.* Mac Keith Press, London, 1990, pp. 127–131.)

Fowler, A.E. (1990) 'Language abilities in children with Down syndrome: evidence for a specific syntactic delay.' *In:* Cicchetti, D., Beeghly, M. (Eds.) *Children with Down Syndrome: a Developmental Perspective.* Cambridge: Cambridge University Press, pp. 302–328.

Gath, A., Gumley, D. (1984) 'Down's syndrome and the family: follow-up of children first seen in infancy.' *Developmental Medicine and Child Neurology*, **26**, 500–508.

Gillberg, C. (1992) 'Subgroups in autism: are there behavioural phenotypes typical of underlying medical conditions?' *Journal of Intellectual Disability Research*, **36**, 201–214.

Green, J.M., Dennis, J., Bennets, L.A. (1989) 'Attention disorder in a group of young Down's syndrome children.' *Journal of Mental Deficiency Research*, **33**, 105–122.

Howlin, P., Wing, L., Gould, J. (1995) 'The recognition of autism in children with Down syndrome: implications for intervention and some speculations about pathology.' *Developmental Medicine and Child Neurology*, **37**, 406–414.

Kerr, R., Blais, C. (1985) 'Motor skill acquisition by individuals with Down syndrome.' *American Journal of Mental Deficiency*, **90**, 313–318.

Krakow, J.B., Kopp, C.B. (1983) 'The effects of developmental delay on sustained attention in young children.' *Child Development*, **54**, 1143–1155.

Lejeune, J., Gautier, M., Turpin, R. (1959) 'Étude des chromosomes somatiques de neuf enfants mongoliens.' *Comptes Rendus de l'Académie des Sciences*, **248**, 1721–1722.

Royston, M.C., Mann, D., Pickering-Brown, S., Owen, F., Perry, R., Raghavan, R., Khin-Nu, C., Tyrer, S., Day, K., *et al.* (1994) 'Apolipoprotein E ε2 allele promotes longevity and protects patients with Down's syndrome from dementia.' *NeuroReport*, **5**, 2583–2585.

Shapiro, B.L. (1994) 'The environmental basis of the Down syndrome phenotype.' *Developmental Medicine and Child Neurology*, **36**, 84–90.

Sinson, J.C., Wetherick, N.E. (1982) 'Mutual gaze in pre-school Down's and normal children.' *Journal of Mental Deficiency Research*, **26**, 123–129.

Wishart, J. (1988) 'Learning to learn: the difficulties faced by infants and young children with Down's syndrome.' *In:* Fraser, W.I. (Ed.) *Key Issues in Research in Mental Retardation.* London/New York: Routledge, pp. 249–261.

DUCHENNE MUSCULAR DYSTROPHY

First description

Meryon (1852) was the first to describe Duchenne muscular dystrophy (DMD) as a familial disease which primarily affects muscle tissue; its association with non-progressive intellectual impairment was first noted by Duchenne (1872).

Incidence/prevalence

DMD has an incidence of approximately 1:3500 male births. The incidence has decreased in recent years due to increased efforts at carrier detection and genetic counselling, and the availability of prenatal diagnosis.

Genetics/aetiology

DMD is an X-linked recessive disorder transmitted via asymptomatic females to 50 per cent of their sons. However, in 30 per cent of cases the condition is the result of a new mutation.

The gene for DMD has been localized to the short arm of the X chromosome at locus Xp21. DMD is caused by deletions, duplications or point mutations at this locus, leading to a disruption in the gene product dystrophin (Hoffman *et al.* 1987). A partial deletion of the dystrophin gene can be detected in approximately 70 per cent of affected males.

Dystrophin is found in muscle fibres and is also expressed in the brain, where it appears to be localized to neurons. Its precise role in muscle and brain is not known, but its absence may well explain the central nervous system defects in DMD as well as the muscle involvement. Alternatively, the association of learning difficulties with DMD may be due to the presence of other unknown genes within the DMD gene, which may be damaged by DNA deletions.

Physical phenotype, natural history and life expectancy

DMD is a degenerative neuromuscular disorder and is the most severe of the muscular dystrophies. However, the condition can be very variable, and it is not always easily differentiated from the more benign Becker muscular dystrophy. The defect in dystrophin causes the breakdown and loss of muscle cells, with resultant progressive muscle weakness and loss of motor function. Onset of the disease is insidious. In the early years motor development is delayed, and in about half the cases walking is not attained before the age of approximately 18 months. Difficulty in walking begins to show at the age of 1 to 3 years. A waddling gait, clumsiness and falling become increasingly obvious, and progressive scoliosis and joint contractures develop. Weakness and wasting of muscles is usually symmetrical, affecting the proximal muscles of the lower extremities, pelvic girdle, trunk and abdomen. Eventually a wheelchair becomes necessary, typically at 10 to 12 years of age. The disease progresses through the upper body, with progressive respiratory muscle weakness and increasing respiratory insufficiency. Death usually occurs in the late teens or early twenties due to respiratory or cardiac failure.

Creatine kinase activity is raised in the serum of boys with DMD, the most likely explanation for this being that the enzyme originates in muscle and escapes into the serum. The level falls as the disease progresses. The characteristic features of muscle histology are necrosis and phagocytosis of scattered individual muscle fibres, which are replaced by fat and connective tissue. Some studies have described morphologic changes in the brains of affected individuals and low brain weight, but this has not been confirmed in other studies. CT and MRI have revealed cerebral atrophy in some affected individuals with low IQ, but they have yielded normal findings in other cases. Abnormal dendritic development and arborization have been noted in at least some cases.

Female carriers of DMD occasionally manifest some features of the disease, which may include varying degrees of muscle weakness.

Psychological and behavioural phenotype

Affected males exhibit a range of developmental and cognitive deficits. These are non-progressive and do not appear to correlate either with the duration or severity of the disorder, or with the site and size of the genetic deletions (Clarke and Miller 1992).

Boys with DMD typically present with general developmental delay, especially in the acquisition of language and in gross motor development. Clumsiness and falling become increasingly obvious. The mean full scale IQ of affected individuals is 85, but IQ is not normally distributed. Approximately 20 per cent of all cases have global learning difficulties, and up to one half of these are in the range of severe impairment. There is a notable discrepancy between verbal and performance abilities, with verbal abilities, and especially verbal expression, being more severely impaired (Dorman *et al.* 1988, Clarke and Miller 1992). This is an unexpected finding in a disorder that is associated with severe and progressive physical disabilities. There is also a high prevalence of specific learning difficulties, with three quarters of affected boys who are of normal intelligence having specific problems with reading, spelling and/or numeracy (Dorman *et al.* 1988). These are often accompanied by specific deficits in auditory processing and phonological skills, and lower scores on tests such as Information, Arithmetic, Digit Span and Coding on the Wechsler Intelligence Scale for Children. Deficits in verbal and non-verbal memory and attentional deficits have also been highlighted.

It is generally agreed that these cognitive deficits represent the central nervous system manifestations of the disorder, rather than reflecting secondary factors such as loss of education or the psychological impact of having a degenerative condition.

Affected boys show high rates of psychological and psychiatric disturbance. In particular, they show more anxiety and depressed mood than controls, and are more often described as having poor peer relationships and being solitary. Affected boys with lower IQs are particularly at risk for such difficulties. Depressive disorder, isolation and withdrawal become even more prominent in older boys, and can be considered an expected psychological response in young people with a disabling, progressive and life-threatening disorder (Fitzpatrick *et al.* 1986). It has been suggested that boys with DMD have a higher incidence of emotional disturbance than other physically impaired children without cerebral involvement, but this finding has yet to be confirmed.

KEY REFERENCES

Clarke, M.A., Miller, G. (1992) 'Xp21-linked muscular dystrophy.' *In:* Miller, G., Ramer, J.C. (Eds.) *Static Encephalopathies of Infancy and Childhood.* New York: Raven Press, pp. 331–341.

Dorman, C., Hurley, A.D., d'Avignon, J. (1988) 'Language and learning disorders of older boys with Duchenne muscular dystrophy.' *Developmental Medicine and Child Neurology,* **30,** 316–327.

Emery, A.E.H. (1993) *Duchenne Muscular Dystrophy. 2nd Edn.* Oxford: Oxford University Press.

Fitzpatrick, C., Barry, C., Garvey, C. (1986) 'Psychiatric disorder among boys with Duchenne muscular dystrophy.' *Developmental Medicine and Child Neurology,* **28,** 589–595.

Iannaccone, S.T. (1992) 'Current status of Duchenne muscular dystrophy.' *Pediatric Clinics of North America,* **39,** 879–894.

ADDITIONAL REFERENCES

Duchenne, G.B. (1872) *De l'Électrisation Localisée et de Son Application à la Pathologie et à la Thérapeutique par Courants Induits et par Courants Galvaniques Interrompus et Continus.* 3rd Edn. Paris: Baillière.

Hoffman, E.P., Brown, R.H., Kunkel, L.M. (1987) 'Dystrophin: the protein product of the Duchenne muscular dystrophy locus.' *Cell,* **51,** 919–928.

Meryon, E. (1852) 'On granular and fatty degeneration of the voluntary muscles.' *Medico-Chirurgical Transactions,* **35,** 73.

15q MARKER CHROMOSOME SYNDROME

Alternative names
Partial trisomy 15; tetrasomy 15.

First description
The syndrome was first described by Parker and Alfi (1972). Gillberg *et al.* (1991) proposed a distinct behavioural phenotype associated with this marker chromosome.

Incidence/prevalence
The incidence of this syndrome is unknown. It has been detected in eight out of 600 cases presenting to an autism clinic in Sweden over a 20 year period (Gillberg 1992). An affected female as well as males have been described (Ghaziuddin *et al.* 1993).

Genetics/aetiology
Affected individuals have a maternally derived supernumerary isodicentric chromosome 15 marker. Although referred to as trisomy 15, Hotopf and Bolton (1995) argue that the syndrome is more accurately labelled tetrasomy 15, since affected individuals have four copies of the chromosome region 15pter–q13.

Physical phenotype, natural history and life expectancy
Affected individuals present a strikingly similar clinical picture, though with some phenotypic variability (Gillberg *et al.* 1991). They have a characteristic facial appearance, with large protruding ears and a high arched palate. Epicanthal folds and hypertelorism, short stature, low weight, muscular hypotonia and kyphoscoliosis are associated features in several cases.

The natural history of the condition is not known. Delayed gross and fine motor development and coordination difficulties are characteristic, and myoclonic epilepsy is common, with onset in late childhood.

Psychological and behavioural phenotype
Affected individuals typically have severe or profound learning difficulties, with IQs below 50. However, two cases with moderate cognitive impairment have been reported (M. King, personal communication 1993).

Early onset autism or autistic-type features have been described in affected individuals, with gaze avoidance, limited language development, stereotypic behaviours, resistance to environmental change, hand flapping, echolalia, and severe deficits in social interaction and communication (Gillberg *et al.* 1991, Hotopf and Bolton 1995). However, it is not clear how characteristic these features are of the syndrome. The two individuals reported by King to have moderate learning difficulties were considered to have language disorders but not to be autistic. Hyperactivity is a common feature, and episodic hyperventilation and hand wringing have been reported in some cases.

A few of the mothers of affected individuals and other relatives are described as showing gaze avoidant behaviour and/or having had speech–language difficulties and specific learning difficulties.

KEY REFERENCES

Ghaziuddin, M., Sheldon, S., Venkataraman, S., Tsai, L., Ghaziuddin, N. (1993) 'Autism associated with tetrasomy 15: a further report.' *European Child and Adolescent Psychiatry*, **2**, 226–230.

Gillberg, C. (1992) 'Maternally derived marker chromosome 15pter–q13 in autism: clinical and epidemiological aspects.' *Paper presented at the 2nd International Symposium of the Society for the Study of Behavioural Phenotypes, Welshpool, November 1992.* (Abstracts available from Dr Gregory O'Brien, Northgate Hospital, Northumberland.)

—— Steffenburg, S., Wahlström, J., Gillberg, I.C., Sjöstedt, A., Martinsson, T., Liedgren, S., Eeg-Olofsson, O. (1991) 'Autism associated with marker chromosome.' *Journal of the American Academy of Child and Adolescent Psychiatry*, **30**, 489–494.

Hotopf, M., Bolton, P. (1995) 'A case of autism associated with partial tetrasomy 15.' *Journal of Autism and Developmental Disorders*, **25**, 41–49.

ADDITIONAL REFERENCE

Parker, C.E., Alfi, O.S. (1972) 'Partial trisomy of chromosome 15.' *Lancet*, **1**, 1073. *(Letter.)*

FRAGILE X SYNDROME

Alternative names

Fra(X) syndrome; Martin–Bell syndrome; Renpenning syndrome.

First description

Martin and Bell (1943) were among the first to describe a pattern of cognitive impairment in males that appeared to be sex-linked. Lubs (1969) identified a fragile site on the long arm of the X chromosome (at Xq27.3) in members of one affected family, and Sutherland (1977) showed that the expression of this fragile site could be induced by culturing blood cells in a folate-deficient medium. More recently, Verkerk *et al.* (1991) described multiple CGG repeat sequences at Xq27.3, producing local hypermethylation and impaired gene expression.

Incidence/prevalence

The fragile X syndrome is the second most common genetic cause of learning difficulties after Down syndrome, and it is the most common inherited form of learning difficulties. It is found across all racial and ethnic groups, affecting 1:1250 males and 1:2000 females. It accounts for approximately 8 per cent of all children with learning difficulties.

Genetics/aetiology

The condition is X-linked but is transmitted atypically: 80 per cent of males who carry the fragile X gene have learning difficulties, while 20 per cent appear to be clinically and cytogenetically unaffected. Up to one third of carrier females also have learning difficulties, and many of the remaining two thirds have specific learning disabilities.

The chromosomal anomaly responsible for the fragile X syndrome has been identified and mapped to the distal end of the long arm of the X chromosome, in the region of Xq27.3. The fragile site is revealed only by culturing lymphocytes in a folate- or thymidylate-deficient medium, and it is found in a variable number (usually 10–40 per cent) of lymphocytes. The fragile X mental retardation–1 (*FMR-1*) gene has been sequenced, and a repeating segment of cytosine guanine guanine (CGG) nucleotides of variable length has been identified within this region (Verkerk *et al.* 1991, Yu *et al.* 1991). The DNA replications grow transgenerationally, the increase being more frequent at female meiosis than during male meiosis. The length of the repeat sequences is correlated with the degree of clinical involvement. It is suggested that when the number of repetitions becomes excesssive, methylation and subsequent silencing of the *FMR-1* gene occurs, disturbing protein synthesis and resulting in the fragile X phenotype. However, the structure and function of the *FMR-1* gene product have yet to be fully determined.

The findings that the chromosomal fragile site is not detectable in up to 50 per cent of females known to be carriers of the fragile X chromosome, and that there are apparently normal male carriers who transmit the fragile X to their daughters, support the claim for a premutation stage which does not express itself phenotypically or yields only subtle anomalies. Premutations have a high risk of transition to full mutations when transmitted by a female, and the size of the premutation has been shown to determine the risk of transition from premutation to full mutation.

Variants of the fragile X syndrome (*FRAXA*) have been identified. *FRAXE* and *FRAXF* are both related to similar abnormal DNA expansions on the X chromosome, slightly nearer the tip of the chromosome's long arm than *FRAXA*. Learning disabilities are found in these variants, though the fragile X behavioural phenotype is probably not present.

Physical phenotype, natural history and life expectancy

A distinctive pattern of physical features is associated with the fragile X syndrome, although there is wide variability in phenotypic expression, and no feature is pathognomonic (Hagerman and Silverman 1991). A triad of physical features, including large or prominent ears, a long face and post-pubertal testicular enlargement, is found in approximately 80 per cent of affected adult males.

The typical facial appearance in adults is long and narrow, with a prominent jaw and large, protruding ears; these features are not always evident in pre-pubertal males. A high arched palate, dental crowding and abnormal dermatoglyphics on hands and feet are common, while epicanthal folds, ptosis and low-set ears have been noted in under 25 per cent of affected children. In female carriers the common facial features are more subtle, and include a high, broad forehead, prominent ears and a long narrow face. These features are observed much more frequently in female carriers who have learning difficulties.

Connective tissue dysplasia has been demonstrated, which produces joint laxity, soft velvety skin, flat feet and mitral valve prolapse. Above average birthweight, overgrowth in the early years, microcephaly, hypotonia and early failure to thrive are further common findings. Life expectancy is probably similar to that in the general population, though there may be some premature deaths due to cardiovascular complications.

Neurological research indicates widespread central nervous system dysfunction, with specific vulnerability arising within the non-dominant hemisphere, parietal areas and posterior fossa. The limited neuropathologic information available to date indicates immaturity of dendritic spines, and decreased areas of synaptic contacts. Reiss *et al.* (1991) found cerebellar vermis hypoplasia, and more recently Reiss (1993) reported enlargement of the caudate nucleus and increased cerebrospinal fluid in the ventricular compartments of affected individuals, indicating cortical atrophy. Seizures occur in some 20 per cent of males (usually generalized tonic–clonic), but they mostly remit with age. EEG findings include high-voltage activity with diffuse spikes and sharp waves and temporal spike activities during sleep in some cases, though non-specific findings are more prevalent.

Psychological and behavioural phenotype

The fragile X syndrome is associated with a distinctive cognitive and behavioural profile, which is often of more help diagnostically than the physical characteristics of the syndrome, particularly in prepubertal males (Hagerman and Silverman 1991, Turk 1992).

Learning difficulties are common, more marked in males than in females, although even in males cognitive abilities span a wide range. Approximately 80 per cent of fragile X males have learning difficulties; these are mostly in the mild to moderate range, but some 30 per cent have severe learning difficulties. Cognitive level appears to be related to the number of CGG repeats present and the degree of methylation (*e.g.* Abrams *et al.* 1994). There is a characteristic uneven profile of abilities, with verbal abilities being superior to performance abilities, and relative strengths in vocabulary, aspects of simultaneous processing and some visual–perceptual tasks. Affected individuals are much weaker on tasks of abstract reasoning, sequential processing, visuospatial abilities, short-term auditory and visual memory, pragmatics, topic maintenance and number concepts (*e.g.* Dykens *et al.* 1987). They tend to have greater difficulty in processing sequential and novel information than in learning school-related verbally based factual material (Reiss and Freund 1990). Even individuals with average or above average IQ have the specific cognitive deficits detailed above, with accompanying learning disabilities. The rate of intellectual development appears to decline with age, the most notable decline being in the early pubertal years, but this may be at least in part because cognitive testing in adolescents and adults relies increasingly on problem solving and reasoning tasks, and on sequential information processing skills, at which individuals with fragile X tend to perform poorly.

Language difficulties range from a complete absence of speech through to mild communication difficulties. A characteristic speech pattern referred to as 'cluttering' is observed, in which the rate of talking is fast and fluctuating, with occasional garbled, repetitive, disorganized and dysrhythmic speech, and in the presence of poor topic maintenance, tangential comments and revisions. Dysfluent conversation is common, with incomplete sentences, echolalia and verbal perseveration. The speech frequently has a jocular quality to it, with swings of pitch ('litany-like'). Articulation problems, too, are a common finding, probably due to the combination of a high arched palate, tempero-mandibular joint laxity and the central processing difficulties.

In the early years many children with fragile X are hypotonic, and motor milestones are likely to be delayed. Gross and fine motor coordination and motor planning remain poor, which affects handwriting.

The behavioural characteristics of fragile X males are equally striking, and are considered to be significant problems in approximately 80 per cent of cases. They include hyperactivity, impulsivity and marked concentration problems, even in higher functioning individuals. Irritability, tantrums and aggressive outbursts are also reported to be characteristic, and are often precipitated by overstimulation in the environment. On the other hand, Einfeld *et al.* (1994) caution that hyperactivity and aggression are not necessarily more common in individuals with fragile X than they are in others matched for cognitive level. A number of studies have shown improved behaviour and attention, and decreased hyperactivity, in a small number of pre-pubertal children with fragile X who were treated with folic acid. Stimulant medication has also been found to be helpful in some cases. Hyperactivity in fragile X tends to decrease with age, but attention difficulties and impulsivity remain problems for many adolescent and adult males. Increased rates of obsessive compulsive behaviours, alcohol abuse and antisocial personality disorder have also been reported in adult male carriers.

There is a spectrum of autistic-like behaviours among fragile X males, including gaze aversion (in up to 90 per cent of cases), stereotypic repetitive behaviours such as hand flapping, repetitive speech, resistance to environmental change, and perseverative preoccupations and interests (*e.g.* Reiss and Freund 1992). However, only a minority of affected individuals have autism. The social indifference and severely disturbed social relations that characterize autistic individuals are in general not found in people with fragile X. Most affected males are affectionate and have an interest in relating socially, but they have notable social interactional deficits and tend to be shy and anxious in social situations. Also, in contrast to the relatively meaningless echolalia associated with autism, the frequent self-repetition seen in individuals with fragile X is felt to serve an important communicatory function, maintaining social interaction in the presence of information processing difficulties (Turk 1992). Affected males are easily overwhelmed by a variety of excessive sensory stimuli. Sensory defensiveness may account for their poor eye contact and gaze avoidance, which can be seen as attempts to avoid excessive stimulation. Other features such as hand-biting and hand-flapping are common, and may be provoked by excitement and/or frustration. In many cases the autistic features become less evident after puberty.

Adult males with fragile X show strengths in daily living skills, relative to their communication and socialization abilities (Dykens *et al.* 1994); nevertheless, independent living is not possible for many.

Symptomatic females with fragile X demonstrate learning and behavioural abnormalities that are similar in quality to, but less severe than, those seen in affected males (*e.g.* Freund *et al.* 1993). Some 25 per cent of females have learning difficulties (IQ < 70), and 25 per cent have borderline intellectual abilities. However, learning disabilities and behavioural and emotional difficulties are common even in carrier females with normal IQ. As is the case in affected males, verbal abilities tend to be better than performance skills, and deficits in arithmetic, visuospatial abilities and short-term auditory memory are common (manifesting as low scores on the Arithmetic, Block Design and Digit Span subtests of the Wechsler adult or child intelligence scales). The spoken language of carrier females may be high pitched, with repetitions and poor topic maintenance. Mazzocco *et al.* (1992) and Sobesky *et al.* (1994) have confirmed findings of deficits on measures of frontal lobe function in affected females with normal IQ, including difficulties with planning, sustaining effort, generating problem-solving strategies, using feedback and self-monitoring. Difficulties with transitions, abstract concept formation and information processing are also apparent, as well as with perseverative thinking, attention (with or without hyperactivity), impulsivity, tangential language and topic maintenance, and motor delay.

Extreme shyness, anxiety, social avoidance, withdrawal and poor eye contact are also commonly reported in females with fragile X (Freund *et al.* 1993). These features may be apparent by the preschool years and persist through adolescence and adulthood. There are also indications of increased prevalence of psychiatric problems in adult females with fragile X, notably depressive disorders and schizotypal features such as odd communication patterns, inappropriate affect, unusual thought content, and increased emotional lability (Reiss *et al.* 1988). Stereotypies are also frequently noted. Parental origin of the fragile X chromosome, and the extent of expressivity are thought to be important determinants of psychopathology, in that females who inherit the fragile X gene from their mothers, and who demonstrate positive fragility, have been found to show greater social, educational and psychological difficulties, when compared with females who inherit the fragile X chromosome from their fathers (Dykens *et al.* 1994).

KEY REFERENCES

Baumgardner, T., Green, K., Reiss, A.L. (1992) 'The psychological effects associated with fragile X syndrome.' *Current Opinions in Pediatrics*, **4**, 609–615
Dykens, E.M., Hodapp, R.M., Leckman, J.F. (1994) *Behavior and Development in Fragile X Syndrome.* London: Sage Publications.
Hagerman, R.J., Silverman, A.C. (Eds.) (1991) *Fragile X Syndrome: Diagnosis, Treatment and Research.* Baltimore: Johns Hopkins University Press.
Reiss, A.L., Freund, L. (1990) 'Fragile X syndrome.' *Biological Psychiatry*, **27**, 223–240.
Turk, J. (1992) 'The fragile X syndrome. On the way to a behavioural phenotype.' *British Journal of Psychiatry*, **160**, 24–35.

ADDITIONAL REFERENCES

Abrams, M.T., Reiss, A.L., Freund, L.S., Baumgardener, T.L., Chase, G.A., Denckla, M.B. (1994) 'Molecular–neurobehavioral associations in females with the fragile X full mutation.' *American Journal of Medical Genetics*, **51**, 317–327.
Dykens, E.M., Hodapp, R.M., Leckman, J.F (1987) ' Strengths and weaknesses in the intellectual functioning of males with fragile X syndrome.' *American Journal of Mental Deficiency*, **92**, 234–236.
Einfeld, S.L., Tonge, B.J., Florio, T. (1994) 'Behavioural and emotional disturbance in fragile X syndrome.' *American Journal of Medical Genetics*, **51**, 386–391.
Freund, L.S., Reiss, A.L., Abrams, M.T. (1993) 'Psychiatric disorders associated with fragile X in the young female.' *Pediatrics*, **91**, 321–329.
Lubs, H.A. (1969) 'A marker X chromosome.' *American Journal of Human Genetics*, **21**, 231–244.
Martin, J.P., Bell, J. (1943) 'A pedigree of mental defect showing sex-linkage.' *Journal of Neurology and Psychiatry*, **6**, 154–157.
Mazzocco, M.M.M., Hagerman, R.J., Cronister-Silverman, A., Pennington, B.F. (1992) 'Specific frontal lobe deficits among women with the fragile X gene.' *Journal of the American Academy of Child and Adolescent Psychiatry*, **31**, 1141–1148.
Reiss, A.L. (1993) 'The contribution of neuroimaging in understanding the biological substrate of the fragile X syndrome.' *Paper presented at the 4th Annual Meeting of the Society for the Study of Behavioural Phenotypes, London, December 1993.* (Abstracts available from Dr Gregory O'Brien, Northgate Hospital, Northumberland.)
—— Freund, L. (1992) 'Behavioral phenotype of fragile X syndrome: DSM-III-R autistic behavior in male children.' *American Journal of Medical Genetics*, **43**, 35–46.
—— Hagerman, R.J., Vinogradov, S., Abrams, M., King, R.J. (1988) 'Psychiatric disability in female carriers of the fragile X chromosome.' *Archives of General Psychiatry*, **45**, 25–30.
—— Aylward, E., Freund, L.S., Joshi, P.K., Bryan, R.N. (1991) 'Neuroanatomy of fragile X syndrome: the posterior fossa.' *Annals of Neurology*, **29**, 26–32.
Sobesky, W.E., Pennington, B.F., Porter, D., Hull, C.E., Hagerman, R.J. (1994) 'Emotional and neurocognitive deficits in fragile X.' *American Journal of Medical Genetics*, **51**, 378–385.

Sutherland, G.R. (1977) 'Fragile sites on human chromosomes: demonstration of their dependence on the type of tissue culture medium.' *Science*, **197**, 265–266.

Verkerk, A.J.M.H., Pieretti, M., Sutcliffe, J.S., Fu, Y-H., Kuhl, D.P.A., Pizzuti, A., Reiner, O., Richards, S., Victoria, M.F., *et al.* (1991) 'Identification of a gene (*FMR-1*) containing a CGG repeat coincident with a breakpoint cluster region exhibiting length variation in fragile X syndrome.' *Cell*, **65**, 905–914.

Yu, S., Pritchard, M., Kremer, E., Lynch, M., Nancarrow, J., Baker, E., Holman, K., Mulley, J.C., Warren, S.T., *et al.* (1991) 'Fragile X genotype characterized by an unstable region of DNA.' *Science*, **252**, 1179–1181.

(CLASSICAL) GALACTOSAEMIA

The three disorders of galactose metabolism, all inherited as autosomal recessive disorders, are classical galactosaemia (galactose-1-phosphate uridyl transferase deficiency), galactokinase deficiency, and epimerase deficiency. This section addresses the most common and most severe of these disorders, classical galactosaemia.

First description
The first detailed description of classical galactosaemia was by Mason and Turner (1935).

Incidence/prevalence
The reported incidence varies considerably in different populations. A large scale survey found a rate of 1:40,000 to 1:60,000 live births in the UK and one of 1:23,500 live births in Ireland (Honeyman *et al.* 1993). Males and females are equally affected.

Genetics/aetiology
Classical galactosaemia is an autosomal recessive inborn error of galactose metabolism caused by a deficiency of the enzyme galactose-1-phosphate uridyl transferase (*GALT*), which participates in the conversion of galactose to glucose. Marked deficiency in transferase activity results in the accumulation of galactose and galactose-1 phosphate in the blood and tissues. The *GALT* gene has now been isolated and cloned (Elsas *et al.* 1993), and a number of gene mutations have been uncovered, the most common of which is *Q188R*. This molecular heterogeneity might explain some of the observed clinical heterogeneity of the disorder.

Physical phenotype, natural history and life expectancy
Affected individuals present in the neonatal period with feeding difficulties, vomiting, lethargy, hypotonia, failure to thrive, hepatocellular damage (jaundice, hepatomegaly), renal tubular damage, hypoglycaemia, brain damage and cataracts. These symptoms may be acute and life threatening, with septicaemia, coagulopathy and encephalopathy, or more chronic with ongoing liver disease and growth problems. There is a high mortality if the disorder is untreated. However, once galactose is removed from the diet, there is rapid clinical and biochemical improvement (Honeyman *et al.* 1993).

Dietary treatment must be life-long. However, it does not ameliorate the long-term complications, which occur in the majority of cases regardless of when treatment was begun, the degree of compliance with the diet, or the severity of neonatal symptoms (Waggoner *et al.* 1990). These complications include ovarian failure in at least 80 per cent of females, motor function abnormalities, developmental delay, and growth retardation in about 20 per cent of cases. The period of growth tends to be prolonged, so that ultimate height and weight are usually satisfactory (Waggoner *et al.* 1990). There are no typical facial characteristics associated with the condition. A third of cases have cataracts, although half of these are mild and resolve with the dietary treatment.

The life expectancy of treated individuals appears to be normal. Some researchers suggest that neurological complications become more prevalent with age, with development of cerebellar ataxia, intention tremor, apraxia and extrapyramidal dysfunction (Friedman et al. 1989, Schweitzer et al. 1993). It is not clear whether this is due to the enzyme defect alone or to other closely linked genetic abnormalities.

MRI and CT scans reveal a lack of normal myelination, multifocal areas of increased signal in the cerebral white matter on T_2-weighted images, ventricular enlargement and mild cerebral and cerebellar atrophy.

Psychological and behavioural phenotype

Even with early diagnosis and immediate treatment, psychological and cognitive difficulties are apparent. Cognitive abilities are on average in the borderline or low-average IQ range. About half of a sample of 177 cases reviewed by Waggoner et al. (1990) were reported to have learning and particularly language difficulties, despite good adherence to the dietary treatment. Overall, verbal abilities tend to be significantly poorer than performance abilities, and even children with IQs in the average range have a high prevalence of speech and language problems (Nelson et al. 1991, Schweitzer et al. 1993, Waisbren et al. 1983). Difficulties are most marked in the area of expressive language, and include verbal dyspraxia, limited vocabulary, word finding difficulties, articulation disorders and deficits in verbal recall. Nelson et al. have described problems with word retrieval, grammar and syntax, transpositions of words in sentences, and deficits in abstract reasoning in over half of their galactosaemic sample. This association of galactosaemia with speech problems, and in particular with verbal dyspraxia, is noteworthy. In contrast, receptive language tends to be age-appropriate. Specific visual–perceptual deficits have also been noted in up to half of the cases, and just under 20 per cent of Waggoner et al.'s sample were further described as having problems with coordination, gait and balance.

Overall, IQ scores and the presence of speech problems and dyspraxia are not highly correlated with the severity of the symptoms, nor with the age at which treatment was begun, nor with the extent of compliance with the dietary treatment. There are a number of reports of slowly progressive encephalopathy in affected adults. Waggoner et al. and Schweitzer et al. further reported a decline in IQ scores with increasing age. This might be regarded as evidence for progressive brain damage, possibly of postnatal origin. Alternatively, it may be explained by the use of different cognitive measures at different ages.

Behavioural characteristics reported to be associated with galactosaemia include lack of confidence, anxiety, social withdrawal and shyness (Sardharwalla and Wraith 1987). These characteristics are not related to level of cognitive ability. Lack of self-esteem and assertiveness continue into adulthood and can lead to difficulty in obtaining independent employment. However, other affected adults are reported to cope well with work, marriage and parenthood.

KEY REFERENCES

Nelson, C.D., Waggoner, D.D., Donnell, G.N., Tuerck, J.M., Buist, N.R.M. (1991) 'Verbal dyspraxia in treated galactosemia.' *Pediatrics*, **88**, 346–350.

Sardharwalla, I.B., Wraith, J.E. (1987) 'Galactosaemia.' *Nutrition and Health*, **5**, 175–188.

Schweitzer, S., Shin, Y., Jakobs, C., Brodehl, J. (1993) 'Long-term outcome in 134 patients with galactos-aemia.' *European Journal of Pediatrics*, **152**, 36–43.

Waggoner, D.D., Buist, N.R.M., Donnell, G.N. (1990) 'Long-term prognosis in galactosaemia: results of a survey of 350 cases.' *Journal of Inherited Metabolic Disease*, **13**, 802–818.

ADDITIONAL REFERENCES

Elsas, L.J., Fridovich-Keil, J.L., Leslie, N.D. (1993) 'Galactosemia: a molecular approach to the enigma.' *International Pediatrics*, **8**, 101–109.

Friedman, J.H., Levy, H.L., Boustany, R-M. (1989) 'Late onset of distinct neurologic syndromes in galac-tosemic siblings.' *Neurology*, **39**, 741–742.

Honeyman, M.M., Green, A., Holton, J.B., Leonard, J.V. (1993) 'Galactosaemia: results of the British Paediatric Surveillance Unit study, 1988–90.' *Archives of Disease in Childhood*, **69**, 339–341.

Mason, H.H., Turner, M.E. (1935) 'Chronic galactosaemia' *American Journal of Diseases of Children*, **50**, 359.

Waisbren, S.E., Norman, T.R., Schnell, R.R., Levy, H.L. (1983) 'Speech and language deficits in early-treated children with galactosemia.' *Journal of Pediatrics*, **102**, 75–77.

HYPOMELANOSIS OF ITO

Alternative names

Ito syndrome; incontinentia pigmenti achromians.

First description

The syndrome was first described by Ito (1952), who termed it incontinentia pigmenti achromians. The name 'hypomelanosis of Ito' was suggested by Jelinek *et al.* (1973) to avoid confusion with the disorder Bloch–Schulzberger incontinentia pigmenti.

Incidence/prevalence

The prevalence of hypomelanosis of Ito is not known, but it is one of the most frequent neuroectodermal disorders. Pascual-Castroviejo *et al.* (1988) reported an incidence of one per 1000 new patients consulting a paediatric neurology service. Some studies report an estimated female:male ratio of 2:1, while others argue for an equal sex ratio. Black people have been over-represented in most of the published reports, which may be because the skin changes typical of the syndrome are more easily detected in people with pigmented skin.

Genetics/aetiology

The aetiology of the syndrome is still not clear. Most cases are sporadic. A variety of different chromosome mosaicisms have been reported, most commonly involving the X chromosome, leading Ritter *et al.* (1990) and others to postulate hypomelanosis of Ito as a non-specific marker for chromosome mosaicism. However, mosaicism cannot be demonstrated in every case. There are a few purported cases of familial transmission of the syndrome, but the diagnosis in some of these cases is doubtful. The mechanisms by which the mosaicism leads to abnormal pigmentation and to the other manifestations of the syndrome are not known.

Physical phenotype, natural history and life expectancy

Hypomelanosis of Ito comprises a heterogeneous group of symptoms. In all cases there are skin pigment abnormalities, which are present at birth or appear during infancy. These consist of unilateral or bilateral streaks, whorls or patches of hypopigmented skin occurring in bizarre patterns anywhere on the body (though seldom on the face), and often following the lines of Blaschko. Histological examination of these areas reveals a reduction in the number of melanin granules in the basal layer of the epidermis. The skin changes typically persist throughout childhood, but are said to become less conspicuous in adulthood. Other skin alterations have been reported in approximately one third of one series of cases, and include café-au-lait spots and angiomatous naevi. Diffuse alopecia and mottled hair have also been reported.

Approximately 90 per cent of affected individuals have additional associated anomalies, including early onset epilepsy, which can be difficult to treat; asymmetry of the body; skeletal abnormalities, notably scoliosis, joint contractures and unequal bone length; eye abnormalities (corneal opacity, microphthalmia and strabismus); malformations of the facial bones and coarse facial features; macrocephaly; hemihypertrophy of part or the entire side of the body; and hypotonia. Other features that have been reported in the literature are genital anomalies, inguinal hernia, congenital heart disease, hypertelorism and cleft palate. Oral anomalies include conical teeth, partial anodontia, dental hypoplasia or dysplasia, and defective enamel.

CT scans may reveal asymmetrical cerebral atrophy, abnormal density of white matter, and neuronal migration defects. MRI is more reliable in showing parenchymal lesions affecting both white and grey matter. Histological findings include pachygyria, multiple grey matter heterotopias and basal ganglia dysplasia in the cerebrum, mild atrophy with heterotopias, Purkinje cells in the granular layer, increase of Bergmann glia in the cerebellum, and non-specific alterations in the brainstem and spinal cord.

Psychological and behavioural phenotype

Psychomotor delay, speech delay and ataxic gait have been reported in at least some affected children. Moderate to severe learning difficulties are characteristic of about 60 per cent of cases; a further 15 per cent have borderline intellectual abilities. There does not appear to be a correlation between the extent of the hypopigmented skin and severity of cognitive impairment.

An association between hypomelanosis of Ito and autism has been frequently noted in the literature. Autism or autistic-like behaviours have been reported in at least 10 per cent of cases (Pascual-Castroviejo *et al.* 1988), while Zappella (1992) reported a prevalence rate of 18 per cent for the syndrome among children with autism. Åkefeldt and Gillberg (1991) found three children with hypomelanosis of Ito in a clinical sample of some 600 cases with autism and autistic-like conditions. These children presented with clinical symptoms of autism or Asperger syndrome (aloof and uninterested in social interactions, with stereotypic behaviours); they became less withdrawn after age 7 years, but continued to show extreme gaze avoidance. The children also displayed self-injurious behaviours, including wrist and knuckle biting. Zappella (1992) has found severe sleep disorders and hyperactivity in affected individuals.

KEY REFERENCES

Åkefeldt, A., Gillberg, C. (1991) 'Hypomelanosis of Ito in three cases with autism and autistic-like conditions.' *Developmental Medicine and Child Neurology*, **33**, 737–743.

Glover, M.T., Brett, E.M., Atherton, D.J. (1989) 'Hypomelanosis of Ito: spectrum of the disease.' *Journal of Pediatrics*, **115**, 75–80.

Pascual-Castroviejo, I., López-Rodriguez, L., de la Cruz Medina, M., Salamanca-Maesso, C., Herrero, C.R. (1988) 'Hypomelanosis of Ito. Neurological complications in 34 cases.' *Canadian Journal of Neurological Sciences*, **15**, 124–129.

Ruiz-Maldonado, R., Toussaint, S., Tamayo, L., Laterza, A., del Castillo, V. (1992) 'Hypomelanosis of Ito: diagnostic criteria and report of 4l cases.' *Pediatric Dermatology*, **9**, 1–10.

Zappella, M.(1992) 'Hypomelanosis of Ito is frequently associated with autism.' *European Journal of Child and Adolescent Psychiatry*, **1**, 170–177.

ADDITIONAL REFERENCES

Ito, M. (1952) 'Studies on melanin. XI. Incontinentia pigmenti achromians. A singular case of nevus depigmentosus systematicus bilateralis.' *Tohoku Journal of Experimental Medicine*, **55**, 57–59.

Jelinek, J.E., Bart, R.S., Schiff, G.M. (1973) 'Hypomelanosis of Ito ('incontinentia pigmenti achromians'). Report of three cases and review of the literature.' *Archives of Dermatology*, **107**, 596–601.

Ritter, C.L., Steele, M.W., Wenger, S.L., Cohen, B.A. (1990) 'Chromosome mosaicism in hypomelanosis of Ito.' *American Journal of Medical Genetics*, **35**, 14–17.

LESCH–NYHAN SYNDROME

First description
The syndrome was first reported in two brothers by Lesch and Nyhan (1964).

Incidence/prevalence
Estimates of incidence range from 1:380,000 live births to 1:10,000 male births. The syndrome occurs almost exclusively in males and is found across many racial and ethnic groups.

Genetics/aetiology
Lesch–Nyhan syndrome is an X-linked recessive disorder. It results from a virtually complete deficiency of the enzyme hypoxanthine phosphoribosyltransferase (HPRT), which is important in purine metabolsim, and this leads to an overproduction of xanthine and uric acid. HPRT is encoded by a single gene on the X chromosome which has been mapped to Xq26–27 (Stout and Caskey 1989). The mutations which result in HPRT deficiency are varied, and include point mutations, deletions and partial deletions and insertions. Most do not represent major gene alterations. Affected males inherit the mutation from asymptomatic carrier females or as the result of *de novo* mutations. A few affected female homozygotes have been reported.

Physical features, natural history and life expectancy
Affected infants appear normal at birth, but motor delay and hypotonia become apparent within the first few months. Involuntary choreoathetoid movements develop between 8 and 12 months, and at about 1 year of age hyperreflexia and clonus appear. Dystonic posturing may be noted, with torticollis, and retrocollis and ballistic movements may occur. The degree of motor disability remains severe. Because of poor muscle control, affected individuals are not able to walk or sit without support; most are unable to keep the head erect. During the first three months of life the infants may be unusually irritable, and most have difficulty feeding. Height and weight generally remain well below the third centile, and bone age is typically delayed. About 50 per cent of cases have seizures, and microcephaly is reported in some cases.

The abnormalities of purine metabolism associated with the syndrome lead to hyperuricaemia, markedly increased excretion of uric acid in the urine, crystalluria and renal stones early in life. Urinary tract infections and haematuria continue to cause problems in many cases.

There is no effective treatment for the severe neurological complications of the syndrome, and death usually occurs in early adulthood, usually as a result of infection or renal failure.

The brains of affected individuals show no specific morphological abnormalities. The characteristics of the syndrome, including the characteristic movement disorder and self-injurious behaviour, are believed to result from central nervous system dysfunction, but the mechanisms of the neurological impairment have not yet been determined. Recent evidence shows that certain motor neurons are in a state of hyperexcitability in affected individuals (Hatanaka *et al.* 1990), and it is thought that metabolic and/or neurological abnormalities cause innervation of muscles, resulting in the self-injurious behaviour. Neuropathologic studies have found reduced dopamine levels in the basal ganglia of affected individuals, and it is suggested that this leads to striatal dopamine D1 receptor supersensitivity. The basal ganglia normally contain a high concentration of HPRT and therefore may be vulnerable to HPRT deficiency. However, the exact relationship between HPRT deficiency and abnormal striatal dopamine function is not known.

Psychological and behavioural phenotype

Severe motor impairment and poor gross and fine motor coordination are characteristic, and represent a mixture of abnormal movements, spasticity and ataxia. Delayed speech development and dysarthria are also common features. Speech is largely unintelligible.

On cognitive testing most affected individuals are found to have moderate or severe learning difficulties. A small number have IQs in the low-average range and attain age-appropriate reading skills. More recently, researchers have suggested that measurement of IQ may seriously underestimate the cognitive abilities of affected individuals because of their limited life experience and severe physical disabilities. Anecdotal reports describe affected children as charming, and with a sophisticated sense of humour. On the basis of structured interviews with the caregivers of 42 children and young adults with Lesch–Nyhan syndrome, Anderson *et al.* (1992) found that their memory for both recent and past events was excellent; they had good awareness of their environment and good concentration, were capable of abstract reasoning, and were highly sociable, with good communication skills. Overall, 13 per cent of the sample could read at their appropriate grade level, and 15 per cent were at their grade level for mathematics. However, in 85 per cent of cases educational attainment was below age level, which may reflect specific learning disabilities in reading and mathematics.

The most striking behavioural characteristic associated with the Lesch–Nyhan syndrome is compulsive self-injurious behaviour, which is reported in over 85 per cent of cases (Christie *et al.* 1982, Anderson and Ernst 1994). This may appear as early as the first year of life or only in adolescence; the mean age of onset is between 2 and $3^1/_2$ years. The self-injurious behaviour has an extensive topography; biting of lips, fingers and the inside of the mouth is the most typical. This is frequently of such severity as to result in extensive loss of tissue, and to require arm splints or teeth extraction to prevent mutilation. Affected individuals may also attempt to injure themselves by hitting their heads against objects, picking with their fingers, or catching themselves in the spokes of their wheelchair (Nyhan 1976). Self-injurious behaviour is a common problem in other clinical populations, but generally not to the extent that is found in Lesch–Nyhan syndrome. Compulsive aggressive behaviour toward others is also common, particularly attempts to hit or bite other people, and verbal aggression.

The self-injurious behaviour can take a variable course; for example, it may manifest for weeks or months, with periods of normal behaviour in between. There appears to be an association between the severity of the self-injury and its age of onset; the earlier the onset, the worse the self-injury eventually becomes. Also, the highest rates of self-injury are associated with stressful physical or emotional events (Anderson and Ernst 1994). Reductions in the frequency of these behaviours are often reported to occur when individuals are engaged in interesting activities and social interactions (Anderson *et al.* 1992). It is now recognized that the self-injury is uncontrollable, not deliberate, and that involuntary contractions of muscles cause these movements. However, most individuals can predict when they will self-injure. Nyhan (1976) has described this paradox of the self-injurious behaviour being uncontrollable but nevertheless very much within the child's consciousness. It is evident that pain accompanies these behaviours. Most affected children want to be restrained most of the time and are happiest when restrained; they may become very agitated when their restraints are removed. With age they appear to develop some degree of control over these behaviours, for example by sitting on their hands or placing them behind their back (Christie *et al.* 1982). Self-mutilation generally becomes less pronounced after ages 10 to 12.

The absence of morphological abnormalities in Lesch–Nyhan syndrome suggests that pharmacological manipulation of central neurotransmitters and receptors may be effective in treating the self-injurious behaviour. Thus far, however, response to medications has been variable. Behaviour modification techniques, including differential reinforcement of incompatible behaviour and punishment, have also been applied, but with inconsistent results. In some cases aversive therapy was found to aggravate the self-injurious behaviour (Nyhan 1976). Stress reduction is generally viewed as a useful and effective method of intervention.

Clinical reports indicate that affected children are often very aware of their aggressive behaviours and are frustrated by their disabilities (Christie *et al.* 1982). Corbett (personal communication, 1994) found very high levels of anxiety in affected individuals, while Anderson *et al.* (1992) reported, on the basis of interviews with caregivers, that one third of a group of affected individuals aged over 11 had talked about committing suicide.

KEY REFERENCES

Anderson, L.T., Ernst, M. (1994) 'Self-injury in Lesch–Nyhan disease.' *Journal of Autism and Developmental Disorders*, **24**, 67–81.
—— —— Davis, S.V. (1992) 'Cognitive abilities of patients with Lesch–Nyhan disease.' *Journal of Autism and Developmental Disorders*, **22**, 189–203,
Christie, R., Bay, C., Kaufman, I.A., Bakay, B., Borden, M., Nyhan,W.L. (1982) 'Lesch–Nyhan disease: clinical experience with nineteen patients.' *Developmental Medicine and Child Neurology*, **24**, 293–306.
Nyhan, W.L. (1976) 'Behavior in the Lesch–Nyhan syndrome.' *Journal of Autism and Childhood Schizophrenia*, **6**, 235–252.
Stout, J.T., Caskey, C.T. (1989) 'Hypoxanthine phosphoribosyltransferase deficiency: the Lesch–Nyhan syndrome and gouty arthritis.' *In:* Scriver, C.R., Beaudet, A.L., Sly, W.S., Valle, D. (Eds.) *The Metabolic Basis of Inherited Disease. 6th Edn.* New York: McGraw-Hill, pp. 1007–1028.

ADDITIONAL REFERENCES

Hatanaka, T., Higashino, H., Woo, M., Yasuhara, A., Sugimoto, T., Kobayashi, Y. (1990) 'Lesch–Nyhan syndrome with delayed onset of self-mutilation: hyperactivity of interneurons at the brainstem and blink reflex.' *Acta Neurologica Scandinavica*, **81**, 184–187.

Lesch, M., Nyhan, W.L. (1964) 'A familial disorder of uric acid metabolism and central nervous system function.' *American Journal of Medicine*, **36**, 561–570.

LOWE SYNDROME

Alternative name
Oculocerebrorenal syndrome of Lowe (OCRL).

First description
Lowe and colleagues made their initial report of this syndrome in 1952.

Incidence/prevalence
The incidence is thought to be around 1:200,000 live births. There are an estimated 60–90 affected boys in the UK and 200–300 in the USA.

Genetics/aetiology
Lowe syndrome is an X-linked recessive disorder, normally affecting only males. All women who are obligate heterozygotes have lens opacities. This forms the basis of carrier detection. The *OCRL* gene has been mapped to Xq24–26, and there are flanking DNA probes. A candidate gene has been isolated (Attree *et al.* 1992). There are at least four girls in the literature who meet rigid diagnostic criteria for the disorder. Two have translocations at the *OCRL* locus, one has a normal unbanded 46,XX karyotype, the other has not been karyotyped. One girl with early features of the condition went on to develop a mitochondrial cytopathy (Moraes *et al.* 1991).

Physical phenotype, natural history and life expectancy
Minimal diagnostic criteria are a history of congenital cataracts, infantile hypotonia, and some evidence of renal tubular dysfunction (renal Fanconi syndrome). Confirmatory criteria are distinctive facies (deep-set eyes, frontal bossing, and a face that becomes progressively elongated), total areflexia, serum enzyme abnormalities, a history of glaucoma, corneal keloid, cryptorchidism, short stature and joint swelling.

There appear to be three distinct phases to the biomedical problems. The neonatal stage is characterized by major eye problems, while the kidneys may appear normal. The second phase, which lasts from a few months of age to mid-childhood, is characterized by increasing renal tubular dysfunction and consequent metabolic problems. The last phase usually has less severe metabolic problems. Deaths at all ages have been reported due to renal failure, dehydration or pneumonia. No survivors beyond age 40 have been reported. There are many musculoskeletal complications. These include joint hyper-mobility, recurrent fractures, scoliosis and recurrent arthritis—particularly in the teenage years. Seizures, including infantile spasms, probably occur in around 30 per cent of patients. The EEG, whenever reported, has always been markedly abnormal.

Psychological and behavioural phenotype
There have been two behavioural studies, both promoted by the US Lowe's Syndrome Association (LSA). Both are cross-sectional. The first is a descriptive study based on an

analysis of the findings from a postal questionnaire devised by the LSA (Dolinsky 1990, McSpadden 1991). The second study (Kenworthy *et al.* 1993) was designed to determine whether behaviours frequently reported among subjects can be explained as secondary to other biological effects of the disorder—*viz.* severe visual impairment and learning disability—or whether there is evidence for a specific biologically determined behavioural phenotype. They conclude cautiously in favour of the latter.

There is great commonality between the two studies which largely tapped into the same population. Most striking is the peaking of maladaptive behaviours in early adolescence. Salient points which emerge are as follows.

Behaviours secondary to visual impairment—specifically hand waving between the eyes and a light source—and self-injurious behaviours have long been recognized as part of the disorder. The recent studies report self-injurious behaviours—notably scratching, chewing the hands and head banging—in around 70 per cent across the age groups, with the highest incidence in early adolescence.

Temper outbursts occur in around 85 per cent of the total population, and in the Kenworthy *et al.* study were found in all subjects in the 12–15 age group. Dolinsky reported that more than half of his total sample had daily outbursts. In the older age groups the proportion with outbursts increased but the number having daily outbursts decreased. Both studies document screaming and yelling in nearly 70 per cent. Anecdotal accounts indicate that the intensity of these outbursts is extreme. The most common triggers for screaming vary with age but may relate to another finding by Kenworthy *et al.*, that 70 per cent of subjects needed to have their demands met immediately. Dolinsky reported that children below age 5 stop visitors' conversation by screaming; those aged 5–13 scream when they are angry; and those age 13–18 scream when people talk or stand up. Screaming and yelling become less frequent after age 18.

Stereotypies (notably repetitive shaking of limbs) interfere with more appropriate behaviours in around 80 per cent. The incidence of these falls off sharply after age 18.

Preoccupations occur in around 60 per cent. They cover a wide range of objects and situations but each child tends to have his own individual set of proccupations. Incapacitating fears, reported in 50 per cent of Dolinsky's sample, cover an even wider range but again tend to be child-specific.

70 per cent of parents of those aged 13–18 years report that difficult behaviours interfere with being able to take their child out in public.

Kenworthy *et al.* found that boys with Lowe syndrome exhibited significantly higher levels of maladaptive behaviours when compared with two control groups (non-learning-disabled children with severe visual impairment and normally sighted subjects with learning disability from other causes). Notable elevations in temper tantrums, stubbornness and stereotypy appeared on all three maladaptive measures used. They noted that the peak in maladaptive behaviours in their 12–15 year age group reflected changes in aggressive (including self-injurious) behaviours, not stereotypies.

Most importantly this study has estimates of IQ for many of the children. 25 per cent lie within the normal range, challenging the previously held consensus that the disorder is always associated with moderate or severe learning disability. Analysis of behaviour difficulties by IQ reveals that IQ accounts for only 12 per cent of the total variance in behaviour, a finding which supports the view that some at least of the behaviours may have primary biological determinants.

This investigation also addressed the possibility that parental stress might determine maladaptive behaviours but there were no correlations. Self report on one of the instruments used suggested that the parents were unusually well adjusted considering their children's problems.

Charnas and Gahl (1991) and Kenworthy *et al.* (1993) reference metabolic, neuro-anatomical and neuroimaging studies which may be relevant to mechanisms underlying the behavioural phenotype.

KEY REFERENCES

Charnas, L.R., Gahl, W.A. (1991) 'The oculocerebrorenal syndrome of Lowe.' *Advances in Pediatrics*, **38**, 75–107.
Kenworthy, L., Park, T., Charnas, L.R. (1993) 'Cognitive and behavioral profile of the oculocerebrorenal syndrome of Lowe.' *American Journal of Medical Genetics*, **46**, 297–303.
Lowe, C.U., Terrey, M., MacLachlan, E.A. (1952) 'Organic aciduria, decreased renal ammonia production, hydrophthalmos, and mental retardation: a clinical entity.' *American Journal of Diseases of Children*, **83**, 164–184.

ADDITIONAL REFERENCES

Attree, O., Olivos, I.M., Okabe, I., Bailey, L.C., Nelson, D.L., Lewis, R.A. McInnes, R.R., Nussbaum, R.L. (1992) 'The Lowe's oculocerebrorenal syndrome gene encodes a protein highly homologous to inositol polyphosphate-5-phosphatase.' *Nature*, **358**, 239–242.
Dolinsky, Z. (1990) 'Behavioural problems in Lowe's syndrome.' *Paper presented at the Behavioural Phenotypes Study Group Symposium, Welshpool, November 1990.* (Abstracts available from Dr Gregory O'Brien, Northgate Hospital, Northumberland.)
McSpadden, K. (1991) *Report of the Lowe's Syndrome Comprehensive Survey.* West Lafayette, LA: Lowe's Syndrome Association.
Moraes, C.T., Zeviani, M. Schon, E.A., Hickman, R.O., Vlcek, B.W., DiMauro, S. (1991) 'Mitochondrial DNA deletion in a girl with manifestations of Kearns–Sayre and Lowe syndromes: an example of phenotypic mimicry?' *American Journal of Medical Genetics*, **41**, 301 – 305.

MARFAN SYNDROME

First description
A French paediatrician, Antoine Marfan (1896), was the first to describe this syndrome.

Incidence/prevalence
Marfan syndrome is one of the most common inherited connective tissue disorders, with an estimated incidence of between 1:10,000 and 1:20,000 (Morse *et al.* 1990). It has an equal sex ratio and occurs across all racial and ethnic groups. There is considerable variability of clinical expression, and individuals with mild forms of the syndrome may be missed. As a result, the actual prevalence may well be greater than the estimated figure.

Genetics/aetiology
Approximately 75–85 per cent of cases of Marfan syndrome are familial, with an autosomal dominant mode of inheritance and with close to complete penetrance. The remaining cases have a negative family history and probably represent new mutations. Morse *et al.* (1990) suggest that individuals representing sporadic cases may be more severely affected than individuals with familial transmission of the syndrome.

The fibrillin gene has been mapped to the long arm of chromosome 15 at 15q21.1, and a variety of mutations have been identified in this gene (Dietz *et al.* 1993). Hollister *et al.* (1990) reported consistent abnormalities of dermal microfibrils in many individuals with Marfan syndrome. The glycoprotein fibrillin, a major constituent of microfibrils, is not synthesized normally in cultured dermal fibroblasts from many affected individuals (Milewicz *et al.* 1992). Microfibrillar fibres are widely distributed in many tissues of the body which are involved in Marfan syndrome, supporting the conclusion that fibrillin is aetiologically linked to the syndrome. Further research is needed into the pathogenesis of the disorder and the nature of the fibrillin gene mutation.

Physical phenotype, natural history and life expectancy
Marfan syndrome is a connective tissue disorder in which the tensile strength of supporting tissue is reduced. There is considerable variability in clinical expression, both between and within families. Affected individuals are characteristically tall and thin-muscled, with little subcutaneous fat. They show abnormalities of the skeletal, ocular and cardiovascular systems. On average, one in ten affected children shows serious abnormalities in these areas.

Most of the skeletal anomalies involving the extremities are the result of excessive bone growth. They include limbs which are extremely long as compared with the trunk, joint laxity, kyphosis/scoliosis (40–60 per cent of cases), flat feet, chest deformities with a protruding or indenting breast bone (due to excessive bone growth of the ribs), and a disproportionately longer lower part of the body compared with the trunk. Affected individuals tend to have a characteristic facial appearance, with a narrow face, large deep-set eyes, malar hypoplasia and a prominent forehead. A narrow high arched palate and dental overcrowding are commonly found. Cardiac anomalies occur in over 90 per cent of cases and include a dilated ascending aorta, aortic aneurysm, aortic regurgitation and mitral valve prolapse. Ocular anomalies include myopia, dislocation of the ocular lens, detachment of the retina and glaucoma. Inguinal and/or femoral hernias are common, and pulmonary malformation may be present, contributing to spontaneous collapse of the lung and/or emphysema, with an increased susceptibility to respiratory tract infection. Sleep apnoea appears to be common, possibly due to a floppy, easily collapsible pharynx.

Life expectancy is markedly reduced. Early studies reported the mean age at death to be in the early thirties, mostly as a result of cardiac complications (primarily disease of the aorta leading to heart failure or aortic dissection). In recent years survival rates have improved significantly as a result of regular echocardiographic surveillance, beta blockade and prophylactic repair or replacement of the dilated aortic root.

Psychological and behavioural phenotype

Gross motor development and cognitive abilities of children with Marfan syndrome typically fall within the average range, and there is no relationship between the severity of the physical features and IQ.

Very few studies have investigated the cognitive abilities of affected individuals; these suggest a high prevalence of learning disabilities and attentional problems within this population. In one investigation, 30 per cent of the children with Marfan syndrome showed significantly lower visuospatial and fine motor coordination abilities, as compared with their verbal abilities (Hofman *et al.* 1988). This discrepancy was significantly related to severity of hand–wrist hypermobility (which is likely to result in motor incoordination), but possible deleterious effects of beta-blocking medication on performance cannot be ruled out. Significant learning disabilities were found in 13 per cent of this series of cases, and attentional deficits with or without hyperactivity in 17 per cent of the cases.

Short-sightedness, and clumsiness due to loose joints and a long thin body build, contribute to learning and motor difficulties. These, and the excessive height of affected children, may also result in difficulties in peer relationships, although Schneider *et al.* (1990) found good psychosocial adjustment in a small group of affected adolescents. A higher incidence of depressed mood has been reported in some children and young adults with Marfan syndrome. Further studies are needed to clarify whether the above findings constitute cognitive and behavioural characteristics of the syndrome.

KEY REFERENCES

Hofman, K.J., Bernhardt, B.A., Pyeritz, R.E. (1988) 'Marfan syndrome: neuropsychological aspects.' *American Journal of Medical Genetics*, **31**, 331–338.
Pyeritz, R.E. (1990) 'Marfan syndrome.' *New England Journal of Medicine*, **323**, 987–989.
Tsipouros, P. (1992) 'Marfan syndrome: a mystery solved.' *Journal of Medical Genetics*, **29**, 73–74.

ADDITIONAL REFERENCES

Dietz, H.C., McIntosh, I., Sakai, L.Y., Corson, G.M., Chalberg, S.C., Pyeritz, R.E., Francomano, C.A. (1993) 'Four novel FBN1 mutations: significance for mutant transcript level and EGF-like domain calcium binding in the pathogenesis of Marfan syndrome.' *Genomics*, **17**, 468–475.

Hollister, D.W., Godfrey, M., Sakai, L.Y., Pyeritz, R.E.(1990) 'Immunohistologic abnormalities of the microfibrillar-fiber system in the Marfan syndrome.' *New England Journal of Medicine*, **323**, 152–159.

Marfan, A-B. (1896) 'Un cas de déformation congénitale des quatre membres, plus prononcée aux extremités, caractérisée par l'allongement des os avec un certain degré d'amincissement.' *Bullétins et Mémoires de la Société Médicale des Hôpitaux de Paris*, **13**, 220–226.

Milewicz, D.M., Pyeritz, R.E., Crawford, E.S., Byers, P.H. (1992) 'Marfan syndrome: defective synthesis, secretion, and extracellular matrix formation of fibrillin by cultural dermal fibroblasts.' *Journal of Clinical Investigation*, **89**, 79–86.

Morse, R.P., Rockenmacher, S., Pyeritz, R.E., Sanders, S.P., Bieber, F.R., Lin, A., MacLeod, P., Hall, B., Graham J.M. (1990) 'Diagnosis and management of infantile Marfan syndrome.' *Pediatrics*, **86**, 888–895.

Schneider, M.B., Davis, J.G., Boxer, R.A., Fisher, M., Friedman, S.B. (1990) 'Marfan syndrome in adolescents and young adults: psychosocial functioning and knowledge.' *Journal of Developmental and Behavioral Pediatrics*, **11**, 122–127.

THE MUCOPOLYSACCHARIDE DISORDERS

The mucopolysaccharidoses are a group of inherited lysosomal storage disorders with a degenerative course. Their mode of inheritance, clinical features and natural history vary from disorder to disorder.

Alternative names
The mucopolysaccharide (MPS) disorders are categorized according to both their clinical features and the particular enzyme deficiencies involved. They have eponymous as well as numerical designations, and comprise:
* Hurler (MPS IH), Scheie (MPS IS) and Hurler/Scheie (MPS IH/S) syndromes;
* Hunter syndrome (MPS II);
* Sanfilippo syndrome types A,B,C and D (MPS IIIA, IIIB, IIIC, IIID);
* Morquio syndrome (MPS IVA) and variant Morquio (MPS IVB);
* Maroteaux–Lamy syndrome (MPS VI); and
* Sly syndrome (MPS VII).

First description
Hunter (1917) and Hurler (1919) published the first clinical descriptions of the MPS syndromes, but it was only in the 1950s and 1960s that their biochemical basis was fully elucidated.

Incidence/prevalence
The MPS disorders occur across all ethnic groups. In the UK, Sanfilippo syndrome is the commonest of the disorders, with an incidence of about 1:25,000 live births (Cleary and Wraith 1993), although some reports have cited a lower incidence (1:200,000). The incidence of Hunter and Hurler syndromes is approximately 1:100,000 (a higher incidence of Hunter syndrome has been reported in the Ashkenazi population); of Morquio syndrome, 1:200,000 to 1:300,000; and of Scheie syndrome, 1:500,000 live births. The Maroteaux–Lamy and Sly syndromes are the rarest forms of MPS.

Genetics/aetiology
The MPS disorders are lysosomal storage diseases caused by deficiencies of lysosomal enzymes which catalyse the degradation of glycosaminoglycans (mucopolysaccharides). These latter are structural components of cartilage, bone, cornea, skin, blood vessel walls, and other connective tissues. In the absence of specific enzymes, non-degraded or partially degraded mucopolysaccharides such as dermatan, heparan or keratan sulfate accumulate in many tissues, eventually resulting in cell, tissue and organ dysfunction. They are also excreted to excess in the urine. To date, ten enzyme deficiencies that give rise to MPS have been identified. They include iduronate sulfatase in Hunter syndrome, α-L-iduronidase in Hurler and Scheie syndromes, and heparan-N-sulfatase in Sanfilippo A syndrome (Neufeld and Muenzer 1989).

Except for Hunter syndrome, the MPS disorders are all inherited as autosomal recessive disorders. The loci of several autosomal genes encoding enzymes of glycosaminoglycan degradation have been identified; for example, the Morquio A gene has been localized to chromosome 16q24, and the Sanfilippo D gene to 12q14. Multiple allelism at each locus has been proposed to explain the clinical variability within each enzyme deficiency; indeed, the identification of a number of mutations in individuals with Hurler and Scheie syndromes has already been linked to differences in their clinical presentation.

In contrast to the other MPS disorders, Hunter syndrome is X-linked, affecting one of every two males born to a carrier female. Up to one third of all cases represent new mutations. The Hunter gene has been cloned and sequenced (Wilson *et al.* 1990) and mapped to the tip of the long arm of the X chromosome, at Xq28. A variety of mutations of the gene have been identified, including complete deletion in some cases, partial deletions or other structural alterations, and point mutations (Wilson *et al.* 1991). In general, the more severely affected individuals appear to have larger deletions of the Hunter gene; however, there is no absolute correlation between the severity of the phenotype and the presence of deletions.

Physical phenotype, natural history and life expectancy
The MPS disorders share many clinical features involving various organs, though other physical characteristics and aspects of natural history vary from syndrome to syndrome. The disorders are all chronic and clinically progressive, but vary in the degree and rate of specific organ deterioration. There is also a wide spectrum of clinical severity within each disorder.

Individuals with MPS I display a wide range of clinical symptoms, with Hurler syndrome and Scheie syndrome representing the two extremes in a spectrum of clinical severity. Features of Hurler syndrome present early, often in the first year, with an enlarged liver and spleen, corneal clouding, stiff joints, severe skeletal deformities and dwarfism. Coarse facial features, an enlarged tongue, prominent forehead, some degree of hearing loss and hirsutism are further features, as well as recurrent respiratory infections, otitis media, upper airway obstruction, heart disease, persistent rhinorrhea and obstructive hydrocephalus. The joints stiffen, and gradually, with motor and cognitive deterioration, the children become more and more sedentary. They lose weight and there is muscle wasting. Death typically occurs in the first decade as a result of neurological and cardiorespiratory complications.

In Scheie syndrome the biochemical findings are identical to those found in Hurler syndrome, but there is a milder phenotype. Scheie syndrome is also characterized by corneal clouding and stiff joints, especially of the hands, with carpal tunnel syndrome, possible mild skeletal deformities and aortic incompetence. However, in this disorder stature is normal and survival to adult life is usual.

Hurler/Scheie syndrome has features intermediate between the two syndromes. It is characterized by progressive somatic involvement, including skeletal abnormalities, corneal clouding, joint stiffness, deafness, valvular heart disease and compression of the cervical cord. The onset of symptoms is usually between 3 and 8 years, and survival to adulthood is common.

In common with other MPS-affected individuals, boys with Hunter syndrome may appear to be normal in early infancy, but their phenotypic appearance is soon modified by the accumulation of mucopolysaccharides in many tissues (Adinolfi 1993). The onset of the disease usually occurs between 2 and 4 years of age. Affected boys acquire a typical coarse facies, with a large nose with flattened bridge and flared nostrils, and a large tongue protruding between thick lips. The abdomen is prominent with umbilical and other hernias, the liver and spleen are enlarged, and joints are progressively affected with restricted movement. Digital clawing is often apparent at about 3 years of age. Most affected children have unusually large heads, with ridges along the saggital suture. Hydrocephalus may be a complication of pachymeningitis. Hirsutism is common at older ages, but kyphosis and corneal clouding are rare. In over half the cases the cardio-vascular system is affected, and most individuals have recurrent respiratory infections and persistent mucopurulent rhinorrhoea. Chronic diarrhoea, recurrent ear infections, progressive hearing impairment and retinal dysfunction are reported in most cases. Some writers recognize a severe and a mild form of the Hunter syndrome; others argue for a continuum of severity spanning a wide spectrum. In the more severe cases there is an early onset, with both physical and mental deterioration and wasting. Growth retardation is prominent from the age of 4–5 years. The children show increasingly reduced physical activity, they have progressive difficulty ingesting solid food, they lose weight and they have more frequent and severe respiratory infections. Death occurrs in the first or second decade as a result of obstructive airway disease and cardiac failure superimposed on severe neurological disease. Milder cases have a later onset, with physical but not mental deterioration at a very slow rate of progression, and typically survival into adult life. Hearing impairment, carpal tunnel syndrome and joint stiffness are common and can result in loss of function. No differences have been found between the mild and severe forms in levels of α-iduronate sulphate sulphatase in serum and cells.

Sanfilippo syndrome is associated with mild skeletal and visceral changes, but severe progressive central nervous system involvement. Early development tends to be slightly or moderately delayed. Onset of symptoms occurs between 2 and 6 years of age, and presenting features include hyperactivity with aggressive behaviour, a slowing down in development and loss of acquired skills. Speech is typically first and most severely affected; it becomes slurred and eventually all language is lost. Hirsutism, mild hepato-splenomegaly, severe hearing loss, recurrent ear, nose and throat infections and episodes of diarrhoea are common. The children are often strikingly attractive, but coarse facies develop late in the disorder in most individuals. Stature is not significantly affected, skeletal involvement is minimal, and there is good physical growth. Cardiac abnormalities are rare. Severe neurological degeneration occurs by 6 to 10 years of age, accompanied by rapid deterioration of social and adaptive skills. Falls are common as balance is lost. Feeding difficulties due to swallowing incoordination result in increasing episodes of aspiration, and food consistency has to be altered. Ultimately most children require tube feeding. Increasing spasticity combined with joint stiffness from the connective tissue deterioration severely impairs mobility, and most children are wheelchair-dependent by their mid-teens. They become withdrawn and lose contact with the environment. Generalized tonic–clonic seizures may develop after age 8 (Cleary and Wraith 1993). Death ensues in the second or third decade, usually as a result of a respiratory infection complicating the severe debility. However, cases have been reported with late and mild deterioration, and with survival into at least the fourth decade. The four subtypes of Sanfilippo syndrome (A,B,C,D) are difficult to distinguish clinically, but they differ biochemically in the specific enzyme deficiency causing the disorder. Cranial CT at the onset of deterioration demonstrates mild to moderate cortical atrophy, with progression to severe cortical atrophy in the late stages of the disease.

Morquio syndrome is also clinically heterogeneous. The classical form (IVA) is associated with growth retardation with short trunk and neck, a waddling gait with a tendency to fall, mild corneal clouding, hepatomegaly, aortic valve disease and severe and progressive skeletal deformities, including dwarfism, kyphosis, odontoid hypoplasia, joint hypermobility and compression of the cervical cord, leading to either acute quadriplegia or myelopathy of slower onset, and in some cases to death by the age of 20 or 30. Survival beyond the third decade is possible providing the skeletal problems are dealt with. There are no central nervous system abnormalities. Morquio IVB (variant) is similar to classical Morquio syndrome but of later onset, milder, with no heart murmurs. Mild variants of Morquio IVA and severe variants of Morquio IVB are occasionally reported.

Maroteaux–Lamy syndrome is clinically similar to Hurler syndrome, except that the facial features are not so markedly abnormal, cognitive abilities are normal, and life expectancy is longer. Severe skeletal abnormalities and restriction of joint mobility develop in the first years of life, and the children assume a crouched stance. Corneal clouding, umbilical and/or inguinal hernias and hepatomegaly are common after age 6 Growth can be normal for the first few years, but seems to virtually stop after age 6–8. Neurological complications include cord compression, carpal tunnel syndrome and hydrocephalus. Death usually occurs in the second or third decade of life, often resulting from cardiopulmonary complications. Milder forms are found, however, with a slower disease course and a longer life span.

Characteristic features of Sly syndrome include moderate skeletal abnormalities, inguinal and/or umbilical hernias, hepatosplenomegaly, coarse facies, short stature, recurrent respiratory infections and developmental delay. There is a wide spectrum of severity, spanning from severe psychomotor delay and progressive disease leading to death in the first years of life to a normal phenotype in the second decade.

CT and MRI scans have revealed cerebral atrophy and white matter low density in some MPS individuals with learning difficulties, as well as in some older individuals with normal intelligence. Progression to severe cortical atrophy occurs with progression of the disorders. Other common findings are delay in myelination, and thickening of dura mater at the cranio-cervical junction, causing narrowing of the subarachnoid space.

Since there is as yet no specific treatment for MPS, management of affected individuals consists of supportive care and treatment of complications. Enzyme replacement by bone marrow transplantation has been attempted, with some encouraging results, which include reversal of various systemic manifestations of MPS and even reversal of some central nervous system findings. However, there is as yet an uncertain long-term outcome to this high-risk procedure.

Psychological and behavioural phenotype

Patterns of cognitive ability and behavioural characteristics vary in the different MPS disorders.

Moderate to severe learning difficulties with progressive mental deterioration are characteristic of Hurler syndrome, Hunter syndrome and all subtypes of Sanfilippo syndrome, although cognitive abilities can vary greatly from one affected individual to another, even in the same family. Poor attention span and distractibility are prominent features, and speech development is particularly delayed when compared with other skills. Some children never acquire speech; others have delayed speech and language and lose these skills as the disorder progresses. In Hunter syndrome, developmental regression becomes noticeable from an average age of about 8 years, and loss of speech occurs at an average age of 10 or 11 years, along with the loss of other cognitive and social skills as the child becomes increasingly disabled. In Sanfilippo syndrome, the severe neurological degeneration occurring by 6–10 years of age is accompanied by rapid deterioration of language and memory function and loss of social and adaptive skills. In contrast to these profiles of learning difficulties, Scheie syndrome, some milder cases of Hunter syndrome, Morquio and Maroteaux–Lamy syndromes are associated with normal intelligence or mild learning difficulties.

Children with MPS show high rates of behaviour problems, which present major difficulties in management for their families (Bax and Colville 1995a). The behaviour problems vary between the different types of MPS; they may be at least partly concomitants of low cognitive levels and degenerative aspects of the disorders, but they also occur in affected individuals with normal development.

Children with Hurler syndrome are often described as anxious and fearful, particularly in the preschool years, but they are rarely aggressive or destructive (Bax and Colville 1995a).

Boys with Hunter syndrome may be overactive and restless, with a short concentration span. They can also be stubborn and difficult to discipline, and display outbursts of destructive and aggressive behaviour and attacks on other people (Bax and Colville 1995a). Fear of such attacks causes many families to curtail social activities and outings. As the disease progresses, the hyperactivity gradually decreases, and the children become increasingly sedentary and apathetic as they near the end of their life.

There is a high prevalence of night-time restlessness and sleep problems in children with Hunter and Hurler syndromes (Bax and Colville 1995a). These are at least partly caused by obstructive sleep apnoea with severe hypercapnia which has been demonstrated in many affected individuals, and is probably due to a combination of factors including glycosaminoglycan accumulation in the soft tissues of the upper airway and skeletal malformations of the skull, cervical spine and rib cage. Suggested treatments include nasal continuous positive airway pressure, nocturnal oxygen administration and bone marrow transplantation.

Children with Sanfilippo syndrome show major behavioural problems, which commonly begin around the age of 3 or 4 years and are associated with regression (Cleary and Wraith 1993, Bax and Colville 1995a). Characteristically the children show increasingly frequent and severe temper tantrums, obstinacy, bouts of aggression and destructiveness, increasing restlessness and hyperactivity, and rapid diminution in attention span. They are often reported to lunge at people and strike them for no apparent reason, and often with no malice intended. Bax and Colville (1995a) hypothesize that these behaviours may represent a reaction to invasion of the child's personal space. Another form of destructive behaviour frequently exhibited is mouthing, chewing and biting clothing and objects (Bax and Colville 1995a). Some parents provide the child with a 'teething ring' to reduce this biting behaviour. The often unpredictable aggressive and destructive behaviours, coupled with good physical growth and strength, make managing these children particularly difficult for families. Drug treatment aimed at controlling the hyperactivity and aggression has a variable effect, and there may even be a temporary worsening of the behaviour. At best, it is only partially successful (Cleary and Wraith 1993). Behavioural approaches to management are occasionally effective, but many families report having to curtail outside activities and social visits, and trying to create a 'safe' environment for their child at home, with soft furnishings, toughened glass on doors and windows, wall padding, and the removal of breakable articles (Bax and Colville 1995a).

During this phase sleep is severely disturbed in over 80 per cent of children with Sanfilippo syndrome (Watters 1988). Typically, the onset of sleep is resisted and there are frequent night wakings, during which the child may wander about the house and disrupt the parents' sleep. Inappropriate laughing or singing in the night have been reported in some affected children. Other unusual and distressing night-time behaviours include staying up all night, chewing the bedclothes and sudden crying out. These features place great strain on families, who often resort to physical restraint at night (Cleary and Wraith 1993). Sleep-inducing medication can be useful as a last resort for short periods, but it can have paradoxical effects. Watters (1988) has shown that the sleep difficulties can be significantly improved with behavioural management advice. Obstructive sleep apnoea does not appear to be a feature in Sanfilippo syndrome.

From the age of about 10 years children with Sanfilippo syndrome enter a third, quieter phase, and their behaviour becomes easier to manage due to increasing immobility. However, there is also rapid deterioration in social and adaptive skills. The children can become very withdrawn and lose contact with the environment as a result of the progressive dementia. Mood swings and bouts of crying are very common in this phase, although it is not clear to what extent these may be a response to pain (Cleary and Wraith 1993).

Bax and Colville (1995a,b) emphasize the enormous strain the behavioural difficulties of affected children place on families, particularly given that MPS disorders are at present incurable, degenerative and disfiguring.

KEY REFERENCES

Adinolfi, M. (1993) 'Hunter syndrome: cloning of the gene, mutations and carrier detection.' *Developmental Medicine and Child Neurology*, **35**, 79–85.

Bax, M.C.O., Colville, G.A. (1995*a*) 'Behaviour in mucopolysaccharide disorders.' *Archives of Disease in Childhood*, **73**, 77–81.

Cleary, M.A., Wraith, J.E. (1993) 'Management of mucopolysaccharidosis type III.' *Archives of Disease in Childhood*, **69**, 403–406.

Hopwood, J.J., Morris, C.P. (1990) 'The mucopolysaccharidoses: diagnosis, molecular genetics and treatment.' *Molecular and Biological Medicine*, **7**, 381–404.

Neufeld, E.F., Muenzer, J. (1989) 'The mucopolysaccharidoses.' *In:* Scriver, C.R., Beaudet, A.L., Sly, W.S., Valle, D. (Eds.) *The Metabolic Basis of Inherited Disease. 6th Edn.* New York: McGraw-Hill, pp. 1565–1587.

Nidiffer, F.D., Kelly, T.E. (1983) 'Developmental and degenerative patterns associated with cognitive, behavioural and motor difficulties in the Sanfilippo syndrome: an epidemiological study.' *Journal of Mental Deficiency Research*, **27**, 185–203.

ADDITIONAL REFERENCES

Bax, M., Colville, G.A. (1995*b*) 'Early presentation in the mucopolysaccharide disorders: A report of a parental survey.' *Journal of Inherited Metabolic Disease. (In press.)*

Hunter, C. (1917) ' A rare disease in two brothers.' *Proceedings of the Royal Society of Medicine*, **10**, 104–116.

Hurler, G. (1919) 'Ueber einen Typ multipler Abartungen, vorwiegend am Skelettsystem.' *Zeitschrift für Kinderheilkunde*, **24**, 220–234.

Watters, J.P. (1988) 'Sleep in children with Sanfilippo syndrome. Report of a parental questionnaire and a behavioural intervention.' MSc thesis, Institute of Psychiatry, University of London.

Wilson, P.J., Morris, C.P., Anson, D.S., Occhiodoro, T., Bielicki, J., Clements, P.R., Hopwood, J.J. (1990) 'Hunter syndrome: isolation of an iduronate-2-sulfatase cDNA clone and analysis of patient DNA.' *Proceedings of the National Academy of Sciences of the USA*, **87**, 8531–8535.

Wilson, P.J., Suthers, G.K., Callen, D.F., Baker, E., Nelson, P.V., Cooper, A., Wraith, J.E., Sutherland, G.R., Morris, C.P., Hopwood, J.J. (1991) 'Frequent deletions at Xq28 indicate genetic heterogeneity in Hunter syndrome.' *Human Genetics*, **86**, 505–508.

NEUROFIBROMATOSIS TYPE 1

The neurofibromatoses comprise a number of different but overlapping conditions, the two best-defined being neurofibromatosis type 1 (NF1) and neurofibromatosis type 2 (NF2). Both have in common a predisposition to the development of tumours of the nerve sheath, but they are distinctly different clinical disorders with different genetic origins. This section focuses on neurofibromatosis type 1.

Alternative names
Von Recklinghausen neurofibromatosis; multiple/peripheral neurofibromatosis.

First description
The first documented descriptions of NF1 appeared in the 18th century, though there are even earlier descriptions. Von Recklinghausen (1882) elaborated upon these, and showed that the skin tumours characteristic of the condition, which he named neurofibromas, arose from the fibrous connective tissue sheaths of small nerves.

Incidence/prevalence
NF1 has an incidence of between 1:2500 and 1:4000 live births (Huson 1989). It occurs with equal frequency in males and females, and has been diagnosed across all racial and ethnic groups.

Genetics/aetiology
NF1 is inherited as an autosomal dominant trait. It also has a very high mutation rate; approximately half of all cases represent new mutations, and in 92 per cent of these it is the paternally derived NF1 allele that is mutated. The penetrance of NF1 is believed to be virtually 100 per cent by the age of 5 years.

The gene for NF1 has been identified and localized to the proximal long arm of chromosome 17 at locus 17q11.2 (Ledbetter *et al.* 1989); it has been cloned and sequenced (Marchuk *et al.* 1991). The gene product is termed neurofibromin and is thought to be a tumour suppressor gene. Several mutations of the NF1 gene have been described: insertions, base alterations and deletions. The result is a truncated or altered form of the NF1 protein with aberrant function. However, there appears to be no clear relationship between the site of the NF1 mutation and the clinical phenotype. Moreover, the pathogenesis of the disorder and the mechanisms responsible for tumours, cognitive deficits and other manifestations in NF1 have yet to be elucidated (Gutman and Collins 1992).

Physical phenotype, natural history and life expectancy
NF1 affects cells derived embryonically from the neural crest and causes abnormal cell growth in the central and peripheral nervous system (Frank-Stromberg 1992). The manifestations of the disorder are extremely variable, even in members of the same

144

family, and may include minor dermatological features or major cosmetic disfigurement, varying levels of physical disability, neurological deficits and malignancy. The major defining features of NF1 are café-au-lait spots, cutaneous neurofibromas and Lisch nodules (Riccardi 1992, Huson and Hughes 1994). The café-au-lait spots are the first to appear and are usually present by 1 year of age, and always by 5 years. They are areas of dark pigmentation on the skin with well-defined borders, and their size and number tend to increase throughout childhood. These lesions occur predominantly on the trunk. Axillary freckling also occurs, though not in all cases. Lisch nodules, which are benign hamartomas on the iris, usually brown and dome-shaped, are seen in over 90 per cent of cases, and appear in middle childhood. They have no effect on vision. The dermal neurofibromas are benign tumours of the nerve tissue and surrounding fibrous tissue. They typically begin to appear at the onset of puberty and tend to increase in number throughout life. These features rarely cause problems, other than cosmetic ones. Subcutaneous neurofibromas may be painful or compress a nerve or the spinal cord, causing neurological deficit.

About one third of affected individuals develop one or more complications of the disorder, some of which may be life-threatening. These include plexiform neurofibromas (in about 30 per cent of cases), which are diffuse tumours along the course of nerves or nerve trunks that usually present in infancy. Because of their size and invasive nature they may cause functional as well as cosmetic problems, and they may be associated with hypertrophy of the surrounding connective tissue and other structures. They may also undergo malignant change. Other complications are skeletal anomalies (in about 14 per cent of cases), including scoliosis, bowing and thinning of long bones and pseudo-arthrosis, and less often central nervous system tumours (in 4 per cent of cases), disease associated malignancy (in 3 per cent of cases), and hypertension. MRI scans reveal optic gliomas in about 15 per cent of affected individuals, but these are mostly asymptomatic. The occurrence of these complications is very variable and cannot be predicted, even within families. This suggests that the severity and range of complications are determined by factors other than just the inherited mutation.

Short stature and macrocephaly have been reported in 32 and 45 per cent of cases respectively, but are of unknown aetiology. Characteristic facial features have been reported in some affected individuals, including mild hypertelorism, ptosis, down-slanting palpebral fissures and posteriorly rotated ears.

Management of NF1 is aimed at early detection of treatable complications. Neurofibromas that are life-threatening, functionally compromising or disfiguring, may be surgically removed. Life expectancy depends on the occurrence of the complications described above. Sørensen et al. (1986) found lower survival rates compared with the general population, especially in affected females.

Studies of the histology of the brains of individuals with NF1 report disorders of the cortical architecture and neuronal heterotopias in cerebral white matter. T_2-weighted MRI scans have shown increased intensity lesions in the basal ganglia, brainstem and cerebellum in approximately 60 per cent of affected individuals (Duffner et al. 1989, Ferner et al. 1993). The nature of these lesions is as yet unclear; their presence shows no obvious relationship with IQ and they appear to be benign. MRI is also effective in showing optic glioma, spinal and other neurological lesions,

Psychological and behavioural phenotype

It is only recently that studies have been undertaken to examine the cognitive and behavioural characteristics associated with NF1.

Up to 50 per cent of children with NF1 present with speech and language difficulties. Speech defects include excessive nasality, breathiness, poor articulation and distortions of prosody. Possible causative factors are neurofibromas and dyspraxia. Speech delay and slow acquisition of vocabulary are also often reported. The pathogenesis of these features is unclear.

The majority of affected individuals have an IQ in the low-average range, while about 8–10 per cent have moderate or severe learning difficulties (IQ <70) (Riccardi 1992, Ferner 1994). A further 40–60 per cent have specific learning difficulties, particularly visuospatial deficits, perceptual organization difficulties, clumsiness and poor coordination, poor spatial and verbal memory, impaired constructional skills, reading and writing difficulties, and problems with numeracy (Riccardi 1992, Spaepen et al. 1992, Ferner 1994, Legius et al. 1994). Overall, verbal abilities tend to be higher than non-verbal abilities. Distractibility, impulsivity and poor concentration are further common features, particularly in children who are more cognitively able (Legius et al. 1994). Huson (1989) found that 10 per cent of a sample of affected children in Wales attended special schools, and a further 17 per cent required remedial teaching. Higher figures have been reported in some American studies, and Riccardi (1992) suggests that up to 40 per cent or more of children with NF1 may require special education, speech therapy, physical therapy, and/or treatment for visual or auditory disabilities.

Many adults with NF1 have unskilled jobs, and the population as a whole manifests a tendency to move down in socio-economic status in relation to their parents (Ferner 1994).

The pathogenetic mechanisms to account for the above difficulties are not known. No correlation has been found between cognitive level and structural abnormalities in the brain, or disease severity.

NF1 further imposes a significant psychological burden on affected individuals and their families, related to issues such as cosmetic disfigurement, uncertainty regarding prognosis, and problems associated with chronic medical illness. Unhappiness, teasing and bullying at school are often reported, and increased rates of behaviour problems have been found in a number of studies, particularly in terms of hyperactivity, disruptive behaviour, anxiety, poor self-confidence, social withdrawal and other psychosocial problems (e.g. Spaepen et al. 1992). These will often result in restricted social contacts and difficulties in interpersonal relationships for older people, as well as for children (Benjamin et al. 1993). A few studies have reported an excess of psychiatric disturbance in individuals with NF1, including anxiety states and depression, particularly in individuals with cosmetic disfigurement (Ferner 1994).

KEY REFERENCES

Ferner, R.E. (1994) 'Intellect in neurofibromatosis 1.' *In:* Huson, S.M., Hughes, R.A.C. (Eds.) *The Neurofibromatoses: a Pathogenetic and Clinical Overview.* London: Chapman & Hall, pp. 233–252.

—— Chaudhuri, R., Bingham, J., Cox, T., Hughes, R.A.C. (1993) 'MRI in neurofibromatosis 1. The nature and evolution of increased intensity T_2-weighted lesions and their relationship to intellectual impairment.' *Journal of Neurology, Neurosurgery, and Psychiatry,* **56**, 492–495.

Frank-Stromberg, M. (1992) 'Neurofibromatosis.' *Seminars in Oncology Nursing,* **8**, 265–271.

Huson, S.M., Hughes, R.A.C. (Eds.) (1994) *The Neurofibromatoses: a Pathogenetic and Clinical Overview.* London: Chapman & Hall.

Nativio, D.G., Belz, C.. (1990) 'Childhood neurofibromatosis.' *Pediatric Nursing,* **16**, 576–580.

Riccardi, V. (1992) *Neurofibromatosis: Phenotype. Natural History and Pathogenesis. 2nd Edn.* Baltimore: Johns Hopkins University Press.

ADDITIONAL REFERENCES

Benjamin, C.M., Colley, A., Donnai, D., Kingston, H., Harris, R., Kerzin-Storrar, L. (1993) 'Neurofibromatosis type 1 (NF1): knowledge, experience, and reproductive decisions of affected patients and families.' *Journal of Medical Genetics,* **30**, 567–574.

Duffner, P.K., Cohen, M.E., Seidel, F.G., Shucard, D.W. (1989) 'The significance of MRI abnormalities in children with neurofibromatosis.' *Neurology,* **39**, 373–378.

Gutmann, D.H., Collins, F.S.. (1992) 'Recent progress toward understanding the molecular biology of von Recklinghausen neurofibromatosis.' *Annals of Neurology,* **31**, 555–561.

Huson, S.M. (1989) 'Recent developments in the diagnosis and management of neurofibromatosis.' *Archives of Disease in Childhood,* **64**, 745–749.

Ledbetter, D.H., Rich, D.C., O'Connell, P., Leppert, M., Carey, J.C. (1989) 'Precise localization of NF1 to 17q11.2 by balanced translocation.' *American Journal of Human Genetics,* **44**, 20–24.

Legius, E., Descheemaeker, M.J., Spaepen, A., Casaer, P., Fryns, J-P. (1994) 'Neurofibromatosis type 1 in childhood: a study of the neuropsychological profile in 45 children.' *Genetic Counseling,* **5**, 51–60.

Marchuk, D.A., Saulino, A.M., Tavakkol, R., Swaroop, M., Wallace, M.R., Andersen, L.B., Mitchell, A.L., Gutmann, D.H., Boguski, M., Collins, F.S. (1991) 'cDNA cloning of the type1 neurofibromatosis gene: complete sequence of the *NF1* gene product.' *Genomics,* **11**, 931–940.

Sørensen, S.A., Mulvihill, J.J., Nielsen, A. (1986) 'Long-term follow-up of von Recklinghausen neurofibromatosis. Survival and malignant neoplasms.' *New England Journal of Medicine,* **314**, 1010–1015.

Spaepen, A., Borghgraef, M., Fryns, J-P. (1992) 'Von Recklinghausen neurofibromatosis: a study of the psychological profile.' *Birth Defects,* **28**, 85–91.

von Recklinghausen, F. (1882) *Ueber die Multiplen Fibroma der Haut und ihre Beziehung zu den Multiplen Neuromen.* Berlin : A. Hirschwald.

NOONAN SYNDROME

Alternative names
Ullrich–Noonan syndrome (Turner phenotype); Ullrich–Turner syndrome.

First description
In 1963 Noonan and Ehmke identified a group of children with valvular pulmonary stenosis associated with short stature, a characteristic physical appearance and mild learning difficulties.

Incidence/prevalence
A high incidence has been estimated, of between 1:1000 and 1:2500 live births (Allanson *et al.* 1985). However, given the wide phenotypic variability in the syndrome and the lack of a definitive marker, the incidence rate cannot be accurately determined. The syndrome has an equal sex ratio.

Genetics/aetiology
Noonan syndrome is inherited as an autosomal dominant condition, with variable penetrance and expressivity. Direct parent-to-child transmission is documented in between 30 and 75 per cent of cases; the remaining cases are sporadic. But since Noonan syndrome features may be subtle, even in the latter cases some of the parents could be affected. Maternal transmission of the syndrome is far more common than paternal transmission, which is likely to be due to associated cryptorchidism and male infertility. The gene for Noonan syndrome has been localized to chromosome 12q22-qter (Jamieson *et al.* 1994).

Physical phenotype, natural history and life expectancy
There is wide phenotypic variability in Noonan syndrome, and manifestations in adults in particular may be rather subtle. The cardinal features are short stature (found in over 80 per cent of cases), characteristic facies, congenital heart defects, a short or webbed neck (in over 70 per cent), and a peculiar chest deformity with pectus carinatum superiorly and pectus excavatum inferiorly (in about half of affected individuals).

Birthweight is normal in about 40 per cent of cases, but it can be high, secondary to subcutaneous oedema. Thereafter, weight gain is often slow, and early feeding difficulties, vomiting, poor sucking and failure to thrive are often documented. Prepubertal growth tends to parallel the third centile, with a relatively normal growth velocity. The pubertal growth spurt is often delayed or absent. Final height approaches the lower limits of normal and is not reached until the end of the second decade of life. In some cases growth hormone treatment is given to boost growth levels, but its effectiveness has yet to be evaluated. Delayed bone age has been reported in up to 20 per cent of cases.

The facial appearance changes predictably with age (Allanson *et al.* 1985). In infancy the head appears relatively large with turricephaly and prominent eyes with thick hooded eyelids. Common features present in 70 to over 90 per cent of infants include hypertelorism with downward-slanting palpebral fissures, arched eyebrows, low-set posteriorly rotated ears with a thick helix, and a deeply grooved philtrum with a pronounced top lip. The nose has a depressed root, wide base and bulbous tip. A high arched palate and excess nuchal skin with low posterior hairline have been noted in about half the cases, and micrognathia in one quarter. In childhood, the face often appears coarse or myopathic. The contour of the face becomes more triangular with age and the facial features sharpen. In the adolescent and young adult the eyes are less prominent and the nose has a pinched root, a thinner, higher bridge, and a wide base. The neck lengthens, accentuating the webbing or prominent trapezius. In the older adult there are prominent nasolabial folds, a higher anterior hairline, and transparent, wrinkled skin. Hair may be wispy in the toddler, but is often curly or woolly in the older child and adolescent.

Hypotonia and skeletal abnormalities (*e.g.* scoliosis, kyphosis) are common findings. Congenital heart defects are seen in one half to two thirds of cases, and include pulmonary stenosis, atrial and septal defects, and hypertrophic cardiomyopathy. Ophthalmic abnormalities and hearing difficulties (mostly due to otitis media) are common.

Undescended testes are reported in over 70 per cent of males, and puberty is delayed in both sexes. Infertility occurs in all males and in some females.

Various skin manifestations have been noted, including café-au-lait spots (in about 10 per cent of cases) and pigmented naevi (in about one quarter). Several cases of neurofibromatosis in association with the Noonan phenotype have been documented, but the relationship between the two syndromes is not clear. Bleeding abnormalities such as factor XI deficiency are found in 50 per cent of cases, and congenital dysplasia is common. Life expectancy is generally normal, unless the cardiac complications are serious.

Psychological and behavioural phenotype
Little is known about the cognitive and behavioural characteristics of individuals with Noonan syndrome. Approximately two thirds have at least low-average cognitive abilities, and one third have mild learning difficulties. Sharland *et al.* (1992) found that only 11 per cent of the affected children they studied attended special schools. Motor delay, clumsiness and specific learning disabilities are common, even in the more able individuals, and difficulties in visual–constructional abilities and motor coordination are often evident. Language delay is found in about 20 per cent of cases, and articulation difficulties in over 70 per cent. There are anecdotal accounts of difficulties with naming and word finding.

Behaviour problems have been reported by significant numbers of parents, including stubbornness, perseverative behaviours, preoccupations, immaturity, and difficulties in social interactions with peers. In contrast, there are also anecdotal descriptions of children with Noonan syndrome having a 'lovable and affable nature', and being over-emotional and overconcerned about the well-being of others.

KEY REFERENCES

Allanson, J.E. (1987) 'Noonan syndrome.' *Journal of Medical Genetics*, **24**, 9–13.
—— Hall, J.G., Hughes, H.E., Preus, M., Witt. R.D. (1985) 'Noonan syndrome: the changing phenotype.' *American Journal of Medical Genetics*, **21**, 507–514.
Mendez, H.M.M., Opitz J.M., (1985) 'Noonan syndrome: a review.' *American Journal of Medical Genetics*, **21**, 493–506.
Sharland, M., Burch, M., McKenna, W.M., Paton, M.A. (1992) 'A clinical study of Noonan syndrome.' *Archives of Disease in Childhood*, **67**, 178–183.

ADDITIONAL REFERENCES

Jamieson, C.R., van der Burgt, I., Brady, A.F., van Reen, M., Elsawi, M.M., Hol, F., Jeffery, S., Patton, M.A., Mariman, E. (1994) 'Mapping a gene for Noonan syndrome to the long arm of chromosome 12.' *Nature Genetics*, **8**, 357–360.
Noonan, J.A., Ehmke, D.A. (1963) 'Associated noncardiac malformations in children with congenital heart disease.' *Journal of Pediatrics*, **63**, 468–470. *(Abstract.)*

(CLASSICAL) PHENYLKETONURIA

Classical phenylketonuria (PKU) is the most severe form of phenylalanine hydroxylase deficiency.

Alternative name
Hyperphenylalaninaemia.

First description
PKU was first described by Fölling (1934, cited in Fishler *et al.* 1987) in ten learning disabled children who excreted phenylpyruvic acid, a phenylalanine metabolite. Subsequently the condition was identified in many institutionalized individuals with learning difficulties.

Incidence/prevalence
The incidence of PKU varies widely across different geographical areas and ethnic groups, and is highest (about 1:5,000 births) in Ireland and western Scotland. In the UK overall the incidence is 1:10,000 live births.

Genetics/aetiology
PKU is an inborn error of metabolism caused by an absence of the enzyme phenylalanine hydroxylase which converts the amino acid phenylalanine into tyrosine in the liver. As a result of this enzyme deficiency, phenylalanine accumulates in the blood as well as in the cerebrospinal fluid and tissues, and is excreted to excess in the urine as phenylpyruvic acid. These elevated levels of phenylalanine are toxic to the body's tissues. Altered myelin and neurotransmitter metabolism may result and have been proposed as possible pathogenic mechanisms.

PKU is inherited as an autosomal recessive disorder and is a consequence of many different mutations in the gene that encodes the enzyme phenylalanine hydroxylase (*PAH* gene) (Eisensmith and Woo 1992). The gene has been localized to the q22–q24.1 region of chromosome 12 (Lidsky *et al.* 1985). Most affected individuals are compound heterozygotes, their clinical state being determined by the combined effect of two mutant *PAH* genes.

Physical phenotype, natural history and life expectancy
Individuals with PKU show wide variability in biochemical and clinical expression. Most affected infants appear normal at birth, although an increased frequency of vomiting and a poor appetite have been noted in some cases. Malar flush, widely spaced teeth and subtle facial features are further characteristics. Many affected children have reduced pigmentation resulting in fair skin, blonde hair and blue eyes.

If left untreated, the accumulation of phenylalanine and its metabolites leads to neuropsychiatric symptoms, the most significant of which are learning difficulties. Other symptoms include a slowness in attaining motor milestones, some degree of eczema or other skin conditions, an aromatic, musty odour associated with the presence of phenylacetic acid in the sweat and urine, insufficient head growth and seizures. Tremor or other movement disorders, hypertonia or spasticity may also be in evidence.

Treatment of PKU involves reduction in phenylalanine intake. Dietary management appears to be most effective when initiated shortly after birth and maintained over the period of most rapid myelinization. In this way damage to the central nervous system is minimized. There is uncertainty about how long treatment should be continued. This issue is discussed further in the following section.

Psychological and behavioural phenotype
The most important clinical characteristic of untreated PKU is severe learning difficulties. Typically, untreated babies are clinically normal at birth, but by 4–6 months of age they present with developmental delay and begin to lose interest in their surroundings; by age 2–3 years a significant proportion have IQs below 50. Behavioural characteristics associated with untreated PKU include poor attention; restlessness and hyperactivity; stereotypic behaviours; erratic and unpredictable behaviour including irritability, negative mood and outbursts of aggression; sleep disturbances; and self-injury.

Provided dietary treatment is introduced shortly after birth, cognitive abilities can be maintained within normal limits. However, there is evidence to suggest that, even so, many children exhibit subtle and often very varied cognitive deficits and behavioural difficulties. A cohort of early-treated children born in the 1970s was found to have a mean IQ eight points below the population norm (Smith *et al.* 1990). The IQs of such children and their reading and arithmetic abilities are often significantly lower than those of their parents and siblings. Neuropsychological assessments have revealed specific deficits of higher cognitive and integrative functions (including visuospatial and conceptual abilities, visual motor coordination, higher level reasoning and problem solving, and attention span) in early treated children when compared with various control groups (Pennington *et al.* 1985, Fishler *et al.* 1989). Welsh *et al.* (1990) proposed a prefrontal lobe deficit caused by dopamine depletion in PKU, resulting in deficits in executive function (problem solving abilities and planning for the attainment of future goals). According to Welsh *et al.*, this would explain the specific relative difficulties found in early treated individuals with PKU in problem solving, planning, sustained attention and perceptual–motor functions.

Ozanne *et al.* (1990) and others have additionally found that between one third and one half of early treated PKU children under 5 years have specific language impairment. In the case of older children, speech and language deficits are especially apparent in those who have poor dietary control. However, there does not appear to be any typical pattern of linguistic deficits.

Children with early treated PKU also tend to have a higher frequency of behaviour difficulties than classroom controls, especially in terms of fidgetiness, poor concentration, mannerisms, and being more solitary, anxious and unpopular (Smith *et al.* 1988). Nevertheless, reporting on the progress of a group of early treated young adults with

PKU, Koch *et al.* (1985) described most as functioning productively in society, living independently and working in skilled or semi-skilled occupations.

The levels of cognitive and behavioural difficulties that have been reported are directly related to age at the initiation of dietary treatment, to the average level of phenylalanine exposure in childhood, and to the age at loss of dietary control (*e.g.* Azen *et al.* 1991, Smith *et al.* 1991). Extending dietary treatment until age 8 years or beyond results in levels of IQ, reading and spelling that are more similar to those of family members and higher than those of children who discontinue their diets earlier (*e.g.* Fishler *et al.* 1989, Azen *et al.* 1991). Thus, it would appear that optimal intellectual and academic achievement is attained by the earliest possible initiation of treatment and strict control of blood phenylalanine levels throughout childhood.

It is uncertain how long children should be continued on the diet. Recent studies have identified some decline in IQ scores and neuropsychological and behavioural performance (including deficits in cognitive vigilance and task persistence, and in social functioning and communication), and a rise in concentration problems, irritability, aggression and forgetfulness in adolescents and young adults with PKU in whom the diet was discontinued (Fuggle and Graham 1991). Symptoms of anxiety or depression, emotional lability, thought disorder, tics, compulsive eating, sleeplessness and poor social relationships have also been reported (Waisbren and Levy 1991). These changes appear to be related to current phenylalanine levels. In some cases they are subtle, in others they are more evident. Overt neurological deterioration has been reported in a few early treated young adults (Thompson *et al.* 1990). These symptoms are at least partly reversible by return to a low phenylalanine diet, with resulting increases in attention and reaction time, and decreases in aggression and irritability (Koch *et al.* 1985). Many clinicians are now recommending continuation of the diet at least through adolescence or even beyond for optimal physical, mental, emotional and educational development (Azen *et al.* 1991). Women must return to a strict low phenylalanine diet before conception, since children born to affected women with high phenylalanine levels almost always show learning difficulties and microcephaly, and have an increased frequency of congenital heart disease and intrauterine growth retardation. In contrast, paternal PKU results in offspring with normal growth and development.

KEY REFERENCES

Fuggle, P., Graham, P. (1991) 'Metabolic/endocrine disorders and psychological functioning.' *In:* Rutter, M., Casaer, P. (Eds.) *Biological Risk Factors for Psychosocial Disorders.* Cambridge: Cambridge University Press, pp. 175–198.

Medical Research Council Working Party on Phenylketonuria (1993) 'Phenylketonuria due to phenylalanine hydroxylase deficiency: an unfolding story.' *British Medical Journal,* **306**, 115–119.

Ozanne, A.E., Murdoch, B.E., Krimmer, H.L. (1990) 'Linguistic problems associated with childhood metabolic disorders.' *In:* Murdoch, B.E. (Ed.) *Acquired Neurological Speech/Language Disorders in Childhood: Brain Damage, Behaviour and Cognition.* London: Taylor & Francis, pp. 625–632.

ADDITIONAL REFERENCES

Azen, C.G., Koch, R., Friedman, E.G., Berlow, S., Coldwell, J., Krause, W., Matalon, R., McCabe, E.,

O'Flynn, M., *et al.* (1991) 'Intellectual development in 12-year-old children treated for phenylketonuria.' *American Journal of Diseases of Children*, **145**, 35–39.

Eisensmith, R.C., Woo, S.L.C. (1992) 'Molecular basis of phenylketonuria and related hyperphenylalaninemias: mutations and polymorphisms in the human phenylalanine hydroxylase gene.' *Human Mutation*, **1**, 13–23.

Fishler, K., Azen, C.G., Henderson, R., Friedman, E.G., Koch, R. (1987) 'Psychoeducational findings among children treated for phenylketonuria.' *American Journal of Mental Deficiency*, **92**, 65–73.

—— —— Friedman, E.G., Koch, R. (1989) 'School achievement in treated PKU children.' *Journal of Mental Deficiency Research*, **33**, 493–498.

Koch, R., Yusin, M., Fishler, K. (1985) 'Successful adjustment to society by adults with phenylketonuria.' *Journal of Inherited Metabolic Disease*, **8**, 209–211.

Lidsky, A.S., Law, M.L., Morse, H.G., Koo, F-T., Rabin, M., Ruddle, F.H., Woo, S.L.C. (1985) 'Regional mapping of the phenylalanine hydroxylase gene and the phenylketonuria locus in the human genome.' *Proceedings of the National Academy of Sciences of the USA*, **82**, 6221–6225.

Pennington, B.F., van Doorninck, W.J., McCabe, L.L., McCabe, E.R.B. (1985) 'Neuropsychological deficits in early treated phenylketonuric children.' *American Journal of Mental Deficiency*, **89**, 467–474.

Smith, I., Beasley, M.G., Wolff, O.H., Ades, A.E. (1988) 'Behavior disturbance in 8-year-old children with early treated phenylketonuria. Report from the MRC/DHSS Phenylketonuria Register.' *Journal of Pediatrics*, **112**, 403–408.

—— —— Ades, A.E. (1990) 'Intelligence and quality of dietary treatment in phenylketonuria.' *Archives of Disease in Childhood*, **65**, 472–478.

—— —— —— (1991) 'Effect on intelligence of relaxing the low phenylalanine diet in phenylketonuria.' *Archives of Disease in Childhood*, **66**, 311–316.

Thompson, A.J., Smith, I., Brenton, D., Youl, B.D., Rylance, G., Davidson, D.C., Kendall, B., Lees, A.J. (1990) 'Neurological deterioration in young adults with phenylketonuria.' *Lancet*, **336**, 602–605.

Waisbren, S.E., Levy, H.L. (1991) 'Agoraphobia in phenylketonuria.' *Journal of Inherited Metabolic Disease*, **14**, 755–764

Welsh, M.C., Pennington, B.F., Ozonoff, S., Rouse, B., McCabe, E.R.B. (1990) 'Neuropsychology of early-treated phenylketonuria: specific executive function deficits.' *Child Development*, **61**, 1697–1713.

PRADER-WILLI SYNDROME

Alternative names
Prader–Labhart–Willi syndrome; HHHO (*h*ypotonia, *h*ypogonadism, *h*ypomentia, *o*besity) syndrome

First description
The syndrome was first described by Prader, Labhart and Willi in 1956.

Incidence/prevalence
The incidence is estimated at about 1:15,000 live births. The syndrome occurs across all racial and ethnic groups, and males and females are equally affected.

Genetics/aetiology
Prader–Willi syndrome is usually sporadic, and results from abnormality or loss of chromosomal material on the paternal copy of chromosome 15. Approximately 70–85 per cent of cases have a deletion or complex rearrangement of the proximal long arm of chromosome 15 (15q11–13) (Ledbetter *et al.* 1987), which is of paternal origin. Most if not all of the remaining cases are caused by maternal uniparental disomy for chromosome 15. This contrasts with Angelman syndrome, which occurs in individuals with the same interstitial chromosome deletion but in the maternally derived chromosome 15, or with paternal uniparental disomy for chromosome 15. A few familial cases of Prader–Willi syndrome have been documented, and various theories of gene mutation have been postulated to account for these (Donaldson *et al.* 1994). In general, recurrence risk for siblings is below 1 per cent in deletion cases, and unknown (still probably below 2 per cent) in disomy cases. It is not yet known how the molecular abnormality in Prader–Willi syndrome accounts for the neurological, psychological and behavioural characteristics seen clinically. Recently, a small nuclear ribonucleoprotein polypeptide N (*SNRPN*) gene was mapped to the critical region for Prader–Willi syndrome. *SNRPN* is highly expressed in the brain, and is a candidate gene for involvement in the pathophysiology of the syndrome (Ozçelik *et al.* 1992).

Physical phenotype, natural history and life expectancy
Prader–Willi syndrome is characterized by a typical facial appearance (a flat face, prominent forehead with bitemporal narrowing, almond-shaped eyes and a triangular mouth); short stature with absence of a pubertal growth spurt; hypogenitalism and delayed, precocious or incomplete sexual maturation; small hands and feet; severe neonatal hypotonia; feeding difficulties; and delayed developmental milestones (Butler 1990). These features are found in over 90 per cent of cases.

There is an increased prevalence of scoliosis and other orthopaedic abnormalities. Growth hormone deficiency has been documented, and growth hormone intervention is being used successfully in some cases. Fairer skin and lighter hair compared to other family members is observed in about 50 per cent of cases (thought to be the deletion cases), and there is a tendency to easy bruising. Refractive errors, hyperopia and non-familial myopia are often encountered in older children, and speech articulation defects are common, especially hypernasality.

Two stages of the syndrome have been differentiated. In the first phase, after birth and in early infancy, the most noticeable characteristic is severe muscle hypotonia. Babies with Prader–Willi syndrome are limp, floppy, sleepy and non-responsive. They tend to have delayed motor milestones and severe feeding difficulties (including swallowing and sucking difficulties) because of the severe hypotonia. Failure to thrive is common, and special feeding techniques are often needed. The hypotonia begins to improve toward the end of the first year, and this is accompanied by increased motor activity and alertness, and increased appetite and weight gain.

The second phase is characterized by hyperphagia, which develops insidiously between 1 and 4 years of age and is accompanied by excessive or rapid weight gain (Greenswag 1987). In the absence of successful intervention, the hyperphagia may cause life-threatening obesity, with significant numbers of affected people weighing more than double their ideal body weight. The hyperphagia is due either to an insatiable hunger drive or to a decreased perception of satiety. The behavioural and pathophysiological basis for this observed failure to satiate is not known. Hypothalamic dysfunction has been postulated by several authors in an attempt to account for the hyperphagia, and for other features found in this syndrome, including hypogonadism, hypotonia and short stature. Medications to suppress appetite have thus far proved largely unsuccessful.

Life expectancy is related to weight control. Without intervention, the obesity often leads to increased morbidity and mortality, with high blood pressure, cardiovascular symptoms, respiratory difficulties and diabetes mellitus being frequent complications. Heart failure is the commonest cause of death. Good weight control is likely to increase life expectancy, and people with Prader–Willi syndrome who have survived into their sixties have been reported.

Psychological and behavioural phenotype

Prader–Willi syndrome is characterized by a number of distinctive psychological and behavioural features. In early childhood, motor and language development are significantly delayed. Difficulties with gross motor skills, coordination and balance typically persist through childhood. The major language problems identified are multiple articulation errors resulting in reduced intelligibility, language difficulties (with expressive skills often being considerably poorer than receptive skills), and voice problems (primarily hypernasality). The speech production problems are likely to be due at least partly to the early hypotonia and also the facial abnormalities associated with the syndrome. Cognitive impairment is mostly in the borderline to moderate range, though average IQ or above is reported in at least 3 per cent of cases. Severe learning difficulties are unusual. Recent research suggests that many more individulas with Prader–Willi syndrome may in fact have an IQ within the borderline or low-average range of abilities, but that most of them demonstrate multiple learning disabilities.

People with Prader–Willi syndrome are reported to have an unusual cognitive profile, with particular strengths in visual organization and perception, and in academic achievement tasks such as reading and vocabulary. Unusual skill with jigsaw puzzles is often noted. In contrast, auditory information processing and sequential processing are relatively weak, and most individuals have specific deficits in arithmetic, writing, visual and auditory short-term memory and auditory attention. More information is needed on the cognitive profiles and educational attainment of affected individuals.

About half the adults with Prader–Willi syndrome surveyed by Greenswag (1987) worked in sheltered settings, and over a third did not work at all. Fewer than 10 per cent were in open employment. Even among individuals whose IQ is within the normal range, very few achieve a fully independent lifestyle, most probably because of the severe behavioural difficulties that are characteristic of the syndrome.

In the first two to three years children with Prader–Willi syndrome tend to be quiet and passive, and they are often described as easy-going, friendly and affectionate. However, behavioural difficulties become increasingly apparent and severe with age and are much more frequent in this population when compared with other children matched on age and ability levels. Some of these problems are related to the insatiable appetite of affected individuals, which is physically, emotionally and socially debilitating. Excessive intake of food starts in early childhood, and relentless foraging for food, stealing and hoarding of food, as well as consumption of inedible food (such as frozen food or rotten food) is common. Research shows that individuals with Prader–Willi syndrome think a lot more about food than other people, and fight for food; they have been shown to continue to eat at a steady rate as long as food is available.

Dietary management is the cornerstone of managing the obesity. Typically, carers have to respond by limiting access to food and taking over total control of food intake. Such approaches to weight control, and behaviour modification methods which rely on reinforcement and self-monitoring as part of weight control and exercise programmes, have been effectively used with Prader–Willi individuals (*e.g.* Descheemaeker *et al.* 1994). However, long-term maintenance of weight loss is difficult to achieve. Problems with weight control often become worse in adult life when, with increased independence, food is more readily available. Greenswag (1987) found that adults living at home with their parents were significantly heavier than those living away from their families, for example in group homes where they were more closely supervised.

Over 90 per cent of affected individuals self-injure by deliberately picking or scratching their skin, which may lead to infection or cellulitis. The reason for this is not clear. Carers often note that the pain threshold of people with Prader–Willi syndrome is higher than usual.

Emotional lability, outbursts of rage and aggression, stubbornness and belligerence are reported in at least 50 per cent of cases, beginning around age 3–5 years and becoming more marked later in childhood. Aggression may be directed particularly against those who are perceived to be withholding or preventing access to food, but it typically extends also to situations unrelated to food, and may occur with little provocation. Surveys of carers (Greenswag 1987, Clarke *et al.* 1989) confirm that these difficulties persist into adulthood, with a continuing high incidence of belligerence (both food and non-food related), stubbornness, irritability and impulsiveness, as well as compulsive/obsessive behaviours and anxiety-based difficulties, excessive worry and skin picking. These behaviours are believed to be the result of the combination of the physical aspects of the syndrome (*i.e.* central nervous system abnormalities, metabolic defects), the relentless hunger, and the psychosocial pressures of being obese, sexually immature and cognitively limited. Psychiatric symptoms such as hallucinations, paranoia, agitation and anxiety, depression and suicidal tendencies have also been reported in some studies.

Between episodes of difficult behaviour, however, individuals with Prader–Willi syndrome are described as being good natured, placid and cooperative. They may be overfriendly, with impulsive chatter. They tend to have difficulties in social relationships with peers and are often described as being immature, lonely and isolated. This may be at least partly because of sensitivity about the presence of such physical features as obesity, genital underdevelopment and delayed secondary sexual characteristics.

Physical inactivity and passivity are common. In addition, a variety of sleep disorders are found in this population, including sleep apnoea, which may contribute to excessive daytime sleepiness (in over 90 per cent of cases). Both of these may be secondary to obesity (Clarke *et al.* 1989). The sleep apnoea may also be due to both anatomical narrowing of the upper airway and severe muscle hypotonia. Abnormal sleep patterns are common, and cataplexy and sleep-onset REM periods, which are typical of the narcoleptic syndrome, have also been reported in some cases. Antisocial behaviour, passivity and sleepiness are most common in the most obese adults.

KEY REFERENCES

Butler, M.G. (1990) 'Prader–Willi syndrome: current understanding of cause and diagnosis.' *American Journal of Medical Genetics*, **35**, 319–332

Curfs, L.M.G., Fryns, J-P. (1992) 'Prader–Willi syndrome: a review with special attention to the cognitive and behavioral profile.' *Birth Defects: Original Article Series*, **28**, 99–104.

Donaldson, M.D.C., Chu, C.E., Cooke, A., Wilson, A., Greene, S.A., Stephenson, J.B.P. (1994) 'The Prader–Willi syndrome.' *Archives of Disease in Childhood*, **70**, 58–63.

Greenswag, L.R. (1987) 'Adults with Prader–Willi syndrome: a survey of 232 cases.' *Developmental Medicine and Child Neurology*, **29**, 145–152.

—— Alexander, R.C. (Eds.) (1988) *Management of Prader–Willi Syndrome.* New York: Springer-Verlag.

ADDITIONAL REFERENCES

Clarke, D.J., Waters, J., Corbett, J.A. (1989) 'Adults with Prader–Willi syndrome: abnormalities of sleep and behaviour.' *Journal of the Royal Society of Medicine*, **82**, 21–24.

Descheemaeker, M.J., Swillen, A., Plissart, L., Borghgraef, M., Rasenberg, S., Curfs, L.M.G., Fryns, J-P. (1994) 'The Prader–Willi syndrome : A self supporting program for children, youngsters and adults.' *Genetic Counseling*, **5**, 199–205

Ledbetter, D.H., Greenberg, F., Holm, V.A., Cassidy, S.B. (1987) 'Conference Report: second annual Prader–Willi Syndrome scientific conference.' *American Journal of Medical Genetics*, **28**, 779–790.

Ozçelik, T., Leff, S., Robinson, W.L., Donlon, T., Lalande, M., Sanjines, E., Schinzel, A., Francke, U. (1992) 'Small nuclear ribonucleoprotein polypeptide N (SNRPN), an expressed gene in the Prader–Willi syndrome critical region.' *Nature Genetics*, **2**, 265–269.

Prader, A., Labhart, A., Willi, H. (1956) 'Ein Syndrom von Adipositas, Kleinwuchs, Kryptorchismus und Oligophrenie nach myatonieartigen Zustand im Neugeborenenalter.' *Schweizerische Medizinische Wochenschrift*, **86**, 1260–1261

RETT SYNDROME

First description

Rett syndrome was originally described by Andreas Rett in 1966, and gained wide recognition following an article by Hagberg *et al.* in 1983.

Incidence/prevalence

Rett syndrome has a prevalence of 1:10,000 to 1:15,000 females, and is found across all ethnic groups.

Genetics/aetiology

The disorder is restricted to females, and most cases are sporadic, although it has been observed in sisters, half-sisters, monozygotic twins, and cousins. There is also a report of the birth of an affected girl to an affected mother. The genetic data are consistent with a dominant mutation located on the X chromosome, which is lethal to males, although other genetic mechanisms have been suggested, including skewed X inactivation. A gene locus has not as yet been identified; nor has there been any convincing evidence for a specific biochemical abnormality, though an early amine neurotransmitter defect seems likely.

Physical and psychological phenotype, natural history and life expectancy

Rett syndrome is a neurodegenerative disorder with a highly characteristic clinical picture. To ensure a coherent overview, the physical, psychological and behavioural characteristics of the syndrome are described together.

Hagberg and Witt-Engerström (1986) proposed a four-stage outline for the clinical course of the disorder: (i) early stagnation in development after initial progress; (ii) rapid regression; (iii) a pseudostationary or plateau stage; and (iv) a late motor deterioration stage.

There is no striking evidence of pre- or perinatal complications, and affected girls appear normal at birth, with weight and occipitofrontal head circumference within the normal range. The girls progress within the accepted norms in the early months and acquire infant skills to the 9–12 month level. Thus smiling, reaching out and examining objects, transferring objects, babbling, developing words, crawling and walking have all been reported. The girls are also described as cuddly and sociable. However, some abnormalities do in fact exist from a very early age. Early development tends toward the lower limit of normal, particularly with respect to balance; also, placidity, relative immobility with excessive patting movements, lack of initiative and poor tone may be noted in the first year, though these rarely attract concern. Imaginative and imitative activities are seldom demonstrated. By about 15 months of age about half of the girls show obvious developmental deviations and abnormal neurological signs. All girls are symptomatic by 2 years of age.

Stagnation of psychmotor development occurs from about the end of the first year, with accompanying hypotonia and deceleration of head growth, perhaps indicating defective late infancy cortical development. Regression begins at around 1–3 years of age and may be sudden or gradual, lasting weeks or months. It encompasses deterioration in purposeful hand use and speech, associated with communication dysfunction and social withdrawal. Motor development is severely impaired, with poor muscular coordination and difficulty in planning and coordinating movement. Jerky truncal and gait dyspraxia appear between 1 and 4 years of age. Involuntary jerking and writhing movements, poor balance and tremors are characteristic. About half of those affected learn to walk independently and frequently show an unsteady, wide-based, stiff-legged gait. Feeding problems are common, including difficulty in chewing and swallowing, with choking and regurgitation. Constipation is often reported. Expressive and receptive language are also severely impaired. Profound learning difficulties are evident and remain stable.

During regression, sleep disturbance, bouts of crying and screaming, and autistic-like withdrawal are common. Continuous, repetitive hand stereotypies gradually appear, often toward the end of the regression period. They include hand wringing, patting, clapping, tapping and mouthing of the hands. These do not appear to be self- stimulatory behaviours but rather involuntary movements which increase with arousal. They are typically midline motions with the hands placed together; in other cases the squeezing, patting or rolling patterns occur with the hands apart.

After regression, extreme agitation with alternating cycles of hyperventilation and breath-holding occur whenever the child is alerted, and are linked to the repetitive movements of the whole musculature, including the hands, limbs, trunk, mouth and face. There is a remarkable incapacity for voluntary movement, with purposeful hand use and fine finger control remaining particularly impaired. Grinding of teeth, facial grimacing, and breathing abnormalities such as disorganized breathing, breath-holding spells and forced gulping and swallowing of air are reported in 70 per cent of cases or more. Kerr (1992) suggests that these behaviours may represent a group of repetitive movement patterns latent in the nervous system and normally modulated by higher centres, but in Rett syndrome released from inhibition due to incompetent control of the cerebral cortex. Breathing control appears to be normal during sleep, suggesting that brainstem respiratory control is not at fault.

After the initial period of rapid loss of skills, the course is marked by a much slower progression of motor neurological signs that extend insidiously into adult life. By this stage autistic traits are uncommon and the girls may regain some of their original abilities, including some communication. Although expressive and receptive language are mostly absent, there is improved eye contact and improved recognizing, memorizing, nonverbal communication and interpersonal skills (Hagberg 1992). Eye-pointing is adopted in 80 per cent of cases, and babbling or even sudden use of complete or fractured words is found in 55 per cent of cases. Many affected females are able to help with their feeding, dressing and toileting. Studies which have used standardized infant intelligence and language tests and adaptive behaviour scales indicate that most girls function at a mental age below 8 months, with receptive and expressive language and socialization skills in the 4–11 month range, and with self-help skills somewhat better at approximately a 12–14 month level (Perry 1991).

The physical disabilities of affected girls tend to increase with age. Early hypotonia gives way to hypertonia, with progression of scoliosis, muscle wasting, joint contractures, foot deformities and increasing spasticity or rigidity of the lower limbs. Previous walkers may lose ambulation in this stage.

Among the emotional and behavioural difficulties that have been reported are episodes of low mood and of screaming, panic and anxiety in over 70 per cent of affected girls (Coleman *et al.* 1988, Sansom *et al.* 1993). These are often caused by sudden noises, strange people or places, or changes of routine, and they are associated with hyperventilation, self-injury and general distress. Self-injury is reported in over half the cases, usually biting of the wrist, hand or fingers, and self-hitting. Activities which have been found to calm the agitation and self-injury include singing, slow music, holding, cuddling and access to favourite toys. Over 70 per cent of affected girls have sleeping problems, which include delayed sleep onset, night waking, decreased night sleep and night screaming or crying. About 80 per cent have episodes of waking during the night laughing. There is a tendency for these behavioural problems to improve with age.

The clinical picture distinguishes Rett syndrome from primary degenerative diseases and may reflect early dysfunction or damage of certain circuits at cortical and subcortical levels in early development, depriving affected girls of necessary control mechanisms, and leaving access only to very immature behavioural and motor patterns.

Linear growth retardation and poor weight gain are apparent, sometimes to a marked degree. These usually begin in early infancy, more or less in parallel with the deceleration of skull growth. Despite this, most girls are considered to have a good appetite. About half have been reported to have pica (Coleman *et al.* 1988). Endocrine evaluations have not identified any abnormalities to explain the growth failure, though feeding difficulties, including incoordination of chewing and swallowing and regurgitation, inadequate dietary intake and increased energy expenditure (because of their constant repetitive motor movements and episodes of disorganized breathing) may be contributory factors. Some affected girls die in childhood or adolescence—most often the poorly nourished and deformed individuals, who have recurrent chest infections. The majority survive well into adulthood.

Focal or generalized seizures have been reported in at least three quarters of cases. Other brief interruptions of awareness ('vacant spells') of unknown origin are also common. Recent neuropathological findings indicate defective neuronal branching in specific frontal, motor and hippocampal regions of the cortex, and depigmentation of the basal ganglia (Oldfors *et al.* 1993). EEG recordings reveal paroxysmal slow wave abnormality from the time of regression, and most investigators have reported a characteristic progression of EEG abnormalities to a relatively unresponsive theta pattern. Epileptic discharges are common, especially in middle childhood. The brain is slightly reduced in size, with diminished cortical thickness. Early defective neuronal branching, especially in the frontal and temporal cortex, and later depigmentation of the basal ganglia are described.

KEY REFERENCES

Hagberg, B. (Ed.) (1993) *Rett Syndrome – Clinical and Biological Aspects. Clinics in Developmental Medicine No. 127.* London: Mac Keith Press.

Perry, A. (1991) 'Rett syndrome: a comprehensive review of the literature.' *American Journal on Mental Retardation*, **96**, 275–290.

Sansom, D., Krishnan, V.H.R., Corbett, J., Kerr, A. (1993) 'Emotional and behavioural aspects of Rett syndrome.' *Developmental Medicine and Child Neurology*, **35**, 340–345.

Sekul, E.A., Percy, A.K. (1992) 'Rett syndrome: clinical features, genetic considerations and the search for a biological marker.' *Current Neurology*, **12**, 173–200.

ADDITIONAL REFERENCES

Coleman, M., Brubaker, J., Hunter, K., Smith, G. (1988) 'Rett syndrome: a survey of North American patients.' *Journal of Mental Deficiency Research*, **32**, 117–124.

Hagberg, B. (1992) 'The Rett syndrome: an introductory overview 1990.' *Brain and Development*, **14** (Suppl.), S5–S8.

—— Aicardi, J., Dias, K., Ramos, O. (1983) 'A progressive syndrome of autism, dementia, ataxia, and loss of purposeful hand use in girls: Rett's syndrome: report of 35 cases.' *Annals of Neurology*, **14**, 471–479.

Hagberg, B., Witt-Engerström, I. (1986) 'Rett syndrome: a suggested staging system for describing impairment profile with increasing age towards adolescence.' *American Journal of Medical Genetics*, **24** (Suppl. 1), 47–59.

Kerr, A. (1992) 'The significance of the Rett syndrome phenotype.' *Paper presented at the 2nd International Symposium of the Society for the Study of Behavioural Phenotypes, Welshpool, November 1992.* (Abstracts available from Dr Gregory O'Brien, Northgate Hospital, Northumberland.)

Oldfors, A., Sourander, P., Percy, A.K. (1993) 'Neuropathology and neurochemistry.' *In:* Hagberg, B. (Ed.) *Rett Syndrome – Clinical and Biological Aspects. Clinics in Developmental Medicine No. 127.* London: Mac Keith Press, pp. 86–98.

Rett, A. (1966) 'Über ein eigenartiges hirnatrophisches Syndrom bei Hyperammonämie in Kindesalter.' *Wiener Medizinische Wochenschrift*, **116**, 723–726.

162

RING CHROMOSOME 15 SYNDROME

First description
The syndrome was first reported by Jacobsen (1966).

Incidence/prevalence
Just over 30 cases have been identified thus far, with a female:male ratio of 3:1.

Genetics/aetiology
Ring chromosome 15 is caused by breakages of both end segments of chromosome 15, followed by fusion of the broken ends. This results in the loss of chromosomal material, particularly from the terminal segments (the 15q26.2 region). It has been suggested that the severe growth retardation associated with the syndrome may be due to a deletion of the insulin-like growth factor receptor gene at this site. If this is found to be the case, different extents of chromosome deletion, ring instability or mosaicism may explain phenotypic variability in the syndrome.

The birth of an affected child to an affected parent has been reported rather infrequently, possibly because of the fragility of the ring chromosome, the extent of cognitive and growth retardation, and the tendency for affected males to be infertile.

Physical phenotype, natural history and life expectancy
The syndrome is characterized by severe pre- and postnatal growth retardation, and mild dysmorphic features (Borghgraef *et al.* 1988). Microcephaly and delayed bone age are found in 88 per cent and 75 per cent of cases respectively, while a triangular face with hypertelorism is noted in just under half of the reported cases. Other features found in up to one third of cases include frontal bossing, a small mouth and thin lips, micrognathism, small hands and feet with clinodactyly of the fifth fingers, anomalous ears, café-au-lait spots, a short neck, cryptorchidism and cardiac anomalies (Butler *et al.* 1988). Specific tongue motor abnormalities have been reported in some individuals, which may affect articulation and speech, as well as eating and swallowing.

The sexual development and function of affected males is impaired, including hypogonadism and primary sterility. In affected females sexual development appears to be normal and they may reproduce, but there is a high risk for complications during pregnancy due to physical growth failure and uterine hypoplasia.

Neurological complications are rare, but epileptic seizures do occur in some of the severely learning disabled individuals.

Psychological and behavioural phenotype
About one quarter of affected individuals have moderate learning difficulties, and over half have severe learning difficulties (IQ <50) (Borghgraef *et al.* 1988). IQs in the borderline or low-average range have been reported in a few cases. Language abilities tend to be poorer than visuospatial and motor abilities, and expressive speech tends to be

significantly delayed compared with receptive language, at least in the early years (Butler *et al.* 1988). The speech rhythm can be very fast. Butler *et al.* reported difficulties in lateralization of the tongue in two cases, which may partly account for the observed speech difficulties. Marked deficits in attention and concentration are further common features.

Affected children are mostly described as cooperative and docile, somewhat shy and reserved, but with good social skills and little sign of aggression or other behavioural difficulties. A poor self-image may be linked to their short stature. However, a few affected individuals with severe learning difficulties have been reported to be aggressive and uncooperative, and to exhibit rapid alterations in mood (Fryns *et al.* 1986).

The above information is based largely on anecdotal descriptions of single cases. There is a need for confirmation of and elaboration on these findings using larger samples of affected individuals.

KEY REFERENCES

Borghgraef, M., Fryns, J-P., van den Berghe, H. (1988) 'Psychological findings in three children with ring 15 chromosome.' *Journal of Mental Deficiency Research*, **32**, 337–347.
Butler, M.G., Fogo, A.B., Fuchs, D.A., Collins, F.S., Dev, V.G., Phillips, J.A. (1988) 'Brief clinical report and review: two patients with ring chromosome 15 syndrome.' *American Journal of Medical Genetics*, **29**, 149–154.
Fryns, J-P., Kleczkowska, A., Buttiens, M., Jonckheere, P., Brouckmans-Buttiens, K., van den Berghe, H. (1986) 'Ring chromosome 15 syndrome. Further delineation of the adult phenotype.' *Annales de Génétiques*, **29**, 45–48.

ADDITIONAL REFERENCES

Jacobsen, P. (1966) 'A ring chromosome in the 13–15 group associated with microcephalic dwarfism, mental retardation and emotional immaturity.' *Hereditas*, **55**, 188–191.

RUBINSTEIN–TAYBI SYNDROME

Alternative name
Broad thumb–hallux syndrome.

First description
In 1963 Rubinstein and Taybi described seven unrelated children with broad thumbs and broad big toes, who all had learning difficulties and a similar facial appearance.

Incidence/prevalence
The incidence is estimated to be 1:125,000 live births, and there is an equal sex ratio (Hennekam *et al.* 1990). Cases have been reported across all racial groups.

Genetics/aetiology
Most cases are sporadic, though a few familial cases have been reported as well as a number of sets of concordant monozygotic twins, suggesting autosomal dominant inheritance (Hennekam *et al.* 1990). The recurrence risk is less than 1 per cent for siblings, but may be as high as 50 per cent for the offspring of affected individuals (Hennekam *et al.* 1990). The aetiology is still uncertain. Recently, Breuning *et al.* (1993) documented microdeletions within chromosome 16 (at 16p13.3) in some affected individuals. If this finding is confirmed, then cytogenetically undetectable deletions, point mutations or mosaicism may explain the apparent absence of cytogenetic or molecular abnormalities in other affected individuals.

Physical phenotype, natural history and life expectancy
Characteristic features of the syndrome include short stature and microcephaly (both often below the fifth centile); broad thumbs and broad big toes which are occasionally also angulated; and a specific facial appearance consisting of a prominent, beaked nose with a broad fleshy bridge, nasal septum well below the alae with an associated short columella, slightly malformed ears, hypertelorism and downward-slanted palpebral fissures—often accompanied by ptosis or thickened eyelids, heavy or highly arched eyebrows, a highly arched narrow palate, a small oral opening and a pouting lower lip. The facial characteristics change in predictable ways with age. Generalized delay of skeletal maturation, frequent fractures and abnormalities of the cervical spine are often reported. Other common characteristics include a stiff gait (in about 80 per cent of cases), hypotonia and hyperextensible joints (in 70 per cent), a small tilted pelvis, extra hairiness, and undescended testicles (in over 80 per cent of affected males).

The course during infancy is marked by feeding difficulties and poor weight gain (in at least 80 per cent of cases), gastro-oesophageal reflux, vomiting, and recurrent respiratory infections (in over one third of cases). Other frequent complications include congenital heart defects (in over one third of cases); dental abnormalities (in two thirds of cases), in particular irregular, crowded teeth; urinary tract abnormalities and infections (in 30 per cent of cases); and constipation (in 74 per cent of cases). Eye infections and abnormalities are also common, including tear duct obstruction, cataracts, refractive errors and glaucoma. In addition, there is susceptibility to fungus infections of the fingernails and toenails, ingrown nails, and a tendency for raised scar formation. Sexual development is mostly normal.

Affected individuals tend to become overweight, particularly the females. There is no information on life expectancy, though people with the syndrome surviving into their sixties have been reported (Rubinstein 1990).

EEG abnormalities are noted in two thirds of cases, but seizures occur in only about one quarter. Neuropathological findings include absence of the septum pellucidum and hippocampal commisure, and abnormally formed and oriented lateral ventricles. The anterior fontanelle is large or late in closing in over half the cases.

Psychological and behavioural phenotype

Children with Rubinstein–Taybi syndrome show similarities in their cognitive profiles and behaviour. Most have poor concentration and distractibility, with moderate to severe learning difficulties, though some have mild learning difficulties. A mean IQ of 51 was reported by Stevens *et al.* (1990), with a range from below 30 to 79. Hennekam *et al.* (1992) reported a decline in IQ with age, although this may be due to the measurement of different abilities at different ages. Overall, Performance IQ tends to be higher than Verbal IQ. Expressive language is particularly limited, and some affected children do not develop speech at all (Clarke and Langton 1992). They can benefit from signing and a 'total communication' approach to language teaching. In general, however, affected individuals are able to use their limited speech communicatively, and they show good overall language competency. Moreover, despite a high frequency of oral anatomic abnormalities, articulation is generally good. Voice quality may be nasal, and some individuals have a rapid speech rhythm (Hennekam *et al.* 1992).

Children with Rubinstein–Taybi syndrome are described anecdotally as happy, loving and easy to get on with. They are very sociable, even overfriendly, and love adult attention (Stevens *et al.* 1990, Baxter and Beer 1992, Clarke and Langton 1992). They are particularly responsive to music, and are very interested in manipulating objects such as electronic appliances and dials. Most become self-sufficient in eating, dressing and toileting. Severe sleep disturbance is reported in about 10 per cent of cases, possibly due to the combination of a narrow palate, micrognathia, and easy collapsibility of the laryngeal walls, leading to sleep apnoea.

Over half of affected children are said to engage in self-stimulatory behaviours such as rocking, hand flapping and spinning. Resistance to environmental change is reported in over three quarters of children, and intolerance to loud noises and self-injurious behaviours in about half (Stevens *et al.* 1990, Hennekam *et al.* 1992). Older individuals often show sudden changes in mood and temper tantrums.

KEY REFERENCES

Baxter, G., Beer, J. (1992) 'Rubinstein–Taybi syndrome.' *Psychological Reports*, **70**, 451–456

Hennekam, R.C.M., Baselier, A.C.A., Beyaert, E., Bos, A., Blok, J.B., Jansma, H.B.M., Thorbecke-Nilsen, V.V., Veerman, H. (1992) 'Psychological and speech studies in Rubinstein–Taybi syndrome.' *American Journal on Mental Retardation*, **96**, 645–660.

Rubinstein, J.H. (1990) 'Broad thumb–hallux (Rubinstein–Taybi) syndrome 1957–1988.' *American Journal of Medical Genetics*, Suppl. 6, 3–16.

Stevens, C.A., Carey, J.C., Blackburn, B.L. (1990) 'Rubinstein–Taybi syndrome: a natural history study.' *American Journal of Medical Genetics*, Suppl. 6, 30–37.

ADDITIONAL REFERENCES

Breuning, M.H., Dauwerse, H.G., Fugazza, G., Saris, J.J., Spruit, L., Wijnen, H., Tommerup, N., van der Hagen, C.B., Imaizumi, K., *et al.* (1993) 'Rubinstein–Taybi syndrome caused by submicroscopic deletions within 16p13.3.' *American Journal of Human Genetics*, **52**, 249–254.

Clarke, D., Langton, J. (1992) 'The Rubinstein–Taybi behavioural phenotype: a postal questionnaire survey.' *Paper presented at the 2nd International Symposium of the Society for the Study of Behavioural Phenotypes, Welshpool, November 1992.* (Abstracts available from Dr Gregory O'Brien, Northgate Hospital, Northumberland.)

Hennekam, R.C.M., Stevens, C.A., Van de Kamp, J.J.P. (1990) 'Etiology and recurrence risk in Rubinstein–Taybi syndrome.' *American Journal of Medical Genetics*, Suppl. 6, 56–64.

Rubinstein, J.H., Taybi, H. (1963) 'Broad thumbs and toes and facial abnormalities. A possible mental retardation syndrome.' *American Journal of Diseases of Children*, **105**, 588–608

THE SEX CHROMOSOME ANEUPLOIDIES (SCA)

This section deals with conditions involving anomalies of the sex chromosomes. The commonest and best researched of these is Turner syndrome, which will be discussed first. Conditions involving the presence of extra X chromosomes in phenotypic males, colectively known as Kleinfelter syndrome, are considered next, followed by the 47,XYY, 47,XXX and 48,XXXX syndromes.

TURNER SYNDROME

First description
Turner (1938) described a syndrome in females with sexual infantilism, small stature and skeletal abnormalities. The genetic abnormality—an absent or abnormal second X chromosome—was identified by Ford in 1959.

Incidence/prevalence
Current estimates are higher than was originally thought, at around 1:2000 to 1:2500 live female births. The anomaly is much more common at conception, with approximately 99 per cent of affected fetuses miscarrying.

Genetics/aetiology
Turner syndrome is a sporadic condition in females due to loss or abnormality of one of the X chromosomes. In 75 per cent of affected individuals the intact X is of maternal origin. Approximately 50 per cent show karyotype 45,XO (though a current view is that a tiny number of undetected normal cells may be present which prevents spontaneous abortion); 13–17 per cent show isochromosome of X; 30–40 per cent show mosaicism, 10–15 per cent of the total group having karyotype 45,XO/45,XX. In mosaic forms the phenotype is milder. 4–5 per cent have a mosaicism including partial Y chromosome material: in these cases there is a risk of gonadoblastoma. Other abnormalities of the second X which may be present in mosaicism or in all cells are partial deletions of X and ring chromosomes.

Physical phenotype, natural history and life expectancy
The essential features are short stature, normally obvious in the early school years (adult height 120–150 cm), and premature ovarian failure *in utero* giving rise to streak ovaries and hence failure of normal pubertal development. Dysmorphic features may be subtle but include webbed neck (54 per cent); low posterior hairline (73 per cent); broad chest with widely spaced nipples (60 per cent); increased carrying angle at the elbow (56 per cent); small nails; and multiple pigmented naevi. Approximately 20 per cent have coarctation of the aorta, and a minority may have renal abnormalities. Hormone treatment for secondary sexual development is often now preceded by growth hormone therapy.

Life expectancy is not affected, although there is a risk of hypertension developing in adult life.

Psychological and behavioural phenotype

Turner's original description of the syndrome concerned seven girls aged 15–23 years who presented at an endocrinology clinic in Oklahoma with short stature and failure of secondary sexual development. Interestingly, three of these were treated with anterior pituitary growth hormone extract. The only comments Turner made about intellectual or behavioural functioning (four cases) were as follows:

- 'she had always made excellent grades in school and at this time was taking a secretarial course';
- 'there was no mental retardation';
- 'she was mentally alert and ahead of her class in school—an honor student';
- 'she was considerably disturbed because of the fact that her associates treated her as a little girl and because she feared she would never be able to marry and have a home'.

The stereotype of the 'normally functioning' girl, only occasionally beset by secondarily determined problems of psychosocial adjustment, is still frequently promoted. Certainly there are girls with the syndrome who do function in this way, but as with many genetically determined disorders there is wide variability. It is a disservice to those with the syndrome if the often subtle psychological attributes are not acknowledged so that appropriate educational and general supportive input can be available from an early age.

Cognitive aspects

IQ spans the normal range. A specific cognitive profile including spatial deficit was first postulated by Shaffer (1962). Temple and Carney's (1993) report on intellectual functioning of 19 girls with Turner syndrome aged 9–12 years includes a useful bibliography which covers neuropsychological aspects of the disorder. These authors' findings do support a specific overall intellectual profile, but they stress the considerable interindividual variation in its expression. They demonstrate in the majority of girls a relative deficit in performance skills—notably in the Object Assembly and Block Design subtests of the Wechsler Intelligence Scales. On verbal subtests they find significant depression of Arithmetic and Information scores compared with Similarities. Similar findings were reported for 50 Belgian children (Swillen *et al.* 1993). 13 of 20 adults with the syndrome reported problems with mathematics or 'scientific drawing' (Delooz *et al.* 1993).

In all studies intersubject differences are considerable. This is well illustrated by Downey and Ehrhardt (1990) who say 'one of our patients needed to be accompanied to our office in order to find it, while another, obviously without any space form difficulty, possessed a private pilot's license'. A major contribution of Temple and Carney's study is the demonstration of associations between genotype and intellectual profile; those with predominantly mosaic karyotypes being less deviant than those with apparently pure 45,XO.

An interesting finding from an earlier Temple and Carney study (1992) was that affected girls showed significantly enhanced performance on several verbal measures, *viz.* superior verbal recognition memory (the sex difference was greater than that found for non-affected children); hyperlexia, with significantly higher reading ages than control children; and apparently enhanced vocabularies with a tendency to select for use more elaborate words which are normally low frequency items. This particular characteristic, when present, is likely to confuse teachers who may therefore overestimate such a child's overall abilities.

To some extent the cognitive profile could be interpreted as an exaggeration of normal sex differences but most workers argue against such an hypothesis.

An intriguing observation which might further inform this area concerns a 21-year-old woman with the syndrome who could not kinematically represent extrapersonal space. Her dreams appeared to be without visual representation, and her accounts of these were remarkably similar in form to those reported by congenitally blind people. She dreamed not as she saw her waking world, but as she was able to think about it (Kerr *et al.* 1978).

Behavioural and psychiatric aspects

A number of reports over the past 20 years have drawn attention to apparent psychosocial difficulties including immaturity, problems with social relations, lack of assertiveness, argumentativeness and hyperactivity. Swillen *et al.* (1993) showed that for 4- to 6-year-olds hyperactivity was universal. The girls were very distractible and unable to complete tasks. They were 'quiet' children who tended to settle down as they got older. Many of those aged 6–11 years showed poor social skills, while those aged 12–16 showed 'social withdrawal'. McCauley *et al.* (1986) noted that, compared to children with constitutional short stature, girls with Turner syndrome had fewer friends, needed more structure to socialize and to complete tasks, and had more difficulty understanding social cues. They also had problems to do with social ineptitude and isolation.

Currently, findings are being reported from by far the largest study to date, a postal survey of 274 girls with the syndrome recruited through the Child Growth Foundation in the UK (Skuse *et al.* 1994). The aim is to determine whether there are indeed social, emotional and behavioural characteristics of the condition which are not simply a reflection of the associated impairment of linear growth. The study used a control group of girls with normal short stature recruited through the same organization. Data from the Child Behaviour Checklist show significant differences on the Anxious–Depressed and Attention Problems subscales; also on Thought Problems. Differences are also reported which reflect a degree of immaturity and difficulties in peer relationships. Overall they find 'up to one quarter suffering from psychiatric disorders of such severity that they are equivalent to referred cases requiring clinical intervention' and 'a rate of disorder nearly six times as high as in the age matched comparison group of girls with normal short stature'. They conclude that the differences in adjustment between the Turner syndrome and control groups are highly likely to be related to the genotypic characteristics of the Turner syndrome subjects. They do not relate their findings to cognitive level.

They find that those girls identified by parents as having a mosaic karyotype are more disturbed than those with 45,XO but acknowledge that the information source is suspect.

The same group have also reported preliminary findings using an instrument devised for the study—the Emotional and Behavioral Characteristics Checklist. Here the Turner syndrome girls appear to be distinguished from controls, often at highly significant levels, by difficulty picking up on social cues; persistently repeating questions; difficulty following instructions; repeating words and phrases; overanxiety; difficulty maintaining concentration; and fidgety, overactive behaviour. They are also reported to be relatively obsessional, with a set routine, and to become distressed if this is interrupted (Skuse *et al.* 1993).

The question of inter–individual and genotypic variation does not as yet appear to have been systematically investigated in the behavioural field. As with the cognitive findings one would expect considerable variability, and the narrow path between the dangers of stereotyped labelling and recognition of often occurring attributes has to be negotiated with care.

Sexual adjustment
Downey and Ehrhardt (1990) have reviewed information—including an excellent bibliography—about adult behaviour in Turner syndrome. Many of the women have problems related to sexual behaviour—high rates of inexperience and low marriage rates—although these are by no means universal. Several studies have suggested no lack of sexual drive but that physical problems to do with sexual immaturity and oestrogen replacement therapy, together with possibly more fundamental problems of social withdrawal may underpin this aspect.

Psychiatric disorder and social functioning
In the second decade the timing of induced puberty may be crucial in determining the level of psychosocial risk. Delooz *et al.* (1993) reported that ten of 20 women with Turner syndrome had a history of depressive illness as recorded by the Schedule for Affective Disorders and Schizophrenia (SADS) questionnaire. By contrast, Downey and Ehrhardt (1990)—also using the SADS—and other studies including one from the Danish centre (see Nielsen 1990) have shown that women with Turner syndrome and controls do not differ significantly in the number who have ever had a psychiatric disorder or in the number who are currently ill. However, in respect of psychosocial functioning in adult life Downey and Ehrhardt point out that mental health comprises more than psychopathology: it also includes social functioning, and in this respect their work suggests impairments in this area. In addition to the sexual problems already discussed, they found that women with Turner syndrome reported having fewer friends and placing less reliance on their closest friend; also, despite comparable verbal IQ, women with Turner syndrome had lower educational and occupational attainment than controls.

In summary, Downey and Ehrhardt say: 'An important clinical implication is that professionals who are consulted about Turner individuals need to be aware that the problems these patients have do not tend to be of the acting-out kind which are most likely to distress family members, school personnel, and employers. Rather, these patients, when having difficulty, tend to become socially withdrawn and isolated, and their lack of attention-getting behaviour and complaint may lead to oversight that any help is needed.'

KEY REFERENCES

Ford, C., Jones, K.W., Polani, P.E., de Almeida, J.C., Briggs, J.H. (1959) 'A sex chromosomal anomaly in a case of gonadal dysgenesis (Turner's syndrome).' *Lancet*, **2**, 711–713.
Temple, C.M., Carney, R.A. (1993) 'Intellectual functioning of children with Turner syndrome: a comparison of behavioural phenotypes.' *Developmental Medicine and Child Neurology*, **35**, 691 – 698.
Turner, H.H. (1938) 'A syndrome of infantilism, congenital webbed neck, and cubitus valgus.' *Endocrinology*, **23**, 566–574.

ADDITIONAL REFERENCES

Delooz, J., van den Berghe, H., Swillen, A., Kleczkowska, A., Fryns, J-P. (1993) 'Turner syndrome patients as adults: a study of their cognitive profile, psychosocial functioning and psychopathological findings.' *Genetic Counseling*, **4**, 169–179.
Downey, J.W., Ehrhardt, A.A. (1990) 'The long-term behaviour of patients with Turner syndrome.' *In:* Rosenfeld, R.G., Grumbach, M. (Eds.) *Turner Syndrome.* New York: Marcel Decker, pp. 483–492.
Kerr, N.H., Foulkes, D., Jurkovic, G.J. (1978) 'Reported absence of visual dream imagery in a normally sighted subject with Turner's syndrome.' *Journal of Mental Imagery*, **2**, 247–264.
McCauley, E., Ito, J., Kay, T. (1986) 'Psychosocial functioning in girls withTurner's syndrome and short stature: social skills, behavior problems, and self-concept.' *Journal of the American Academy of Child Psychiatry*, **25**, 105–112.
Nielsen, J. (1990) 'Mental aspects of Turner syndrome and the importance of information and Turner contact groups.' *In:* Rosenfeld, R.G., Grumbach, M. (Eds.) *Turner Syndrome..* New York: Marcel Decker, pp. 451–461.
Shaffer, J. (1962) 'A specific cognitive deficit observed in gonadal aplasia (Turner's syndrome).' *Journal of Clinical Psychology*, **18**, 403–406.
Skuse, D., Percy, E., Stevenson, J. (1993) 'Psychosocial functioning in the Turner syndrome: a national survey.' *Paper presented at the 4th Annual Meeting of the Society for the Study of Behavioural Phenotypes, London, December 1993.* (Abstracts available from Dr Gregory O'Brien, Northgate Hospital, Northumberland.)
—— —— —— (1994) 'Psychosocial functioning in the Turner syndrome: a national survey.' *In:* Stabler, B., Underwood, L.E. (Eds.) *Growth, Stature, and Adaptation. Behavioral Social, and Cognitive Aspects of Growth Delay.* University of North Carolina at Chapel Hill, pp. 151–164.
Swillen, A., Fryns, J-P., Kleczkowska, A., Massa, G., Vanderschueren–Lodeweyckx, M., van den Berghe, H. (1993) 'Intelligence, behaviour and psychosocial development in Turner syndrome. A cross-sectional study of 50 pre-adolescent and adolescent girls (4–20 years).' *Genetic Counseling*, **4**, 7–18.
Temple, C.M., Carney, R.A. (1992) 'Cognitive skills in Turner's syndrome: specific deficits and talents.' *Paper presented at the 2nd International Symposium of the Society for the Study of Behavioural Phenotypes, Welshpool, November 1992.* (Abstracts available from Dr Gregory O'Brien, Northgate Hospital, Northumberland.)

OTHER ANEUPLOIDIES

General background
Much of the information about this group of disorders derives from the prospective study of seven birth cohorts of children identified through general programmes of cytogenetic testing of newborn infants set up in the 1960s and '70s. Six of these are now closed. These studies identified 307 children with SCA among 199,898 births. The methods of

ascertainment of subjects and controls and the outcome measures used were different for each study. International collaborative meetings to share follow-up information have been supported by the March of Dimes Birth Defects Foundation, and many of the findings from these cohort studies are published in the proceedings of these meetings (Ratcliffe and Paul 1986, Evans *et al.* 1991). Hereafter, each study will be referred to by the name of its place of origin as follows:

• *The Denver study*, 1964–1974. Identification based principally on X chromatin examination. 69 SCA cases (eight neonatal deaths) identified in 40,371 live births. Mainly sibling controls.
• *The Boston study*, 1970–1974. Male infants only. Heel-prick blood. 23 boys with SCA identified among 13,751 male births. Controls were children with balanced familial autosomal anomalies.
• *The Toronto study*, 1969–1971. Mainly X chromatin examination. 74 SCA cases identified among 71,004 infants. Sibling controls.
• *The Winnipeg study*, 1970–1973. Chromosome analysis of cord blood. 20 SCA cases identified among 14,069 newborn infants. Three control groups: matched newborn infants, plus siblings of cases and controls.
• *The New Haven study*, 1967–1968. One-year births cohort in a single hospital. Matched newborn infant controls.
• *The Danish study*, 1969–1974; restarted in 1990. 58 SCA cases among 20,222 newborn infants.
• *The Edinburgh study*, 1967–1979. Either sex chromatin screening (X and Y) or chromosome analysis of heel-prick blood. 70 SCA cases among 34,380 infants. Matched newborn infant controls.

The early literature on the psychological and psychiatric consequences of sex chromosome abnormalities suffers greatly from ascertainment bias as most affected individuals were identified by screening of mental subnormality hospitals, mental/penal institutions or psychiatric clinics. This led to assumptions that criminality was to be expected. The birth cohort studies have provided an opportunity to redress much misinformation. The fine line between the dangers of stereotyped labelling and the proper use of behavioural phenotypic information to inform practice to the advantage of the subject is nowhere better illustrated than among this group of disorders.

Nevertheless, progress has to some extent been bedeviled by the small numbers recruited to each study (*e.g.* 73 XXY boys are spread between six studies) and by methodological differences, particularly in the selection of controls. However, an enormous strength is that these studies are longitudinal and changes over time are now becoming apparent. Inter-karyotype comparisons are reported by the Denver group (Bender *et al.* 1993) and the Boston group (Walzer *et al.* 1991). Netley (1986) attempted to collate the overall picture on behalf of the various groups involved but clearly ran into difficulties pooling data from the different control samples. Nevertheless, a more or less consistent picture does emerge from the individual studies, and most authors argue strongly in favour of karyotype-specific differences.

In general, significant global learning disability is not a major feature of this group of disorders, but problems with speech and language development, specific learning difficulties and sometimes difficult behaviours occur. The possibility of an underlying sex chromosome aneuploidy should always be born in mind and investigated when a tall boy or girl presents with such difficulties.

KLINEFELTER SYNDROME (47,XXY; 48,XXYY; 48,XXXY; 46,XY/47,XXY; PLUS OTHERS)

'Klinefelter syndrome' includes all sex chromosome anomalies characterized by a surplus of X chromosomes in phenotypic males.

Alternative names
The precise karyotype in question is usually stated.

First description
The endocrinological syndrome (breast development, small testicles, aspermia, raised gonadotrophins) was first described by Klinefelter *et al.* (1942). The cytogenetic abnormality was identified by Jacobs and Strong (1959).

Incidence/prevalence
The estimated incidence is 1:500 to 1:1000 live male births, of whom two-thirds are 47,XXY.

47,XXY

An excellent review of many aspects of this karyotype is provided by Mandoki *et al.* (1991).

Genetics/aetiology
Karyotype 47,XXY arises by meiotic non-disjunction during gametogenesis of the ovum or sperm. The extra X chromosome is maternally derived in 60–70 per cent of cases.

Physical phenotype, natural history and life expectancy
Height, weight and head circumference are small at birth. From age 3 years there is increased growth velocity, the major component of this being increased leg length. The mean adult height is 185 cm (75th centile), affected individuals being on average 13 cm taller than their fathers. However, there is no head growth catch-up—head circumference remains below controls. The extra X chromosome seems to inhibit brain growth *in utero*. Weight is around the 50th centile. Affected individuals may also have poor muscle development.

Most 47,XXY children enter puberty normally. Testosterone levels fall off in adolescence and early adulthood. Adults have a normal sized penis but small testes. They are

174

nearly always infertile because of failed sperm production, but may occasionally produce sperm for a short period. Around 60 per cent show gynaecomastia (*vs* 30 per cent in controls). This is often transient but very occasionally necessitates mastectomy. There is no specific predisposition to homosexuality.

47,XXY individuals tend to be awkward and have mild neuromotor deficit. Life expectancy is probably unaffected.

Psychological and behavioural phenotype

Cognitive aspects

As with most aspects of the 47,XXY syndrome, the cognitive phenotype is very variable. Full scale IQ ranges from the 60s to the 130s. However, there is no doubt that for the group as a whole the IQ distribution is skewed downwards—presumably a consequence of the extra X chromosome-determined constraint on fetal brain growth. In the Edinburgh study average Verbal (V) IQ (93.3) and Performance (P) IQ (97.6) were significantly below those of case controls (V=111.7, P=112.3) and, for the smaller numbers tested, below those of sibling controls. This is in general consistent with findings from other studies. In the Boston and Toronto studies average V–P discrepancies were greater, in the majority of cases significantly so.

All studies reveal notable effects on speech and language development which are apparent from an early age. The majority, whether or not the chromosome anomaly has been made known to teachers and parents, receive speech and language therapy. Walzer *et al.* (1991) report relatively normal receptive language skills among 9- to 12-year-olds but significantly impaired expressive language with deficits in word retrieval abilities and problems with syntax and narrative formation. There are underlying deficits in auditory rate processing and short-term auditory memory.

Behavioural aspects

Information from the cohort studies presents a picture of the XXY boy as introverted and quiet, less assertive, passive, demonstrating lower levels of activity compared with other children, and tending to withdraw from group activities. Adolescents rate themselves as more 'tender minded', apprehensive and insecure as compared with controls. They report more problems with peer group relationships and less sexual interest in girls. However, the adult and clinical literature suggests antisocial and/or psychopathological behaviours rather than the passivity and inactivity of childhood and adolescence.

Netley (1991) examined the social and emotional characteristics of the Toronto cohort as they progressed through adolescence to see if any evidence emerged for a change in behavioural style for some subjects at this time. Around age 16–18 years the extra X males were more aloof, disregarding of rules and assertive than chromosomally normal youths. A self-completion questionnaire showed them to be less cooperative and respectful and more forceful and sensitive than controls. They expressed greater concerns in relation to tolerating social norms, relating to family members and coping with academic requirements. They were also more likely to have problems with impulse control. Most importantly, individual differences did not relate to the quality of parental management, but there were fairly consistent associations with variables reflecting pubertal development—notably that tendencies toward assertiveness, difficulties in relation to family relationships, impulse control and conforming within social norms were most evident in those with relatively quick pubertal development and high levels of serum testosterone.

It is of great interest here that the behavioural implications of testosterone levels are different in XXY males and controls. Levels which for the chromosomally normal are average or slightly below average and which would be associated with prosocial behaviours are associated with antisocial behaviours among XXY males. Netley speculates about associations between these pubertal anomalies and some aspects of brain maturation. His data also suggest that there may be implications for pharmaceutical manipulation which could smooth the path for some of these young adults.

The issue of testosterone treatment was raised in a report by Miller and Sulkes (1988) which suggested that among firesetters a small number might have Klinefelter syndrome. This provoked concerned correspondence that stereotyped labelling was again being promoted. However, in defense of their position the authors pointed out that if an XXY diagnosis was made, testosterone therapy might be beneficial in counteracting this particular behaviour in these individuals.

Educational aspects
The most consistent finding in the investigation of XXY males is poor school performance. Across all the cohort studies 64 per cent of 58 XXY cases as compared to 26 per cent of controls had educational difficulties requiring remedial input. Walzer *et al.* (1991) emphasize a continuum of language/learning disabilities over many years. Deficits in language production and processing in the preschool years were associated with severe and chronic reading and writing disabilities during the school years. Mathematical skills were unimpaired (Bender *et al.* 1993). However, despite their serious language processing deficits and specific learning disabilities, Walzer *et al.* reported that because they are 'low key' children, who present few behavioural management problems and are well liked by their teachers, the primary importance of their language processing difficulties tends to be overlooked. Their poor academic progress is often ascribed to 'motivational' problems, with typical reports as 'lazy' and 'could do the work if he tried'. This in turn serves to erode self esteem and precipitate secondary behavioural difficulties.

48,XXYY

First description
48,XXYY syndrome was first reported by Muldal and Ockney (1960).

Incidence/prevalence
The incidence is uncertain but around 60 cases have been reported world-wide.

Physical phenotype, natural history and life expectancy
Physical features are similar to those in 47,XXY and 47,XYY syndromes but subjects

may be even taller. Variable mild dysmorphic features reported include macrocephaly and mild craniofacial dysmorphism with brachycephaly and maxillary hypoplasia. Generalized hypotonia and truncal obesity are also recorded. Sexual development is like that of XXY males.

Psychological and behavioural phenotype

All 48,XXYY subjects reported to date have learning disability, usually in the mild/ moderate range. IQs range from the 30s to the 90s, and there is usually severe language delay.

No specific behavioural phenotype has been reported but Borghgraef *et al.* (1991) noted behavioural similarities in four males, aged 4–25 years, who had presented to a specialist clinic with tall stature and behavioural problems. These included autistic features, distractibility, non-conformity, and a tendency to violent and impulsive actions which gravely prejudiced social integration. There was some indication that the behaviours settled down to some extent after puberty.

49,XXXXY

First description

49,XXXXY syndrome was first reported by Fraccaro *et al.* (1960).

Physical phenotype, natural history and life expectancy

Distinctive features include characteristic craniofacial abnormalities, skeletal deformities and microgenitalism. Microbrachycephaly with upward- and outward-sloping eyes, epicanthic folds and short neck give an appearance suggestive of Down syndrome. Gross and fine motor clumsiness is apparent.

Psychological and behavioural phenotype

Curfs *et al.* (1990) presented psychological data on five boys and a useful set of references. Learning disability was the rule, with a range from profound to moderate. All five showed severe articulation defects such that two were able to produce only sounds, and all showed major discrepancy between receptive and expressive language.

All had a low frustration level and a tendency to temper outbursts, but overall adaptive functioning was said to be at a higher level than cognitive functioning. Four were described as extremely timid and shy but one was 'pleasant and cheerful'.

47,XYY

First description

The first report of 47,XYY syndrome was made by Sandberg *et al.* (1961).

Incidence/prevalence

The incidence is estimated at around 1:1000 live male births.

Genetics/aetiology

The anomaly is caused by a primary non-disjunction of the Y chromosome. 10 per cent of cases are mosaic 46,XY/47,XYY.

Physical phenotype, natural history and life expectancy

Height, weight and head circumference are normal at birth. Between age 4 and 9 years there is a greater than normal increase in both body and leg length. Head circumference remains proportionate throughout. At age 18 mean height is around 187 cm, with growth still occurring in some subjects. Most are at least 13 cm taller than their fathers. Ratcliffe (1994) speculates that as this is an amount equivalent to the average male–female difference, the presence of an additional Y chromosome seems to double the magnitude of sexual dimorphism in man implying a quantitative effect of genes on the Y chromosome. Overall, the pattern of accelerated growth, final height achieved and maintenance of head growth differentiate this phenotype from that of 47,XXY syndrome.

All aspects of sexual development are normal, as are testosterone levels. Puberty begins at the normal time or slightly late. Fertility is normal, and offspring rarely have two Y chromosomes.

Motor performance may be somewhat awkward, with minor neuromotor deficit. Mean scores for coordination and balance were lower than for controls in the Edinburgh study.

Psychological and behavioural phenotype

Cognitive aspects

As a group XYY individuals are more intellectually able than those with XXY karyotype. IQ is only slightly below population means but is usually lower than that of siblings. However, some have IQ in the superior range. In the Edinburgh study average verbal IQ (100.2) fell just significantly below that for case controls (109.2) but performance IQ (105.2) did not (case controls 116.6). Findings from the Boston study are similar.

Speech and language difficulties are common. 44 per cent of those in the Edinburgh study received speech therapy as young children. The Boston study (Walzer *et al.* 1991) revealed greater clinical diversity in communication problems than among XXY boys. Only two of 13 boys had no problem. Some showed marked speech dysfluency, some had difficulty understanding complex sentence structures, and some had problems with word finding and narrative formulation. Various combinations of deficits were found, and auditory memory problems were evident in six of the 11.

Behavioural aspects

In the late 1960s it was proposed that males with an extra Y chromosome were predisposed to violent criminal behaviour. Later work found little support for this hypothesis, but it has bedeviled clinical work related to the sex chromosome aneuploidies, posing problems relating to disclosure of karyotype.

Parents often describe XYY boys as 'difficult to rear'. Distractibility, hyperactivity and temper tantrums tend to feature. Disclosure of diagnosis of XYY may afford relief and reduce parents' perceptions that their own inadequacy is to blame.

At age 11–16 the Edinburgh group scored high on the Rutter total and antisocial scales (Walzer *et al.* 1991). Behaviours which featured were speech problems, tempers, solitariness, dislike by peers and stealing. Aggression and bullying did not feature on parental or teacher reports. By contrast with their findings in XXY boys, the Boston study reported higher levels of motor activity than in controls, classroom teachers reporting motor restlessness, fidgetiness and excessive gross motor activity (meandering around the room, running) at times when the boys were expected to sit or stand quietly. Distractibility was reported from an early age in contrast to XXY boys in whom such behaviours did not intrude until their learning difficulties had become manifest. XYY boys frequently posed management problems for their teachers.

At age 13–24 years the rate of court conviction among 13 boys in the Edinburgh study was 0.27 compared with 0.07 for control boys from a similar social background. However, the offences of XYY boys were of a more minor nature.

Educational aspects
While some of the boys are advanced in reading skills, remedial reading was initiated by teachers (with no knowledge of the chromosome constitution) for 54 per cent of those in the Edinburgh study. Walzer *et al.* (1991) give an excellent comparative account of boys with XXY and XYY identified in the Boston study. 85 per cent of XYY boys had persistent reading and spelling difficulties. 55 per cent required special educational support. Compared to XXY boys those with XYY abnormality were more frequently perceived as unteachable in mainstream classes because of management problems, even though they were often less disadvantaged in their learning skills.

47,XXX

Alternative name
Triple X syndrome.

First description
47,XXX syndrome was first reported by Jacobs *et al.* (1959).

Incidence/prevalence
The incidence is around 1:1000 female births, and there are probably 25,000 women in the UK with the triple X anomaly although most are undiagnosed.

Genetics/aetiology
The anomaly is caused by a primary non-disjunction of maternally or paternally derived X chromosome. There is some relationship to increased maternal age.

Physical phenotype, natural history and life expectancy
Length, weight and head circumference are reduced at birth. Some subjects show

increased growth velocity between age 4 and 9 years and have relatively long legs, while others show normal growth velocity. Adult height is usually at or above the 90th centile (171 cm) but some are much shorter. Subjects are usually underweight for height, so appear tall and thin. Head circumference increase with age is normal but there is no catch-up of prenatal retardation of head growth. Head size therefore remains smaller than for controls.

Developmental milestones are usually slightly delayed. There are no distinctive physical features but many subjects show deficits of fine motor coordination, visuomotor coordination and balance. Few participate in sporting activities. Mean age at puberty and menarche is slightly delayed. Fertility is not affected and offspring are usually chromosomally normal. No information is available on life expectancy, but this is unlikely to be affected.

Psychological and behavioural phenotype

Cognitive aspects

All studies show mean IQs in the 80–90 range, which is lower than for XXY males. Most have IQ lower than siblings. In the Edinburgh study IQ ranged from 75 to 117 with a mean of 90.6 (control mean = 110.3). Verbal scores are more depressed than performance scores and more so than for XXY boys. Bender *et al.* (1993) compare children with XXY and XXX and draw attention to the fact that their learning and neuropsychological difficulties are quite different. The majority have expressive language delay—sometimes severe—and require speech therapy. Some show poor short-term auditory memory. However, it is important to recognize that some girls appear neither impaired nor disadvantaged by the aneuploidy.

Educational aspects

Most require remedial help for reading, but reading skills are usually in line with IQ and are on the whole better than for XXY boys.

Behavioural aspects

In the Edinburgh cohort school teachers reported underreaction and withdrawal with no complaints of disruptive behaviour. On the Rutter questionnaire high scores were often achieved, with the excess derived from both antisocial and neurotic subscales; however, the parents did not perceive these girls as being 'difficult'. Psychiatric referral rate was lower than for any other aneuploidy group (25 per cent) but still exceeded that for controls (3 per cent). One girl in the Edinburgh study and one in the Denver group exhibited elective mutism and trichotillomania. Emotional development is relatively slow and there is evidence of increased vulnerability to stress and, in some cases, difficulty with peer relationships and group functioning. There is little useful information about psychiatric disorder among adults. The evidence to date suggests that most adapt to adult life with few problems but, as with Turner syndrome, it may be that since problems are not of an acting-out type they go unnoticed. Further investigation is needed among this group.

48,XXXX

Alternative name
Tetra X syndrome.

First description
The first report was by Carr *et al.* (1961).

Incidence/prevalence
The exact incidence is unknown, but the condition is probably rare. There are only around 40 reported cases.

Physical phenotype, natural history and life expectancy
Reports are inconsistent as to whether there is a characteristic physical phenotype, suggesting that the phenotype is very variable. Borghgraef *et al.* (1991) reported in three patients serious delay in achieving motor milestones, and notable hypotonia in the first years of life which had effects on gross and fine motor development. Growth and general physical development was normal.

Psychological and behavioural phenotype
IQs have been reported between 30 and 90, with the majority in the 55–75 range which is lower than for girls with only three X chromosomes. Borghgraef *et al.* state that their specific findings are in line with the other few reports of the syndrome. All subjects showed speech defects and articulatory problems. They behaved as pleasant, cooperative girls but were shy and timid in new situations. The overall impression is that the presence of four X chromosomes is less severely deleterious to girls than to boys (cf. 49,XXXXY syndrome).

Fryns *et al.* (1983) have reviewed the literature on this syndrome.

KEY REFERENCES

Evans, J.A., Hamerton, J.L., Robinson, A. (Eds.) (1991) *Children and Young Adults with Sex Chromosome Aneuploidy. Follow-up, Clinical, and Molecular Studies. March of Dimes Birth Defects Foundation. Birth Defects: Original Article Series, Vol. 26, No. 4.* New York: Wiley–Liss.
Mandoki, M.W., Sumner, G.S., Hoffman, R.P., Riconda, D.L. (1991) 'A review of Klinefelter's syndrome in children and adolescents.' *Journal of the American Academy of Child and Adolescent Psychiatry,* **30**, 167–172.
Ratcliffe, S.G., Paul, N. (Eds.) (1986) *Prospective Studies on Children with Sex Chromosome Aneuploidy. March of Dimes Birth Defects Foundation. Birth Defects: Original Article Series, Vol. 22, No. 3.* New York: Alan R. Liss.

ADDITIONAL REFERENCES

Bender, B.G., Linden, M.G., Robinson, A. (1993) 'Neuropsychological impairment in 42 adolescents with sex chromosome abnormalities.' *American Journal of Medical Genetics (Neuropsychiatric Genetics),* **48**, 169–173.

Borghraef, M., Fryns, J-P., van den Berghe, H. (1991) 'The 48,XXYY syndrome. Follow-up data on clinical characteristics and psychological findings in 4 patients.' *Genetic Counseling*, **2**, 103–108.

Carr, D.H., Barr, M.L., Plunkett, E.R. (1961) 'An XXXX sex chromosome complex in two mentally defective females.' *Canadian Medical Association Journal*, **84**, 131 137.

Curfs, L.M.G., Schreppers-Tijdink, G., Wiegers, A., Borghgraef, M., Fryns, J-P. (1990) 'The 49,XXXXY syndrome: clinical and psychological findings in five patients.' *Journal of Mental Deficiency Research*, **34**, 277–282.

Fraccaro, M., Kaijser, K., Lindsten, J. (1960) 'A child with 49 chromosomes.' *Lancet*, **2**, 899–902.

Fryns, J-P., Kleczkowska, A., Petit, P., van den Berghe, H. (1983) 'X-chromosome polysomy in the female: personal experience and review of the literature.' *Clinical Genetics*, **23**, 341–349.

Jacobs, P.A., Baikie, A.G., Court-Brown, W.M., MacGregor, T.N., Maclean, N., Harnden, D.G. (1959) 'Evidence for the existence of the human "super-female".' *Lancet*, **2**, 423–425.

—— Strong, J.A. (1959) 'A case of human intersexuality having a possible XXY sex-determining mechanism.' *Nature*, **183**, 302–303.

Klinefelter, H.F., Reifenstein, E.C., Albright, F. (1942) 'Syndrome characterized by gynecomastia, aspermatogenesis without A–Leydigism, and increased excretion of follicle-stimulating hormone.' *Journal of Clinical Endocrinology*, **2**, 615–627.

Miller, M.E., Sulkes, S. (1988) 'Fire–setting behavior in individuals with Klinefelter syndrome.' *Pediatrics*, **82**, 115–117.

Muldal, S., Ockney, C.H. (1960) 'The "double male": a new chromosome constitution in Klinefelter's syndrome.' *Lancet*, **2**, 492–493.

Netley, C.T. (1986) 'Summary overview of behavioural development in individuals with neonatally identified X and Y aneuploidy.' *In:* Ratcliffe, S.G., Paul, N. (Eds.) *Prospective Studies on Children with Sex Chromosome Aneuploidy. March of Dimes Birth Defects Foundation. Birth Defects: Original Article Series, Vol. 22, No. 3.* New York: Alan R. Liss, pp. 293–306.

—— (1991) 'Personality in 47,XXY males during adolescence.' *Clinical Genetics*, **39**, 409–418.

Ratcliffe, S.G. (1994) 'The psychological and psychiatric consequences of sex chromosome abnormalities in children, based on population studies.' *In:* Poustka, F., (Ed.) *Basic Approaches to Genetic and Molecularbiological Developmental Psychiatry.* Quintessenz Library of Psychiatry, pp. 99–122.

Sandberg, A.A., Koepf, G.F., Ishihara, T., Hauschka, T.S. (1961) 'An XYY human male.' *Lancet*, **2**, 488–489. *(Letter.)*

Walzer, S., Bashir, A.S., Silbert, A.R. (1991) 'Cognitive and behavioral factors in the learning disabilities of 47,XXY and 47,XYY boys.' *In:* Evans, J.A., Hamerton, J.L., Robinson, A. (Eds.) *Children and Young Adults with Sex Chromosome Aneuploidy. Follow-up, Clinical, and Molecular Studies. March of Dimes Birth Defects Foundation. Birth Defects: Original Article Series, Vol. 26, No. 4.* New York: Wiley–Liss, pp. 45–58.

SMITH–LEMLI–OPITZ SYNDROME

Alternative name

RSH (*r*etardation, *s*yndactyly, *h*ypotonia) syndrome.

First description

Smith, Lemli and Opitz (1964) described three males with a similar pattern of anomalies, consisting of microcephaly, growth retardation, abnormalities of hands and feet, incomplete development of genitalia in males, and learning difficulties.

Incidence/prevalence

The syndrome is relatively common, with an incidence of 1:20,000 to 1:40,000 live births (Lowry and Yong 1980). It is found in different ethnic groups, and there is a 3:1 male to female preponderance, though this may reflect the easier diagnosis in males due to the presence of genital ambiguity.

Genetics/aetiology

The syndrome has been reported in siblings and is inherited as an autosomal recessive condition. Tint *et al.* (1994) recently described a severe defect in cholesterol biosynthesis in five individuals with the syndrome, resulting in abnormally low plasma cholesterol concentrations and greatly elevated levels of the cholesterol precursor 7-dehydrocholesterol, due to deficiency of the enzyme 7-dehydrocholesterol reductase. This finding might provide a biochemical marker for the syndrome. Tint *et al.* postulate that the defect in cholesterol biosynthesis results in a reduced supply of cholesterol to the embryo and fetus, and an accumulation of abnormal sterols in all plasma membranes and in myelin. These sequelae may explain the organ and tissue malformations and abnormalities found in the syndrome.

Physical phenotype, natural history and life expectancy

The Smith–Lemli–Opitz syndrome is characterized by severe psychomotor retardation and multiple congenital anomalies involving most organ systems. There is wide phenotypic variability even within families, ranging from cases with severe expression and perinatal death, to cases with only minor anomalies. There appears to be a positive correlation between the degree of genital involvement and overall severity of phenotypic expression in the syndrome; individuals with complete external feminization represent extreme severity of the syndrome. Some writers prefer to separate off the more severely affected cases and refer to these as Smith–Lemli–Opitz syndrome type II (Curry *et al.* 1987), while others feel that the two types are part of the same spectrum, since the biochemical defect is the same in both.

Affected children commonly have growth deficiency of prenatal onset, microcephaly, severe feeding difficulties and failure to thrive in infancy, recurrent infections and initial hypotonia, mostly progressing into generalized hypertonia in those children who survive beyond the first year of life. Typical craniofacial anomalies include facial capillary haemangiomata, broad nasal bridge and epicanthal folds, ptosis, strabismus, cataracts, anteverted nares, thick alveolar ridges, a small tongue, cleft palate, micrognathia, and large low-set ears. The facial features change with age; the only characteristic feature that persists is the broad alveolar ridges. Limb anomalies include syndactyly, typically of the second and third toes, and postaxial polydactyly of the hands and/or feet, as well as short, displaced thumbs. In males there are varying degrees of genital anomalies, often with severe or even complete failure of external male genital development, and sometimes with apparent female external genitalia. Affected females do not have major genital abnormalities.

Major organ malformations are often present, involving the central nervous system (*e.g.* microcephaly, internal hydrocephalus), heart (including endocardial cushion defect, Fallot's tetralogy), kidneys (which may be hypoplastic, with small cysts), lungs and gastrointestinal tract. In some affected individuals these anomalies result in death early in life (Bialer *et al.* 1987); other individuals survive into adulthood. Preliminary studies suggest that a high cholesterol diet with bile acids can improve growth and reduce irritability in some cases (Elias *et al.* 1994).

Neuropathologic studies have shown some patients to have mild to moderate internal hydrocephalus, and hypoplasia of the frontal lobes, corpus callosum, cerebellum and brainstem. The frontal lobes have also revealed broad, irregular gyri with excessive formation of secondary transverse sulci.

Psychological and behavioural phenotype

There is little information on the abilities and behaviour of affected individuals. Cognitive abilities apparently span a wide range, from borderline intelligence to severe learning difficulties. Spoken language and communication have been described in some severely affected children, and there is one report of self-injury and aggression in an affected girl (Tint *et al.* 1994).

KEY REFERENCES

Bialer, M.G., Penchaszadeh, V.B., Kahn, E., Libes, R., Krigsman, G., Lesser, M.L. (1987) 'Female external genitalia and Müllerian duct derivatives in a 46,XY infant with the Smith–Lemli–Opitz syndrome.' *American Journal of Medical Genetics*, **28**, 723–731.
Curry, C.J.R., Carey, J.C., Holland, J.S., Chopra, D., Fineman, R., Golabi, M., Sherman, S., Pagon, R.A., *et al.* (1987) 'Smith–Lemli–Opitz syndrome—Type II: muliple congenital anomalies with male pseudohermaphroditism and frequent early lethality.' *American Journal of Medical Genetics*, **26**, 45–57.
Tint, G.S., Irons, M., Elias, E.R., Batta, A.K., Frieden, R., Chen, T.S., Salen, G. (1994) 'Defective cholesterol biosynthesis associated with the Smith–Lemli–Opitz syndrome.' *New England Journal of Medicine*, **330**, 107–113.

ADDITIONAL REFERENCES

Elias, E.R., Irons, M., Nwokoro, N., Abuelo, D.N., Tint, S., Salen, G. (1994) 'Therapy of the cholesterol defect in Smith–Lemli–Opitz (S-L-O) syndrome.' *American Journal of Human Genetics*, **55** (Suppl.), A42. *(Abstract.)*

Lowry, R.B., Yong, S-L. (1980) 'Borderline normal intelligence in the Smith–Lemli–Opitz (RSH) syndrome.' *American Journal of Medical Genetics*, **5**, 137–143.

Smith, D.W., Lemli, L., Opitz, J,M. (1964) 'A new recognised syndrome of multiple congenital anomalies.' *Journal of Pediatrics*, **64**, 210–217.

SMITH–MAGENIS SYNDROME

First description
The syndrome was first reported in 1986 in papers by Smith and co-workers and Stratton and co-workers.

Incidence/prevalence
The exact incidence is not known, but it is estimated to be around 1:50,000 live births (Colley *et al.* 1990).

Genetics/aetiology
The condition is caused by the partial or complete deletion of band 17p11.2. Physical features may depend on the extent of the deletion. DNA markers linked to the gene for Charcot–Marie–Tooth disease type 1A (*CMT1A*) also map to 17p11.2. Moncla *et al.* (1993) have suggested that an unstable region, located between the Smith–Magenis syndrome locus (*SMS*) and *CMT1A*, could be a hot spot for rearrangements leading proximally to *SMS* microdeletions and distally to *CMT1A* duplications. Chevillard *et al.* (1993) have proposed a candidate gene.

Physical phenotype, natural history and life expectancy
Smith–Magenis syndrome is notable in that florid behavioural manifestations may precede and overshadow the learning disability and physical features. The latter may be unremarkable and include brachycephaly; broad face and nasal bridge; flat mid-face; short broad hands; inbent fingers; small toes and a hoarse, deep voice (Greenberg *et al.* 1991). The upper lip characteristically has a cupid's bow shape, and the corners of the mouth may be downturned. Facial features become coarser as the children get older. Abnormalities of ear shape and position, and hearing loss following recurrent otitis infections also are commonly seen. Less consistent features are genital abnormalities, up-slanting palpebral fissures, Brushfield spots and abnormal palmar creases. Finucane *et al.* (1993) have described strabismus, high myopia and retinal detachment as less common features. They note that the combination of high myopia, self-injurious head-banging, aggression and hyperactivity makes subjects particularly susceptible to retinal detachment. Greenberg *et al.* found signs suggestive of peripheral neuropathy—decreased or absent deep tendon reflexes, decreased pain sensitivity and reduced leg muscle mass—in 55 per cent of their sample.

Most ongoing problems relate to behavioural and communication difficulties rather than physical attributes, but hearing and visual impairments may impose additional disadvantage. Three adult females, aged 32, 42 and 65, are reported in some detail in the literature. The 65-year-old is mentioned in a subsequent paper as having reached 72. Two of these women have been institutionalized since childhood. All are profoundly retarded. Two exhibit self-injurious behaviour. Two have been, or still are, receiving antipsychotic medication. All have variable hearing/vision problems. One has hypogonadism, and one has late onset congenital adrenal hyperplasia. Clearly these three cases have been identified because of the severity of their problems. There is currently no published information about less severely affected adults, but it is clear that some teenagers do not exhibit the more distressing features of the disorder.

Psychological and behavioural phenotype
There have been no systematic studies of cognitive function. Case descriptions suggest a variable degree of learning disability spanning the mild, moderate and severe ranges but with the majority moderately affected. Speech may be more retarded than other functional areas. There are no reports of affected people who do not have associated learning disability.

The Smith–Magenis syndrome is a powerful paradigm in the context of behavioural phenotypes. The behavioural attributes can be florid and overwhelming. They are of critical diagnostic importance, but are not universal. Parents have been blamed for the behaviours, and there is at least one documented case of a child being taken into local authority care with a putative diagnosis of deprivation and neglect before the correct diagnosis was made (McNaught and Turk 1993).

Among those cases reported in the literature, behavioural problems are identified in around 70 per cent. It is likely that as case recognition increases, more less severely affected children will be identified and the percentage with florid behavioural problems will fall.

In the various studies hyperactivity has been reported in around 75 per cent of cases, while self-injurious behaviours, which may be present as early as 18 months and which increase with age, are reported in around 66 per cent. These behaviours can be extreme and include head-banging, wrist and hand biting, and pulling out finger- and toe-nails. The severity of these latter manifestations may be explained in some cases by insensitivity to pain, which Greenberg documents in around 25 per cent. Some children fulfil diagnostic criteria for autism (Stratton *et al.* 1986, McNaught and Turk 1993). Sleep disorder can be extreme and has been reported in around 50 per cent. It manifests as difficulty falling asleep and difficulty staying asleep. The children characteristically sleep in short bursts (around two hours) and are then awake and active for a long time. Total hours of sleep are reduced. Some have absence of REM sleep, as demonstrated by polysomnography.

Concluding their report, Colley *et al.* (1990) state: 'A paediatrician, when confronted with a child who has mental retardation, dysmorphic features, sleep disturbance, hyperactivity, and grossly abnormal, often destructive behaviours, should include a search for this small chromosome deletion in investigations.'

KEY REFERENCES

Colley, A.F., Leversha, M.A., Voullaire, L.E., Rogers, J.G. (1990) 'Five cases demonstrating the distinctive behavioural features of chromosome deletion 17(p11.2p11.2) (Smith–Magenis syndrome).' *Journal of Paediatrics and Child Health*, **26**, 17–21.
Greenberg, F., Guzzetta, V., Montes de Oca-Luna, R., Magenis, R.E., Smith, A.C.M., Richter, S.F., Kondo,

I., Dobyns, W.B., Patel, P.I., Lupski, J.R. (1991) 'Molecular analysis of the Smith–Magenis syndrome: a possible contiguous-gene syndrome associated with del(17)(p11.2).' *American Journal of Human Genetics*, **49**, 1207–1218.

Smith, A.C.M., McGavran, L., Robinson, J., Waldstein, G., Macfarlane, J., Zonona, J., Reiss, J., Lahr, M., Allen, I., Magenis, E. (1986) 'Interstitial deletion of (17)(p11.2p11.2) in nine patients.' *American Journal of Medical Genetics*, **24**, 393–414.

Stratton, R.F., Dobyns, W.B., Greenberg, F., DeSana, J.B., Moore, C., Fidone, G., Runge, G.H., Feldman, P., Sekhon, G.S., *et al.* (1986) 'Interstitial deletion of (17)(p11.2p11.2): report of six additional patients with a new chromosome deletion syndrome.' *American Journal of Medical Genetics*, **24**, 421–432.

ADDITIONAL REFERENCES

Chevillard, C., Le Paslier, D., Passage, E., Ougen, P., Billault, A., Boyer, S., Mazan, S., Bachellerie, J.P., Vignal, A., *et al.* (1993) 'Relationship between Charcot–Marie–Tooth 1A and Smith–Magenis regions: snU3 may be a candidate gene for the Smith–Magenis syndrome.' *Human Molecular Genetics*, **2**, 1235–1243.

Finucane, B.M., Jaeger, E.R., Kurtz, M.B., Weinstein, M., Scott, C.I. (1993) 'Eye abnormalities in the Smith–Magenis contiguous gene deletion syndrome.' *American Journal of Medical Genetics*, **45**, 443–446.

McNaught, A., Turk, J. (1993) 'Smith–Magenis syndrome mistaken for emotional abuse: a case report.' *Paper presented at the 4th Annual Meeting of the Society for the Study of Behavioural Phenotypes, London, December 1993.* (Abstracts available from Dr Gregory O'Brien, Northgate Hospital, Northumberland.)

Moncla, A., Piras, L., Arbex, O.F., Muscatelli, F., Mattei, M-G., Mattei, J-F., Fontes, M. (1993) 'Physical mapping of microdeletions of the chromosome 17 short arm associated with Smith–Magenis syndrome.' *Human Genetics*, **90**, 657–660.

SOTOS SYNDROME

Alternative name
Cerebral gigantism.

First description
Sotos *et al.* (1964) described a number of children with large body size, early accelerated growth and advanced bone age, who had a characteristic facial appearance and developmental delay.

Incidence/prevalence
In the absence of a definitive diagnostic marker for the syndrome, its prevalence is difficult to determine. A slight excess of affected males has been documented, but estimates of the ratio of males to females vary.

Genetics/aetiology
Most cases are sporadic, although a few familial cases have been reported. In these, the mode of inheritance is most likely to be autosomal dominant. The aetiology of the syndrome is not known, and thus far chromosomal investigations have failed to yield any consistent findings.

Physical phenotype, natural history and life expectancy
Sotos syndrome is a disorder of growth and development. Body size tends to be large at birth, especially in length, and the children show advanced bone age and accelerated growth, particularly in the first five years. Thereafter, growth usually continues above the 97th centile for a variable period, before gradually falling towards the normal range. Head circumference proceeds above the 97th centile, and hands and feet are often larger than expected for the person's height (Cole and Hughes 1990, 1994).

Individuals with Sotos syndrome have a characteristic facial appearance. In infancy, the face and forehead are round, with a high forehead, frontal bossing, a prominent jaw, antimongoloid slant of the palpebral fissures, anteverted nares, and a high arched palate. These features are present in over 90 per cent of children with the syndrome. Premature eruption of teeth, and sparseness of hair, particularly in the fronto-parietal region, are also common. With time, the face becomes longer and thinner, the jaw becomes more prominent and the features coarsen. The facial features are said to become less obvious with age, but this may be because of lack of familiarity with the typical adult facial appearance.

Jaundice and early feeding problems are found in over 40 per cent of affected neonates, which may be due to asphyxia and difficult deliveries of these large babies, but thereafter appetite and fluid intake tend to be greater than would be expected. Constipation is a common complaint. Persistent drooling and reluctance to chew are found in up to 44 per cent of cases. An atypical pubertal history in females has been reported in several cases, with an early menarche, probably reflecting biological age. In males puberty tends to be delayed.

Joint laxity and pes planus are frequent findings. Hypotonia is present in over 85 per cent of affected individuals during the first year of life and may persist. As a result, delayed motor development and clumsiness are common, affecting gross motor movements more than fine motor abilities. These difficulties tend to improve with age.

Frequent upper respiratory tract infections are common in childhood, often resulting in conductive hearing loss. In general, there are no frequent life-threatening complications in Sotos syndrome which might affect life expectancy. Convulsions occur in up to 50 per cent of cases, although approximately half of these may take the form of febrile convulsions only. Abnormal EEGs are seen in approximately 45 per cent of cases. Radiological investigation of the head has shown ventricular dilation in over 50 per cent of cases.

Psychological and behavioural phenotype
There is only a limited amount of information on the psychological and behavioural characteristics associated with Sotos syndrome. Early motor milestones and language development are usually delayed. Marked clumsiness, unsteady gait and poor gross and fine motor coordination are common, though these tend to improve somewhat with age, while language problems include echolalia, perseverative responding, stammering and oral dyspraxia (Finegan et al. 1994, Scarpa et al. 1994).

Cognitive abilities span a wide range, from severe learning difficulties to average intelligence, with most individuals having mild or borderline learning difficulties. They tend to have an uneven pattern of abilities, with particular difficulties in verbal processing (including long latency responding to verbal stimuli and possibly also word finding problems), and deficits in short-term memory, abstract and practical reasoning, and in numeracy and writing ability. One third to one half of affected children attend ordinary schools, but many require additional help in the classroom because of their specific learning disabilities, There is a suggestion that reading attainment may be advanced for age and ability level.

A few recent studies have found high rates of emotional and behavioural difficulties in children with Sotos syndrome, more evident at home than at school, and primarily related to aggression, mood and social impairment (Rutter and Cole 1991, Finegan et al. 1994). Common problems found in at least 35–50 per cent of children include temper tantrums and aggressive behaviour (often directed against parents and siblings), ritualistic behaviours, sleeping problems, fears, attention deficits and hyperactivity. Cole and Hughes (1994) suggest that the aggression may result from frustration because of communication difficulties and intellectual limitations in affected individuals. Social difficulties, poor peer relationships and emotional immaturity are also characteristic, the latter manifesting for example in difficulties separating from parents. Finegan et al. (1994) found that the rates of behaviour problems reported in a sample of affected children were higher than in normal children, but they were no higher than the rates reported for a comparison group of children with overgrowth and developmental delay who did not have Sotos syndrome. Cole and Hughes (1990) suggest that the developmental and behavioural problems in children with Sotos syndrome may be perceived as being more severe because of enhanced expectations owing to the children's size. A tendency for these difficulties to improve with age has been noted, though some individuals remain severely impaired.

KEY REFERENCES

Cole, T.R.P., Hughes, H.E. (1990) 'Sotos syndrome.' *Journal of Medical Genetics,* **27**, 571–576.
—— —— (1994) 'Sotos syndrome: a study of the diagnostic criteria and natural history.' *Journal of Medical Genetics,* **31**, 20–32.
Dodge, P.R., Holmes, S.J., Sotos, J.F. (1983) 'Cerebral gigantism.' *Developmental Medicine and Child Neurology,* **25**, 248–252.
Finegan, J-A.K., Cole, T.R.P., Kingwell, E., Smith, M.L., Smith, M., Sitarenios, G. (1994) 'Language and behavior in children with Sotos syndrome.' *Journal of the American Academy of Child and Adolescent Psychiatry,* **33**, 1307–1315.
Rutter, S.C., Cole, T.R.P. (1991) 'Psychological characteristics of Sotos syndrome.' *Developmental Medicine and Child Neurology,* **33**, 898–902.
Varley, C.K., Cruic, K. (1984) 'Emotional, behavioural and cognitive status of children with cerebral gigantism.' *Journal of Developmental and Behavioral Pediatrics,* **5**, 132–134.

ADDITIONAL REFERENCES

Scarpa, P., Faggioli, R., Voghenzi, A. (1994) 'Familial Sotos syndrome: longitudinal study of two additional cases.' *Genetic Counseling,* **5**, 155–159.
Sotos, J.F., Dodge, P.R., Muirhead, D., Crawford, J.D., Talbot, N.B. (1964) 'Cerebral gigantism in childhood. A syndrome of excessively rapid growth with acromegalic features and a nonprogressive neurologic disorder.' *New England Journal of Medicine,* **271**, 109–116.

TRISOMY 8

First description
De Grouchy *et al.* published the first observation of chromosome 8 trisomy in 1971.

Incidence/prevalence
Trisomy 8 is a relatively rare syndrome of unknown incidence, with a male:female ratio of 3:1. Affected individuals show extreme variability in clinical expression, and this makes the prevalence difficult to establish.

Genetics/aetiology
Trisomy of chromosome 8 is an autosomal trisomy syndrome. De Grouchy and Turleau (1977) classified two forms of the syndrome: complete trisomy (which occurs *de novo* and may be in homogenic or mosaic state) and partial trisomy (represented by trisomy of different segments of the short and long arm of chromosome 8). Most cases of partial trisomy 8p are the unbalanced product of a parental balanced translocation. The cause of the nondisjunction that results in an extra number 8 chromosome is not known. There have been a number of reports of age-related decreases in the number of trisomy 8 cells in cases of mosaicism, resulting in more cells with a normal number of chromosomes.

Whereas trisomy 8 in the mosaic form is a well delineated clinical syndrome, trisomies of the long and short arm of chromosome 8 are relatively rare. The best documented of the partial trisomy cases is partial trisomy for a specific segment in the short arm of chromosome 8 (8p21.1→8p22).

Physical phenotype, natural history and life expectancy
There is great variability of clinical expression in individuals with trisomy 8 mosaicism. Thus far there appears to be no correlation between the extent of clinical expression and the percentage of trisomic cells, nor many obvious differences between the physical phenotype of individuals with a partial trisomy of chromosome 8 as compared with individuals with full trisomy 8 (in mosaic). The syndrome may be associated with multiple severe congenital malformations; at the other extreme it may result in only small dysmorphic changes.

The typical facial features of affected individuals, particularly those with mosaic trisomy 8, consist of a prominent, bulging forehead, elongated face, hypertelorism, broad nasal bridge with prominent nostrils, deep and widely set eyes, palpebral anomalies, a high arched palate, a large mouth with a thick everted lower lip, dental abnormalities, and abnormally shaped low-set ears with a large auricle and prominent antehelix. Other common features include deep palmar and plantar creases, a short neck and long narrow shoulders. The trunk is usually long and narrow. Osteoarticular anomalies are common and can entail significant articular limitations. They include rib anomalies, vertebral anomalies (bifid vertebrae, extra lumbar vertebrae, spina bifida occulta) and kyphoscoliosis. Limitations of joint movement are common. Hypotonia is a frequent finding, and heart defects occur in over 50 per cent of cases of mosaic trisomy 8. Cryptorchidism, testicular hypoplasia and delayed puberty are also frequent findings.

A number of different hematological disorders have been observed in affected individuals. These include deficiency of clotting factor VII in homogenous trisomy 8, hypoplastic anaemia, and acute lymphocytic leukaemia. An association of trisomy 8 with Wilm's tumour, mixed parotid gland tumour and other smooth muscle tumours has also been reported. There have been reports of agenesis of the corpus callosum, particularly in individuals with trisomy 8p, but the frequency of this finding is uncertain.

Early sucking and feeding difficulties and failure to thrive have been reported in some cases of partial trisomy 8, with persisting growth retardation and weight deficits in some affected adults. In other respects, overall physical development is normal, and life expectancy is thought to be normal.

Psychological and behavioural phenotype

Most individuals with mosaic trisomy 8 have moderate to borderline learning difficulties (IQ 50–80). Speech and language abilities and reasoning tend to be significantly impaired when compared with visuospatial abilities and memory. There is also a tendency toward poor fine motor coordination, whereas attention and concentration tend to be good. In contrast to this, most cases of partial trisomy 8 exhibit marked psychomotor delay and severe or profound learning difficulties (IQ <50) (Borghgraef and Fryns 1987). Neurological signs and symptoms in the population with partial trisomy 8 become more striking with age, probably due to progressive degenerative brain damage. Movements become slow or very limited because of spastic paraparesis or spastic quadriplegia. There appears to be no correlation between the percentage of trisomic cells and the severity of learning difficulties in the syndrome.

Children with mosaic trisomy 8 share distinctive behavioural and personality characteristics. They tend to be shy, anxious and introverted, and are said to be friendly but socially withdrawn, with limited eye contact and lacking in self-confidence. At times they can be demanding and egocentric, with temper outbursts (Borghgraef and Fryns 1987). These findings are based on studies of small numbers of affected children; they require confirmation with larger samples.

KEY REFERENCES

Borghgraef, M., Fryns, J-P. (1987) 'Clinical and psychological findings in three young children with full or partial trisomy of chromosome 8.' *Tijdschrift voor Orthopedagogiek Kinderpsychiatrie en Klinische Kinderpsychologie*, **12**, 9–22.
de Grouchy, J., Turleau, C. (1990) 'Autosomal disorders.' *In:* Emery, A.E.H., Rimoin, D.L. (Eds.) *Principles and Practice of Medical Genetics. Vol. 1. 2nd Edn.* Edinburgh: Churchill Livingstone, pp. 247–271.
Riccardi, V.M. (1977) 'Trisomy 8: an international study of 70 patients.' *Birth Defects, Original Article Series*, **13**, 171–184.

ADDITIONAL REFERENCES

de Grouchy, J., Turleau, C. (1977) *Clinical Atlas of Human Chromosomes.* New York: John Wiley.
—— —— Léonard, C.(1971) 'Étude en fluorescence d'une trisomie C mosaique probablement 8: 46,XY/47,XY,?8+.' *Annales de Génétique*, **14**, 69.

TRISOMY 18

Alternative name
Edwards syndrome.

First description
Trisomy 18 was first recognized as a distinct entity by Edwards *et al.* (1960).

Incidence/prevalence
Trisomy 18 is the second most common trisomy after Down syndrome, with an incidence of 1:3000 to 1:5000 live births. The syndrome occurs with a 3:1 female preponderance at birth.

Genetics/aetiology
Full trisomy 18 signifies an extra chromosome 18 in every cell, and is diagnosed in 95 per cent of abnormalities affecting chromosome 18. In most cases the extra chromosome is of maternal origin. Babies with full trisomy 18 have profound disabilities, while others with mosaicism (diagnosed in about 3 per cent of cases) or with partial trisomy of chromosome 18 (2 per cent of cases) have much less severe disabilities. Individuals with a ring chromosome 18 show features in common with trisomy 18, though these cases are quite rare.

Most cases are sporadic. As with other autosomal trisomies, there is a strong association with increased maternal age. Occasionally partial trisomy 18 occurs because of a balanced translocation in one of the parents.

Physical phenotype, natural history and life expectancy
Many affected cases do not survive pregnancy. Those who do typically have a short life expectancy, with over 90 per cent dying within the first year of life, and only 5 per cent of one cohort surviving to age 10 years (Baty *et al.* 1994*a*). A few live into their teens and twenties. Children who survive beyond infancy are invariably very severely disabled.

Children with trisomy 18 present with characteristic features, including an enlarged occiput, small mouth and jaw, cleft lip and palate (in about 15 per cent of cases), low-set ears, short palpebral fissures, clenched hands, overlapping fingers, club/rocker-bottomed feet, hypoplastic nails and a short sternum. They have low birthweight, microcephaly, and life-threatening malformations such as oesophageal atresia, diaphragmatic hernia and multiple congenital heart defects. These occur in over 90 per cent of cases, and include ventricular septal defects, atrial septal defects and patent ductus arteriosus. Many of these abnormalities require surgical correction during the neonatal period. Cardiopulmonary arrest is the most common cause of death.

Affected infants typically have hyper- or hypotonia, and marked developmental and motor disabilities. Gastro-oesophageal reflux and severe feeding difficulties are common.

Failure to thrive, apnoea and an increased susceptibility to respiratory and urinary tract infections are also frequent complications. Marked growth deficiency, joint contractures, spina bifida and scoliosis are further common features, and sensitivity to changes of temperature and to sunlight are frequently reported. Hearing loss occurs in more than 50 per cent of cases. Eye problems include absence of the eyeball, coloboma and poor development of the eye muscles. Frequent eye infections may be the result of poor eyelid function.

CT scans reveal general enlargement of the ventricular system, especially the lateral ventricles. EEG reports indicate generalized cerebral dysfunction, with semi-rhythmic ground activity with components of slow activity over both hemispheres.

Psychological and behavioural phenotype

Children with trisomy 18 have severe or profound learning difficulties. Their motor milestones are severely delayed, and they are unable to walk unassisted. Verbal communication, too, is severely impaired, and is limited to a few single words at best. However, many older children have a much more extensive receptive vocabulary, and affected individuals continue to acquire new skills over time. Overall, skills in daily living, receptive language and social interaction tend to be higher than motor and expressive language abilities (Baty *et al.* 1994*b*). Affected individuals are mostly aware of their environment and are able to communicate some of their needs non-verbally.

Children with trisomy 18 mosaicism or partial trisomy 18 tend to be less severely disabled; they are able to walk and have moderate or mild learning difficulties. A number of individuals with trisomy 18 mosaicism have been reported who have normal intelligence.

KEY REFERENCES

Bos, A.P., Broers, C.J.M., Hazebroek, F.W.J., Van Hemel, J.O., Tibboel, D., Wesby-van Swaay, E., Molenaar, J.C. (1992) 'Avoidance of emergency surgery in newborn infants with trisomy 18.' *Lancet*, **339**, 913–915.
Robbins, J., Rose, C. (1993) *Facts for Families*. Sutton Coldfield: Support Organisation for Trisomy 13/18 and Related Disorders. (Available from SOFT UK, c/o C. Rose, 48 Froggatts Ride, Walmley, Sutton Coldfield, West Midlands, B76 8TQ.)
Van Dyke, D.C., Allen, M. (1990) 'Clinical management considerations in long-term survivors with trisomy 18.' *Pediatrics*, **85**, 753–759.

ADDITIONAL REFERENCES

Baty, B.J., Blackburn, B.L., Carey, J.C. (1994*a*) 'Natural history of trisomy 18 and trisomy 13: I. Growth, physical assessment, medical histories, survival, and recurrence risk.' *American Journal of Medical Genetics*, **49**, 175–188.
—— Jorde, L.B., Blackburn, B.L., Carey, J.C. (1994*b*) 'Natural history of trisomy 18 and trisomy 13: II. Psychomotor development.' *American Journal of Medical Genetics*, **49**, 189–194.
Edwards, J.H., Harnden, D.G., Cameron, A.H., Crosse, V.M., Wolff, O.H. (1960) 'A new trisomic syndrome.' *Lancet*, **1**, 787–790.

TUBEROUS SCLEROSIS COMPLEX (TSC)

Alternative names
Tuberose sclerosis, epiloia.

First description
The name 'tuberous sclerosis' was first given to the hard cerebral lesions and neurological signs of the condition by Bourneville in 1880. The characteristic facial rash ('angiomatous vegetations') had been illustrated by Rayer in 1835. Vogt (1908) established the diagnostic triad of epilepsy, mental retardation and adenoma sebaceum. He also mentioned the cardiac and renal tumours that can be part of the condition.

Incidence/prevalence
Recent population studies suggest an overall prevalence of at least 1:7000. This is much higher than previously thought and reflects increasing recognition of the multisystem nature of the disorder.

Genetics/aetiology
TSC is an autosomal dominant genetic condition but with very variable clinical expression and, in clinical terms, a high incidence of apparent *de novo* mutation. It is genetically heterogeneous, with about 50 per cent of cases linked to chromosome 9 (9q34—*TSC1*) and 50 per cent to chromosome 16 (16p13—*TSC2*). No clinical differences are apparent between the two groups. The *TSC2* gene has been identified and cloned (European Consortium 1993). It is adjacent to the gene for adult polycystic kidney disorder (*APKD-1*). A single deletion is responsible for those children with TSC who also have polycystic kidneys. The *TSC1* gene has not yet been identified. Clinical disorder has so far been found associated with over 25 different mutations in the *TSC2* gene. These mutations are probably transmitted stably from generation to generation, and further mutations are necessary for the condition to be clinically expressed in different tissues—*i.e.* a two-hit process.

The *TSC2* gene codes for a protein named tuberin which appears to be expressed in all mammals. The *TSC2* gene may act as an oncogene, a deleted tumour suppressor gene.

Physical phenotype, natural history and life expectancy
TSC is a multisystem disorder with variable clinical and intellectual expression. Hamartomatous lesions are found in the brain (90 per cent), skin (96 per cent), kidneys (60 per cent), heart (50 per cent), teeth, eyes (47 per cent), bones and lungs as well as occasionally in other organs. The classical diagnostic triad of Vogt is no longer adequate and leads to underdiagnosis. Currently, diagnosis is based on primary and secondary clinical criteria (Gomez 1988).

Cardiac rhabdomyomata may present *in utero* causing stillbirth or early death but in surviving children they subsequently decrease in size. Depigmented patches, best seen under UV light, are often present at birth and are ultimately found in around 95 per cent of cases. The pathognomonic facial angiofibromata (misnamed adenoma sebaceum) become increasingly obvious with age and are detectable, though not prominent, in many children by age 5 years. Epilepsy occurs in around 80 per cent of people with TSC and may be very severe and refractory. It frequently presents in the first year as infantile spasms. Midline giant cell astrocytoma develop in around 10 per cent of children. A few babies present with polycystic kidney disease, but renal problems on the whole intrude little until the teenage years when characteristic angiomyolipomata may develop, leading to renal failure. Honeycomb lung can lead to respiratory failure in some adults. Retinal hamartomas rarely affect vision.

Many people with TSC have no intellectual impairment or epilepsy, and TSC is diagnosed only when they attend a dermatology department for treatment of the facial rash or a renal clinic for kidney failure, or after the identification of a more severely affected family member.

TSC is not a degenerative condition, and survival into the seventh and eighth decades is recorded even among those whose lesions have caused epilepsy and cognitive impairment. However, functional disruption caused by the cerebral and peripheral hamartomatous lesions leads to an increased incidence of morbidity and mortality before middle age.

Psychological and behavioural phenotype
IQ ranges from below 20 to superior intelligence levels. It is likely that fewer than half of those with the disorder are learning disabled, but among those who are the disability is often profound. Cognitive abilities are associated to some extent with expression of epilepsy but not with any aspect of the physical phenotype. Severe language disorder usually predominates at all levels of disability, including a high proportion with no speech (Hunt and Dennis 1987).

In 1932 Critchley and Earl reported on 29 people resident in psychiatric hospitals who fulfilled the then contemporary diagnostic criteria (Vogt's triad). They stated that 'the essential feature of the psychology of epiloia is a combination of intellectual defect proper with a primitive form of psychosis.' They described 'a certain amount of negativism' and 'a peculiar type of motor restlessness'. Speech is 'usually grossly impaired', 'screaming fits are very common', 'the children usually play with their fingers a good deal', and 'all manner of bizarre attitudes and stereotyped movements occur and these are most striking in the hands and fingers.' These stereotypies, they stated, are different from those seen in 'simple aments of the idiot grade'. Here they address a problem frequently posed today as to whether the autistic features are merely a reflection of the degree of cognitive impairment. Clearly, Critchley and Earl believed that this was not so and that there was some specificity in the behaviours observed. With regard to adult psychosis they observed, 'from the sudden fixation of their gaze and from their air of listening—again to nothing—intently and with a strange and alien smile, it seems possible that they undergo some crude hallucinatory experience.' They recognized also the extent of psychopathology among apparently unaffected or 'forme fruste' relatives.

Throughout Critchley and Earl's paper the toll of institutionalization—and presumably also poor seizure control—in reducing functional competence among adolescents and adults is notable. This classic paper sets the scene for and poses most of the questions currently being addressed with regard to the behavioural characteristics of TSC.

Subsequently, apart from one paper in the *South African Medical Journal* in 1981, no further mention of a possible behavioural phenotype appears in the literature for over 50 years. In 1987 Hunt and Dennis reported on psychiatric disorder at age 5 years among 97 children: 51 per cent rated as autistic, 59 per cent as hyperkinetic, 69 per cent as either autistic or hyperkinetic, and 41 per cent as both. Aggression featured in 13 per cent of cases.

Smalley and Tanguay (1992) reviewed their own and other available data and concluded that 17–58 per cent of TSC subjects manifest autism and 0.4–3 per cent of autistic subjects have TSC. They emphasized that it is the core deficits of social empathic behaviour and language rather than motoric features which distinguish TSC cases. In a West of Scotland prevalence study (Hunt and Shepherd 1993), 43 per cent of children with TSC fulfilled DSM-III-R criteria for autism or pervasive developmental disorder. Using the same criteria in Western Sweden, Gillberg *et al.* (1994) reported autistic disorder in 61 per cent of TSC subjects aged under 20 years, many also rated for attention deficit hyperactivity disorder. They predicted that 9 per cent of children with autism may have TSC.

Many children are severely sleep disturbed. Hunt and Stores (1994) found no correlation between severity of sleep disorder and a diagnosis of pervasive developmental disorder, but the presence of epileptic activity, whether or not this manifested as overt nocturnal seizures, was very highly correlated with sleep problems. Curatolo *et al.* (1992) demonstrated severe abnormalities of sleep architecture in patients with TSC and uncontrolled partial or generalized epilepsies. Given the known associations between sleep disturbance and daytime behaviour, one must postulate that the severe sleep disturbance often seen in TSC must at the least gravely exacerbate other organically determined behavioural difficulties.

In everyday terms children severely affected by TSC can rarely be left unsupervised for a moment. They create chaos aimlessly, picking up, discarding and destroying; all loose objects in the home must be put out of their reach, They do not respond to verbal input or other interpersonal cues. Many parents say that their child is 'in a world of her/his own.' Most children have been thought 'deaf' at some time or other, but on formal testing auditory acuity proves normal. They are likely to resent interference and are very disturbed by changes in routine; they may signal distress by uncontrollable screaming. Trips out of the house pose such problems that parent and child live as virtual prisoners in their own home. They rarely settle to sleep before midnight and thereafter may wander the house for hours during the night being shadowed or diverted by an exhausted parent; they may sleep in a padded room with a mattress on the floor; frequent seizures may intrude through day and night.

There is little information about behaviour in adults. Hunt (1992) reassessed the older children from the 1987 study at age 18+. Only around 30 per cent of those who had shown impaired social–empathic behaviours, hyperactivity, or destructive outbursts at age 5 still showed these behaviours. However, 73 per cent of the whole group were still rated as manifesting some behaviour disorder. There is one published account of an adult who presented with florid psychotic behaviour and subsequently proved to have TSC complex. Beyond that there are anecdotal reports of adults with TSC in psychiatric hospitals with a diagnosis of 'atypical schizophrenia'. It may be that some of these people are adults with autism. On the other hand, some certainly experience hallucinations which would exclude them from this diagnostic category. There is an urgent need for more investigation in this area.

Behavioural correlations
The question arises as to whether there is evidence for specific lesional underpinning of behaviour which is not mediated via seizures or cognitive impairment.

With regard to infantile spasms, Hunt and Dennis (1987) and Gillberg *et al.* (1994) argue against a causal link with subsequent autistic/hyperkinetic behaviour and in favour of both being manifestations of a common underlying brain disorder. Outcome, however, may be poorer among those whose spasms are resistant to treatment.

The evidence as to whether autistic behaviour can develop in the absence of epilepsy lies mainly in single case descriptions. Oliver (1987) gives a well documented account of a child, admitted to a child psychiatric unit at age 3 years with profound language disorder, severe autistic traits and potentially normal intelligence, who did not have a first seizure until age 6 and was not diagnosed as having tuberous sclerosis until age 9.

With regard to associations between autism and cognitive level, Smalley and Tanguay (1992) state that not all autistic TSC subjects are mentally retarded and cite a male autistic TSC subject with an estimated IQ of 106.

A final question is whether there are associations between cerebral lesions and behavioural and cognitive function. Jambaqué and colleagues (1991) demonstrated that both the number and topography of tubers demonstrated on MRI seemed to play an important role in outcome as regards epilepsy and cognitive level. By contrast, Webb *et al.* (1991) found significant numbers of cortical tubers in some individuals with known TSC and normal intellect. They stressed therefore that wrong conclusions may be drawn if the number of cerebral lesions alone is used to predict neurological outcome. This study also suggested that tubers in the posterior temporal, occipital and parieto-occipital areas when coexisting with large bifrontal lesions might predispose to autism.

Conclusion
More children with tuberous sclerosis than ever before are moving into adolescence and adult life due to advances both in seizure control and in general levels of child care. This relentless protean disorder, however, seems always to have a trick up its sleeve to create confusion, distress, morbidity and death. Already too many children have been blinded because of failure to recognize that head-banging may be a response to the severe headache of raised intracranial pressure caused by a rapidly expanding but potentially operable midline giant cell astrocytoma. Too many young adults have been admitted to

hospital in end-stage renal failure because of failure to recognize that postural change, increasing withdrawal, and presumed 'somatization' may be behavioural responses to chronic loin pain as the renal angiomyolipomata so characteristic of the later stages of the disorder enlarge and destroy functional renal tissue.

When behavioural change occurs, against whatever prior psychiatric background, the search for organic factors must be as rigorous as that for possible environmental precipitants. To achieve this, a high level of adequately informed multidisciplinary surveillance has to be made readily available for all those at all ages who are affected by this disorder.

KEY REFERENCES

Gomez, M.R. (1988) *Tuberous Sclerosis, 2nd Edn.* New York: Raven Press.
Hunt, A., Dennis, J. (1987) 'Psychiatric disorder among children with tuberous sclerosis.' *Developmental Medicine and Child Neurology*, **29**, 190–198.
Sampson, J.R., Harris, P.C. (1994) 'The molecular genetics of tuberous sclerosis.' *Human Molecular Genetics*, **3**, 1477–1480.

ADDITIONAL REFERENCES

Bourneville, D.M. (1880) 'Sclérose tubéreuse des circonvolutions cérébrales: idiotie et épilepsie hemi-plégique.' *Archives de Neurologie* (Paris), **1**, 81–91.
Critchley, M., Earl, C.J.C. (1932) 'Tuberose sclerosis and allied conditions.' *Brain*, **55**, 311–346.
Curatolo, P., Bruni, O., Cortesi, F., Giannotti, F. (1992) 'Sleep disorders in tuberous sclerosis.' *Paper presented at the 2nd International Symposium of the Society for the Study of Behavioural Phenotypes, Welshpool, November 1992.* (Abstracts available from Dr Gregory O'Brien, Northgate Hospital, Northumberland.)
European Chromosome 16 Tuberous Sclerosis Consortium (1993) 'Identification and characterization of the tuberous sclerosis gene on chromosome 16.' *Cell*, **75**, 1305–1315.
Gillberg, I.C., Gillberg, C., Ahlsén, G. (1994) 'Autistic behaviour and attention deficits in tuberous sclerosis: a population-based study.' *Developmental Medicine and Child Neurology*, **36**, 50–56.
Hunt, A. (1992) 'A longitudinal study of the behaviour of 23 people with tuberous sclerosis from age 5 to adulthood.' *Paper presented at the 2nd International Symposium of the Society for the Study of Behavioural Phenotypes, Welshpool, November 1992.* (Abstracts available from Dr Gregory O'Brien, Northgate Hospital, Northumberland.)
—— Shepherd, C. (1993) 'A prevalence study of autism in tuberous sclerosis.' *Journal of Autism and Developmental Disorders*, **23**, 323–339
—— Stores, G. (1994) 'Sleep disorder and epilepsy in children with tuberous sclerosis: a questionnaire-based study.' *Developmental Medicine and Child Neurology*, **36**, 108–115.
Jambaqué, I., Cusmai, R., Curatolo, P., Cortesi, F., Perrot, C., Dulac, O. (1991) 'Neuropsychological aspects of tuberous sclerosis in relation to epilepsy and MRI findings.' *Developmental Medicine and Child Neurology*, **33**, 698–705.
Oliver, B.E. (1987) 'Tuberous sclerosis and the autistic syndrome.' *British Journal of Psychiatry*, **151**, 560. *(Letter.)*
Rayer, P.F.O. (1835) *Traité Théorique et Pratique de Maladies de la Peau. 2ème Edn.* Paris: Baillière.
Smalley, S.L., Tanguay, P.E., Smith, M., Gutierrez, G. (1992) 'Autism and tuberous sclerosis.' *Journal of Autism and Developmental Disorders*, **22**, 339–355.
Vogt, H. (1908) 'Zur Diagnostik der Tuberösen Sklerose.' *Zeitschrift für die Erforschung und Behandlung des jugendlichen Schwachsinns auf Wissenschaftlicher*, **2**, 1–12.
Webb, D.W., Thomson, J.L.G., Osborne, J.P. (1991) 'Cranial magnetic resonance imaging in patients with tuberous sclerosis and normal intellect.' *Archives of Disease in Childhood*, **66**, 1375–1377.

WILLIAMS SYNDROME

Alternative names
Williams–Beuren syndrome; idiopathic infantile hypercalcaemia.

First description
Idiopathic infantile hypercalcaemia (IIH) was first described by Fanconi and Girardet (1952). In 1961 Williams *et al.* identified four children with supravalvular aortic stenosis in association with mental retardation and a characteristic facial appearance, and soon after Black and Bonham Carter (1963) associated this facial appearance with that of children with IIH. It has since been assumed that the two conditions are identical.

Incidence/prevalence
The incidence is estimated at 1:20,000 to 1:25,000 live births, with an equal sex ratio.

Genetics/aetiology
Most cases are sporadic; concordant monozygotic twins have been reported, and there are reports of a few cases of parent to child transmission. This supports an autosomal dominant mode of inheritance, with most cases representing new mutations. Recently, a microdeletion on chromosome 7 (at locus 7q11.23) was identified in individuals with Williams syndrome, with resultant disruption of the elastin gene (Ewart *et al.* 1993). Elastin is an important constituent of connective tissue, especially in arterial walls, and reduced or abnormal elastin could explain the vascular and connective tissue pathology found in the syndrome. It is likely that other genes are also involved in the deletion, which could account for the other phenotypic features of Williams syndrome. Further investigations with larger samples are necessary.

Physical phenotype, natural history and life expectancy
Williams syndrome is a developmental disorder involving the vascular, connective tissue and central nervous systems.

The mean birthweight of affected individuals is reduced, and cardiac murmurs and an unusual facial appearance are often noted at birth. Difficulties with feeding are a major problem in infancy. Vomiting, constipation and irritability lead to failure to thrive. A proportion of children are found to have raised levels of blood calcium. This subgroup is generally treated with a low-calcium and vitamin D-restricted diet, and serum calcium levels return to normal and the feeding difficulties improve with dietary treatment or simply with the passage of time. However, other features of the condition persist. Comparisons between cases with and those without documented hypercalcaemia in infancy show very few differences in terms of abilities, behaviour and development (Martin *et al.* 1984, Udwin 1990). It is therefore suggested that hypercalcaemia is linked to the Williams syndrome phenotype but is expressed with variable frequency and penetration.

Physical features of the children include a distinctive 'elfin-like' face with full prominent cheeks, a wide mouth, long philtrum, a retroussé nose with a flat nasal bridge, heavy orbital ridges, medial eyebrow flare and stellate iris pattern; dental abnormalities, including microdontia, missing teeth and enamel hypoplasia; and renal and cardiovascular abnormalities (most commonly supravalvular aortic stenosis and peripheral pulmonary artery stenosis). The cardiovascular symptoms vary in severity and may change over time. Commonly found skeletal abnormalities include radioulnar synostosis, joint contractures and laxity. Gait abnormalities are common and include immature gait and abnormal stress gait, with early hypotonia giving way to hypertonia in older individuals. Growth retardation, short stature and a hoarse voice are further frequent findings, and an early starting and fast progressing puberty has been reported in many cases.

The face becomes thinner and coarser with age. Progressive multisystem medical problems have been identified in at least some adults with Williams syndrome, which can lead to premature death. These include cardiovascular complications, hypertension, gastrointestinal problems, urinary tract abnormalities, and also progressive joint limitations (Morris *et al.* 1988). However, it is not clear how common these problems are.

Studies using MRI, positron emission tomography and other techniques have not found any lesions in the brains of affected individuals, but they have identified significant differences in brain volume in individuals with Williams syndrome when compared with normal individuals and other groups such as autistic individuals (Jernigan *et al.* 1993). The studies indicate relatively normal development of some limbic, frontal cortical and cerebellar structures in affected individuals, which may explain their relative competence in linguistic, affective and face processing functions; however, supratentorial volume in the cerebrum is reduced, as is total cerebral grey matter.

Psychological and behavioural phenotype
Studies have highlighted a distinctive psychological profile and unusual personality and behavioural characteristics that are associated with Williams syndrome (Udwin *et al.* 1987, Udwin and Yule 1990).

Approximately 55 per cent of affected individuals have severe learning difficulties, 40 per cent have moderate learning difficulties, and some 5 per cent fall in the borderline to low-average range of abilities. Most require special schooling (Udwin *et al.* 1987). Language may be slow to develop in the preschool years, but by school-age verbal abilities are in most cases markedly superior to visuospatial abilities and to gross and fine motor skills. Most of the individuals have an unusual command of language: their comprehension is usually far more limited than their expressive language, which tends to be grammatically correct, complex and fluent at a superficial level, but verbose and pseudo-mature. Most individuals have a well developed and precocious vocabulary, with excessive and frequently inappropriate use of clichés and stereotyped phrases. The children tend to be very chatty, and auditory memory, mimicry skills and social use of language are particularly well developed (Bellugi *et al.* 1994). They are also very proficient in theory of mind tasks. In contrast, they show significant deficits in the integration of visual–perceptual information and in constructional tasks. However, even in non-verbal areas there is an uneven profile, with consistent relative strengths on tasks of visual recall and face recognition (Udwin and Yule 1990, Bellugi *et al.* 1994).

Most Williams syndrome children have poor relationships with peers, but are outgoing, socially disinhibited and excessively affectionate toward adults, including strangers. They also appear acutely attentive to the feelings of others. Their relatively good verbal abilities, engaging personalities and excessive sociability can result in an overestimation of their general cognitive abilities.

Affected children show higher rates of emotional and behavioural disturbance when compared with the rates that have been reported for other children with learning difficulties, particularly in terms of overactivity, poor concentration and distractibility, eating and sleeping problems, excessive anxiety and attention seeking behaviours (Udwin *et al.* 1987). They show high rates of preoccupations and obsessions with particular activities, objects or topics. Over 90 per cent of the children are hypersensitive to particular sounds, which may include electrical noises like vacuum cleaners, drills, music and thunder. The basis for this hyperacusis is not clear, but in some cases it becomes less acute in adulthood.

The distinctive psychological characteristics and behavioural and emotional dif-ficulties described above persist into adulthood with similar, and in some cases even increased frequency (Udwin 1990). Despite their relatively good verbal and social skills, most adults with Williams syndrome are unable to live independently and require ongoing support and supervision in everyday activities. A minority work in supervised jobs, but most attend adult training centres or day centres, or remain at home with no daytime occupation. The limited levels of independence they attain are most likely due to their particular psychological profile; their characteristic over-friendliness and social disinhibition, distractibility, and anxiety mitigate against independence in daily living and employment.

KEY REFERENCES

Bellugi, U., Wang, P.P., Jernigan, T.L. (1994) 'Williams syndrome: an unusual neuropsychological profile.' *In:* Broman, S.H., Grafman, J. (Eds.) *Atypical Cognitive Deficits in Developmental Disorders.* Hills-dale, NJ: Lawrence Erlbaum, pp. 22–83.
Martin, N.D.T., Snodgrass, G.J.A.I., Cohen, R.D. (1984) 'Idiopathic infantile hypercalcaemia—a continuing enigma.' *Archives of Disease in Childhood*, **59**, 605–613.
Udwin,O. (1990) 'A survey of adults with Williams syndrome and idiopathic infantile hypercalcaemia.' *Developmental Medicine and Child Neurology*, **32**, 129–141
—— Yule, W. (1990) 'A cognitive and behavioural phenotype in Williams syndrome.' *Journal of Clinical and Experimental Neuropsychology*, **13**, 232–244.
—— —— Martin, N. (1987) 'Cognitive abilities and behavioural characteristics of children with idiopathic infantile hypercalcaemia.' *Journal of Child Psychology and Psychiatry*, **28**, 297–309.

ADDITIONAL REFERENCES

Black, J.A., Bonham Carter, R.E. (1963) 'Association between aortic stenosis and facies of severe infantile hypercalcaemia.' *Lancet*, **2**, 745–749.
Ewart, A.K., Morris, C.A., Atkinson,D., Jin, W., Sternes, K., Spallone, P., Stock, A.D., Leppert, M., Keating, M.T. (1993) 'Hemizygosity at the elastin locus in a developmental disorder, Williams syndrome.' *Nature Genetics.* **5**, 11–16.

Fanconi, G., Girardet, P. (1952) 'Chronische Hypercalcämie, kombiniert mit Osteosklerose, Hyperazotämie, Minderwuchs und kongenitalen Missbildungen.' *Helvetica Paediatrica Acta*, **7**, 314–334.

Jernigan, T.L., Bellugi, U., Sowell, E., Doherty, S., Hesselink, J.R. (1993) 'Cerebral morphologic distinctions between Williams and Down syndromes.' *Archives of Neurology*, **50**, 186–191.

Morris, C.A., Demsey, S.A., Leonard, C.O., Dilts, C., Blackburn, B.L. (1988) 'Natural history of Williams syndrome: physical characteristics.' *Journal of Pediatrics*, **113**, 318–326,

Williams, J.C.P., Barratt-Boyes, B.G., Lowe, J.B. (1961) 'Supravalvular aortic stenosis.' *Circulation*, **24**, 1311–1318.

WOLF–HIRSCHHORN SYNDROME

Alternative name
4p– syndrome.

First description
Wolf *et al.* (1965) and Hirschhorn *et al.* (1965) were the first to describe this syndrome.

Incidence/prevalence
The syndrome is rare, but there are no reliable estimates of incidence. At least one report points to a female:male ratio of 2:1, suggesting differential survival.

Genetics/aetiology
Most cases are sporadic, and result from a *de novo* deletion in the distal part of chromosome 4 (4p16). The size of the deletion varies from approximately one half of the short arm to being so subtle as to be cytogenetically undetectable (Lurie *et al.* 1980), but with no significant differences in syndrome phenotype or in clinical severity. In most cases a paternal origin of the deleted chromosome has been demonstrated, which probably reflects differences in the exposure and susceptibility of male and female germ cells to chromosomal damage (Quarrell *et al.* 1991, Estabrooks *et al.* 1994). There have also been reports of a significant number of familial cases of the syndrome (possibly 13–15 per cent of cases), resulting from parental translocations.

Physical phenotype, natural history and life expectancy
Children with Wolf–Hirschhorn syndrome show severe prenatal growth retardation and low birthweight, continuing profound postnatal growth retardation, and multiple congenital abnormalities. They have characteristic craniofacial dysmorphism, with severe microcephaly, hypertelorism, highly arched eyebrows, epicanthal folds, a beaked nose with a broad base, a carp-shaped mouth with downturned corners, micrognathia, a prominent glabella and a short philtrum. Additional prominent craniofacial anomalies include a cleft lip and palate, large and simple low-set ears, and scalp defects. Hypotonia is common, and skeletal abnormalities that have been noted in most cases include clinodactyly, deformities of the feet, and scoliosis. Eye defects and hearing disorders are also reported in many cases. Congenital heart defects occur in approximately half of the cases (including septal defects), and frequent respiratory infections are noted. Other common features include seizures (which are often difficult to control), overlapping toes, and urogenital abnormalities, including cryptorchidism and hypospadias in affected males. There is a wide spectrum of renal defects, including dysplasia of the kidneys, simple hypoplasia and polycystosis.

About one third of affected individuals are found to have central nervous system defects at autopsy. Findings include hypoplasia and insufficient myelinization of the pyramids, dysplastic and dystopic gyrae in the cerebellum, and hydrocephalus. CT scans show cortical atrophy. Agenesis of the corpus callosum has also been documented.

Life expectancy is dependent on the number and severity of serious malformations. According to one report, approximately one third of affected children die by the age of 2 years, from either cardiac failure or bronchopneumonia. However, significant numbers of children survive beyond infancy, and cases of adults in their thirties have been documented.

Psychological and behavioural phenotype

Children with Wolf–Hirschhorn syndrome show severely delayed psychomotor development, and severe or profound learning difficulties. Typically, they do not develop speech and have minimal communication skills. Some are also unable to stand, walk or feed themselves. Beyond this, no information is available on the behavioural and psychological characteristics of affected children and adults.

KEY REFERENCES

Lazjuk, G.I., Lurie, I.W., Ostrowskaja, T.I., Kirillova, I.A., Nedzved, M.K., Cherstvoy, E.D., Silyaeva, N.F. (1980) 'The Wolf–Hirschhorn syndrome. II. Pathologic anatomy.' *Clinical Genetics*, **18**, 6–12.

Quarrell, O.W.J., Snell, R.G., Curtis, M.A., Roberts, S.H., Harper, P.S., Shaw, D.J. (1991) 'Paternal origin of the chromosomal deletion resulting in Wolf–Hirschhorn syndrome.' *Journal of Medical Genetics*, **28**, 256–259.

Wilson, M.G., Towner, J.W., Coffin, G.S., Ebbin, A.J., Siris, E., Brager, P. (1981) 'Genetic and clinical studies in 13 patients with the Wolf–Hirschhorn syndrome [del(4p)].' *Human Genetics*, **59**, 297–307.

ADDITIONAL REFERENCES

Estabrooks, L.L., Lamb, A.N., Aylsworth, A.S., Callanan, N.P., Rao, K.W. (1994) 'Molecular characterisation of chromosome 4p deletions resulting in Wolf–Hirschhorn syndrome.' *Journal of Medical Genetics*, **31**, 103–107.

Hirschhorn, K., Cooper, H.L., Firschein, I. L. (1965) 'Deletion of short arms of chromosome 4–5 in a child with defects of midline fusion.' *Humangenetik*, **1**, 479–482.

Lurie, I.W., Lazjuk, G.I., Ussova, Y.I., Presman, E.B., Gurevich, D.B. (1980) 'The Wolf–Hirschhorn syndrome. I. Genetics.' *Clinical Genetics*, **17**, 375–384.

Wolf, U., Reinwein, H., Porsch, R., Schrotter, R., Baitsch, H. (1965) 'Defizienz an den kurzen Armen eines Chromosoms Nr. 4.' *Humangenetik*, **1**, 397–413.

X-LINKED α-THALASSAEMIA/MENTAL RETARDATION SYNDROME

Alternative names
ATR-X syndrome; 'non-deletion type' α-thalassaemia/mental retardation syndrome.

First description
The syndrome was first described by Wilkie *et al.* (1990), who distinguished it from cases of α-thalassaemia/mental retardation due to deletions involving the haemoglobin gene complex on the tip of chromosome 16p (ATR-16 syndrome).

Incidence/prevalence
ATR-X syndrome is extremely rare, but its exact incidence is not known. All reported cases are male.

Genetics/aetiology
The syndrome is familial, showing an X-linked recessive pattern of inheritance with complete penetrance in males. Female carriers are of normal intelligence and appearance, though some have been found to have rare haemoglobin H (HbH) inclusions.

ATR-X syndrome is quite distinct from the ATR-16 syndrome, since no abnormality of the α-globin gene complex on chromosome 16p is present in the former condition. Linkage analysis indicates that the disease locus for the ATR-X syndrome lies on the proximal part of the long arm of the X chromosome (Xq12–Xq21.31) (Gibbons *et al.* 1992). It has been suggested that this locus possibly encodes a transacting factor which regulates the expression of the α-globin genes, and that an abnormality of this factor down-regulates the expression of the α genes in affected individuals (Wilkie *et al.* 1990). However, the nature of the underlying abnormality in the syndrome and the mechanism by which the ATR-X mutation down-regulates the expression of the α-globin genes have yet to be elucidated.

Physical phenotype, natural history and life expectancy
Individuals with ATR-X show a strikingly similar phenotype, comprising characteristic facies, global developmental delay, genital anomalies, and a mild form of HbH disease (α-thalassaemia). The phenotype is quite different from that of ATR-16.

The characteristic facial appearance associated with the ATR-X syndrome comprises telecanthus, hypertelorism, epicanthic folds, a flat nasal bridge, mild facial hypoplasia, a small triangular nose with anteverted nares, a triangular open mouth with full lips, and an enlarged tongue that is often protruding. Dental anomalies are common, and the ears may be small and simple, low-set or posteriorly rotated. The facial features appear to coarsen with age, and the nasal bridge often becomes more pronounced.

Affected individuals may also show microcephaly, genital abnormalities (*e.g.* cryptorchidism, hypospadias), growth deficiency of postnatal onset (short stature and delayed bone age) and skeletal abnormalities (kyphoscoliosis, talipes). There is an unusual mild form of HbH disease which involves a defect in the production of the α-globin chains of haemoglobin, but with less hypochromia and lower levels of HbH than are seen in the mendelian forms of HbH disease. Some affected individuals have normal or only marginally abnormal haematological indices. No cases have required treatment for the haematologic abnormality.

Neonatal hypotonia and feeding difficulties are common. Hypotonia usually persists from birth, but some individuals develop spasticity later on. Sitting and walking are usually severely delayed, and seizures occur in about half the cases. Hearing and vision are typically normal, although strabismus has been observed in a third of cases. CT scans reveal cerebral atrophy in at least some cases. Life expectancy is significantly reduced, with nine out of ten deaths occurring in childhood; however, there are also affected individuals in their twenties, and at least one in his mid-thirties (R.J. Gibbons, personal communication 1994).

Female carriers may have subtle haematological changes including HbH inclusions in a small proportion of their red cells, a feature that is diagnostic for the presence of α-thalassaemia.

Psychological and behavioural phenotype

Neonatal hypotonia and severely delayed developmental milestones are characteristic. Affected individuals have severe global learning difficulties (IQ <50), with limited or no speech and very limited comprehension. Information on behavioural characteristics is still largely anecdotal. Gibbons (personal communication 1993) describes affected individuals as sociable, with positive affect and able to enjoy games and music. Episodes of spontaneous uncontrollable laughter have been noted in a few cases. Self-help skills are mostly very limited.

A few individuals display self-induced rumination and regurgitation, which is thought to be behavioural in origin since no organic cause has been found. In some cases, stubbornness, agitated behaviours and head-banging have also been reported.

KEY REFERENCES

Lancet (1991) 'More bad luck for the X chromosome: α-thalassaemia/mental retardation.' *Lancet*, **338**, 1562–1563. *(Editorial.)*

Gibbons, R.J., Wilkie, A.O.M., Weatherall, D.J., Higgs, D.R. (1991) 'A newly defined X linked mental retardation syndrome associated with α thalassaemia.' *Journal of Medical Genetics*, **28**, 729–733.

—— Suthers, G.K., Wilkie, A.O.M., Buckle, V.J., Higgs, D.R. (1992) 'X-linked α-thalassemia/mental retardation (ATR-X) syndrome: localization to Xq12–q21.31 by X inactivation and linkage analysis.' *American Journal of Human Genetics*, **51**, 1136–1149.

ADDITIONAL REFERENCE

Wilkie, A.O.M., Zeitlin, H.C., Lindenbaum, R.H., Buckle, V.J., Fischel-Ghodsian, N., Chui, D.H.K., Gardner-Medwin, D., MacGillivray, M.H., Weatherall, D.J., Higgs, D.R. (1990) 'Clinical features and molecular analysis of the α thalassemia/mental retardation syndromes. II. Cases without detectable abnormality of the α globin complex.' *American Journal of Human Genetics*, **46**, 1127–1140.

INDEX

211

NOTES

NOTES

NOTES